The McGraw-Hill Essential Dictionary of Health Care

A Practical Reference for Physicians and Nurses

The McGraw-Hill Essential Dictionary of Health Care

A Practical Reference
for Physicians and Nurses

Lee Hyde, M.D.

McGraw-Hill Book Company

Healthcare Information Center

New York   St. Louis   San Francisco   Colorado Springs   Oklahoma City
Auckland   Bogotá   Hamburg   Lisbon   London   Madrid   Mexico
Milan   Montreal   New Delhi   Panama   Paris   San Juan
São Paulo   Singapore   Sydney   Tokyo   Toronto

The McGraw-Hill Essential Dictionary of Health Care
A Practical Reference for Physicians and Nurses

1 2 3 4 5 6 7 8 9 0 DOC DOC 8 9 4 3 2 1 0 9 8

ISBN 0-07-031614-7

This book was set in Century Schoolbook by McGraw-Hill Book Company Publishing Center in cooperation with Monotype Composition Company.
The editors were Deborah Glazer and Mariapaz Ramos-Englis.
The production supervisor was Elaine Gardenier.
The text was designed by Carol Woolverton and the cover was designed by Edward Schultheis.
R. R. Donnelley & Sons was printer and binder.

Library of Congress Cataloguing-in-Publication Data

Hyde, Lee, date.
    The McGraw-Hill essential dictionary of health care:
a practical reference for physicians and nurses.

    Bibliography: p.
    Includes index.
    1. Medical care—Dictionaries. 2. Health planning—
Dictionaries. I. Title. [DNLM: 1. Health Services—
dictionaries. W 13 H994m]
RA423.H93   1988   362.1'03'21   87-32497
ISBN 0-07-031614-7

"Ya' gotta serve somebody."
—Bob Dylan

To those I serve
and
to those who raised
and taught me to do it

Contents

Foreword

In a world of high technology and highly evolved bureaucracies, we have come increasingly to depend, in our businesses and professions, on machines, whether those made of steel and microprocessing chips or those fashioned out of human institutions. We have mechanized our transactions, our communications, our interactions. And we have changed our language to express and to accommodate our new relationships.

New words enter our personal and professional lives to capture meaning, to give form to our discoveries, to fill needs created by an expanding universe. The language is dynamic, and those words that are not mere passing fancy help write human history.

The proliferation of technology, of concepts, and of words is overwhelming if it is not organized. Our highways organize our transportation, our laws organize our social institutions, and our dictionaries organize our words and thoughts.

In the field of health care, this proliferation is manifest—for technology, concepts, and words are joined in a crucial endeavor. In the matter of health care, language must be purposeful, useful, and crystal clear. We have medical technology that offers unprecedented opportunities for remedy, rehabilitation, and relief; we have a health care establishment that is vast, powerful, and complex.

The machinery of this enterprise—the sophisticated life-saving devices, the financial inner workings, the social relations, the regulating mechanisms—is under the direction of a cast of players, from administrators and physicians to lawmakers and patients. To direct this enterprise wisely, to keep the machinery tuned and adjustable, and to achieve efficiency and equity, we require a firm grasp on the words and the terms, the acronyms and the abbreviations that serve as our tools. In this way, we can make sure that we understand each other and that we can proceed to shared goals.

No matter what our stake in the health care enterprise, we are constantly being guided—by our peers and by our knowledge. In this process, a dictionary of health care, embodying the values and concepts that have made it necessary to affix the label "modern" to health care, is an essential guide. We refer to it in order to refresh our memories, to reacquaint ourselves with words that we have temporarily lost, and to educate ourselves in new or unfamiliar territory. We may want to refer to it before we make important, perhaps even life-and-death, decisions. We should refer to it when we begin to feel overrun by cliches and jargon. It is to this end that *this* dictionary is written.

Edward F. X. Hughes, M.D., M. P. H.
Director
Center for Health Services and Policy Research
Northwestern University
Professor
J.L. Kellogg Graduate School
of Management and the Medical School

Preface

☐

This is a collection of words. My grandfather collected stamps; I have collected the words, concepts, peculiar recurrent phrases, common and obscure acronyms, and good names for useful ideas from my life as a physician. The collection, a dictionary, is intended for use by anyone interested or involved in efforts to maintain health, including clinicians, managers, and lay people, whether members of Congressional committees concerned with health, consumer members of health program governing boards, or patients. As any good stamp collector knows the history of each stamp in his collection, I know the "history" of my words. I have included references that provide additional, more encyclopedic information about the particular concepts and an annotated bibliography of additional sources. References are generally available, which justify and give the primary sources for the definitions.

The dictionary should be of particular use to clinicians.

Historically, doctors, nurses, and other clinicians knew everybody in the business. The number of other clinicians and managers in one's own town was small enough that one might know all of them. There were no insurance companies, out of town managers, or interested government officials. But, during the last several decades, as the effort to maintain a healthy population has grown in knowledge, technology, size, and complexity, the medical community has also become deeply divided. The internists have never met the neonatologists, let alone a Blue Cross executive or an industrial hygienist. The administrators of the community and profit-making hospitals rarely talk to each other, although both are talking to the health maintenance organization people; none of them understand the psychiatrist.

The most fundamental division separates the clinicians, the physicians, nurses, and other people engaged in direct patient care, from the managers, the hospital administrators, policymakers, insurers, and people who run the system that makes care possible. This book is intended to help bridge the divide, to make it possible for the clinician to understand the manager.

Each division of the health system has its own language. As knowledge and practice become more specialized, so does each division's dialect. If clinicians are to be effective in their caring efforts, to be as good as they would like to be, they must speak the language the managers speak. Actually they don't have to speak it, to actually say those things, but they better understand it. By trying to reduce the language of administrators, insurers, lawyers, and such to plain English I hope to make this possible. While English is spoken herein, this is not watered down; an attempt has been made to define terms with precise and complete definitions reflecting full professional meaning. Discourse has been added to show the terms in use, give examples and alternative or official definitions, and emphasize issues and nuances. In case the managers read this as well, and for the amusement of the clinicians, I have included some of the jargon of clinical medicine leaving out the worst, as (lexicographers say "as" rather than "for example" or "such as," it is briefer) Texas catheter and nun's cap, although I have never met a manager who knew their meaning.

The dictionary defines primarily the language, specialized vocabulary, and jargon of the practice and management of health care, without covering the clinical and technical language used in the direct delivery of services. (The latter is left to the standard medical dictionaries: good sources include *Blakiston's*, 1979; *Dorland's*, 1986; *Friel*, 1985; *Landau*, 1986, and *Stedman's*, 1983.) Alternatively put, the vocabulary defined is that of the institutional and organizational form of health care, rather than of its clinical content. The dictionary's scope is the terminology people working in health care use during, and as a specialized part of, their work. There is naturally some overlap between this work, standard medical dictionaries, and glossaries of other disciplines with which health and its care interact. Where terms are well covered in other works, the treatment here is fairly brief and generic, since the focus is on the language unique to health care.

Some of the terms are truly unique to the health field, as slang, which is included. Some are borrowed from or overlap with those of other disciplines (law, economics, sociology, psychology, insurance, finance, and management, for instance). The former are given greater coverage than the latter, particularly where good dictionaries in the related fields are cited. Coverage of other disciplines focuses on concepts that are particularly generic, useful, commonly misunderstood, or in common use in the health field.

Coverage is limited only by the author's limitations of time, energy, resources, and ability to find contributors to share the load. These limits must explain why some programs, laws, and subjects are included or better covered in preference to others. The same limits also certainly explain any errors; they are not made intentionally. Corrections will be much appreciated. Besides, errors are a lexicographer's way of proving he or she is human. (Throughout the text where male pronouns appear, it should be understood that their use is for convenience and the intention is that their meaning be universal.).

Coverage is also generally and preferentially exhaustive (although brief definitions with cross-references may be used for large families of related terms and other minor variants). Historical events and entities are included, and specialized or infrequently used terms are covered, particularly where they have distinct or useful meanings.

Each definition in the McGraw-Hill Essential Dictionary of Health Care starts with a formal statement of the term's meaning. Except for the initial article, most definitions are given in a form that will replace the term defined in use in a sentence. Multiple meanings are numbered. Terms defined within a larger definition are preceded by an asterisk (*) where they are actually defined.

Wherever it is helpful to the reader, definitions contain discourse on the concepts they define. This goes beyond simple definition to examples, exclusions, limitations, suggestions on usage, cross-references, and so forth. Terms are defined as they are used by most workers in the field. This is in preference to defining them as may have been done in law or by other formal means, or as they ought to be used according to researchers, lexicographers, or other pedants. Where "official" or "proper" definitions are known, particularly by competent bodies or recognized organizations, they may be quoted or cited in addition to the definition given.

Cross-references are given in italics to generic terms in the family of concepts to which a term belongs, as "see *malpractice*" in the case of "good samaritan law," and where otherwise less than obvious or likely to be useful. A list of defined related terms will typically be found in the Conspectus at the location given in a definition. References are included, not for source or justification of a definition (often available from the author), but for further expansion on the term. They locate the kind of material the reader would seek in an encyclopedia or text rather than in a dictionary.

No effort is made to cover the pronunciation or etymology of the terms defined except in the unusual circumstance that the term is regularly mispronounced or an understanding of its origin is necessary to understand its meaning.

Many of the great array of acronyms and abbreviations encountered in health care are listed in their own section with their full meanings given so they may be found in the vocabulary, where most are defined. Finally, an annotated bibliography is supplied. It gives references on the language of medicine, about lexicography, concerning medical writing and resources, and to numerous other glossaries and encyclopedias related to health and health care. The bibliography is indexed by subject using the Conspectus. In the interests of brevity, citations in the Conspectus and text are given, as in anthropology, with only the principal author's last name and the year of publication.

In addition to defining the vocabulary, the dictionary uses several means to help the reader organize, map, and connect the covered vocabulary. Some have already been described: the cross-references within the text that suggest related terms, guide the reader to more generic or basic concepts and indicate useful if not obvious connections, references cited to more exhaustive material suitable to an encyclopedia or text, and the indexed bibliography of additional sources.

The most important organizing tool is the Conspectus. The terms in a specialized vocabulary like that of health care naturally have their own hierarchy and structure. Many of the terms form families of related concepts and these families are related to each other in ways that can be loosely but helpfully described with an outline or taxonomy. An attempt was made in the dictionary's first edition (*Discursive, 1976*) to describe these families for the reader's use, but it was inconsistently and inadequately done (*Viseltear, 1977*). In this edition the families of related concepts are listed more carefully, along with lists of the members of the families, in an outline locating the various families in relationship to each other in health care. This takes the form of a subject outline, known as the Conspectus, which lists essentially all the terms defined in the dictionary. Conspectus locations in each term's definition guide the reader to its family and place in the taxonomy and thus allow an understanding of the term's role and place in health care. The mapping of a language, attempted in the Conspectus, is more difficult than might have been expected, as I am sure the authors of MeSH and other indices are aware. Critical feedback on this part of the effort would be particularly appreciated.

This volume does not contain my whole collection. A fair amount of incomplete, uncertain, peripheral, and obscure material has been left out but is available from the author.

Stamp collectors trade through newsletters and collector's magazines; we shall have to trade through correspondence. I would appreciate any comments or contributions from users of this vocabulary.

Write me

Lee Hyde, M.D.
Hygeia—A Practice of Family Medicine
1425 Patton Avenue
Asheville, N.C. 28806

I shall attempt to respond, perhaps with a new definition in a new edition. Please provide complete references and information about new material: for a program or organization, an address, the year founded (and ended, if no longer in existence), a statement of purpose(s), a size indicator (budget, membership, whatever), and a reference to a history, an independent evaluation, or major products; for people, their birth and death years, nationality, profession, and contributions; and for plain concepts, one good reference enlarging on the subject and the actual text of any official, legal, or technical definitions with proper citations.

Writing this has helped me understand health and health care, what I am doing as a physician, and the health system in which I do it. I hope it serves you similarly.

Thank you.

Lee Hyde

Acknowledgments

☐

Acknowledging help with a dictionary may be done by telling its story.

My conscious interest in health care began with public health while doing anthropological field work in Africa during college, for which I thank the National Science Foundation and Harvard Department of Anthropology. In medical school my concern for health policy was nurtured by a generally receptive faculty and, particularly, Deans Fred Robbins and Jack Caughey. Medical school and internship were followed by my years as a *yellow beret*. These were especially exciting because of a large group of powerful peers — Brian Biles, Rick Carlson, Merle Cunningham, Joe Fortuna, George Goldberg, Bob Graham, Dave Kindig, Fitz Mullen, Patrick O'Donoghue, Budd Shenkin, Bill Waters, Pete West — a wonderful group (no offense intended to anyone omitted).

Suddenly I went to Capitol Hill, where I particularly appreciate those who gave and taught me my job — Harley Staggers, Paul Rogers, James Menger, David Meade, Steve Lawton. There I took an incredible crash course in law, health policy, and the U.S. health system and community. I find a lot of parallels between defining terms and legal drafting.

The dictionary itself began in 1975 when the U.S. House of Representatives Committee on Interstate and Foreign Commerce and, particularly, its Subcommittee on Health and the Environment were studying national health insurance. As the Committee's professional staff member for health, I undertook a glossary of terms relevant to the debate. This produced the first edition, which the Committee published as a staff background document, *The Discursive Dictionary of Health Care*, in February 1976. The acknowledgment printed then is repeated here, but it does not tell the whole story. Most of the organizations cited actually had all the work done by individuals whose names were omitted because of personal preference, organizational policy, or courtesy. These people are remembered with appreciation, many did lots of good work. Karen Nelson was the best office mate I've ever had and the only person I've known who understood Title XIX of the Social Security Act. If Anne Jordan hadn't been professionally trained as a secretary, I'm not sure I'd have ever found or finished anything. Anne also began the second edition by cutting up the first and taping each word on its own 5x8 index card (*Safire, 1978*, prefers 5x7 cards?!).

The 5x8 card file, known as "old words," grew to three twelve-inch boxes that were gradually edited at home, of course, but also at my mother's basement desk, Barb and Dale Schumacher's Rockburn Institute, Camp Sequin on the Maine Coast, Gloria O'Dell's place in Silver Lake, Pinewoods Folk Camp, and a number of other such kind, comfortable, and memorable places.

During most of the preparation of the second edition I made my professional home in the Department of Family Medicine of East Tennessee State University's Quillen-Dishner College of Medicine, i.e., in the beautiful Tennessee mountains. The Department's various chairmen, particularly David Doane, faculty, and staff have provided invaluable time and friendship for the effort. James Mitchell and Craig Haire worked well as medical student research fellows both in the library and at the word processor keyboards. Dawn Connor, Debbie Norton, Kim Griffith, and Vivian Love deciphered the incredibly elaborate editorial scrawling on large shares of the 5x8 cards, turning old words into a manuscript known as "new words." The 5x8's are gone now; I've moved on to a remarkably handy portable pc and software.

From time to time I've sought help from a group of friends that I've thought of as an "Editorial Board." Especially diligent and helpful among these have been Joe Newhouse, John Dirk, Dan Pettengill, Art Viseltear, and David Willis. McGraw-Hill's "Washington Health Letters" newsletters have been a long-time major source, and former editor of the newsletters, Jerry Brazda, has for years been a particular friend and supporter. Stephanie Tames, Deborah Glazer, Mariapaz Ramos-Englis, Elaine Gardenier, and Jim Fullerton of the McGraw-Hill staff have been very supportive and responsive.

Gail Hyde-Pike has proofread more than anyone, helped particularly with the family medicine vocabulary, and, finally, given her study to housing the effort.

Kate and Zack Hyde learned to alphabetize and file at early ages, and Kate proved she was ready for college by making most of McGraw-Hill's editorial changes while her father was being a doctor. (Caleb, True, and Leah certainly face similar fates as they grow.) Jane Hyde enjoyed more requests to "read a good definition" and related enthusiasm than anyone. At least lexicographers are well known to be harmless and are usually friendly.

Enduring thanks go to the people who have given generously of their time for writing definitions, suggesting terms, locating existing glossaries, and criticizing the various drafts of the 1976 edition of the dictionary. All of their efforts are still much appreciated. Particular appreciation is due to the staff of the Congressional Research Service of the Library of Congress: Ira Raskin, John Gallicchio, and other staff of the National Center for Health Services Research; Dan Pettingill of the Aetna Life & Casualty Company; Catherine Lyon, Joe Newhouse, and other staff of the Rand Corporation; Irv Wolkstein and Steve Sieverts of the American Hospital Association; Joe Manes of the House Committee on the Budget; David Banta of the Office of Technology Assessment; Jane Murnaghan and Kerr White of the Department of Health Care Organization of the School of Hygiene and Public Health of the Johns Hopkins University; Steve Summers of the Association of American Medical Colleges; Edwin Tuller and other staff of the Blue Cross Association; Linda Horton and other staff of the Food and Drug Administration; Ruth Johnson and other staff of the Bureau of Health Manpower of the Health Resources Administration; the staff of Spectrum Research, Inc.; the staff of the Health Policy Program of the University of California, San Francisco; Ruth Hanft and other staff of the Institute of Medicine of the National Academy of Sciences; the staff of the American Medical Association; and the staff of the Office of the Assistant Secretary for planning of HEW. Special thanks also go to Anne Jordan, Susan Tomasky, and Bill Burns of the Committee staff for doing much of the real work. Without the assistance of these and other people the job simply would never have been done. The responsibility for the results of course remains with the Committee professional staff, who would like to add to Samuel Johnson's explanation of errors in his dictionary, "Ignorance, sir, ignorance!", only "and laziness."

Thank you, everyone. Thank you.

The McGraw-Hill Essential Dictionary of Health Care

A Practical Reference
for Physicians and Nurses

Conspectus of Health and Health Care

CONSPECTUS OF HEALTH AND HEALTH CARE: A PREVIEW

1

AN EXPLANATION

A conspectus is "a general view or comprehensive survey (with the mind's eye)";[1] an outline or subject index; a synopsis or thesaurus. What follows is a conspectus of the vocabulary in this dictionary. A conspectus is not really a taxonomy, which is a classification according to natural relationships, although this conspectus does generally serve as such and the concepts of necessity overlap. While a conspectus must show some logic, it must be an arbitrary structuring of a whole, particularly if it is to include the whole. Further, its scope and coverage, or breadth and depth, are bound to be uneven, as are those of this dictionary and the language of health and health care itself.

This Conspectus includes essentially all the concepts defined in the dictionary. Each individual definition ends with where the concept is located in the Conspectus; this is often an arbitrary choice, no matter how sophisticated the outline. It is useful as an index, a source of cross-references, a guide to concepts' places in larger contexts, and a collection of lists of defined terms related to a given general subject. A reader interested in a particular subject should find it in the Conspectus and explore the terms listed with it.

The model of health and health care underlying the outline is sketched in the following two simple figures. Health, our well-being (Figure 1), is determined (I) by a host of factors and may be described (II) by a variety of characteristics.

The first part of the Conspectus or subject outline, I, is therefore concerned with individual, cultural, and environmental determinants of health. The next section, II, deals with the description of health and health status.

Health care encompasses all conscious efforts to influence events so

---

[1] *The Compact Edition of the Oxford English Dictionary.* New York: Oxford University Press, 1971.

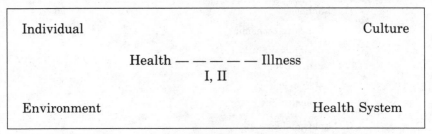

Figure 1
Health: Its Determinants (I) and Description (II).

that individual health, the collective health of the community, and the healthfulness of the environment are raised to and maintained at the greatest feasible level. The individuals and institutions engaged in providing health care together constitute the health system (Figure 2) in its broadest definition. The system and its various constituent subsystems use resources (listed in III, the third section) to deliver the many different services (VII) which together are the product of the caring effort. The people and activities of the system may be separated into those who actually provide the services (practicing, V) and those who make it possible (management, VI). Financing (IV) specifies the value of the effort and distributes its burden. All of this is itself the subject of much study (VIII).

Dictionaries and other references cited in the annotated Bibliography are shown in the Conspectus as a means of cross-referencing the Bibliography by subject matter. The citations are given in italics with their publication date to distinquish them from defined terms. See *Heyel, 1973,* for another example of a conspectus.

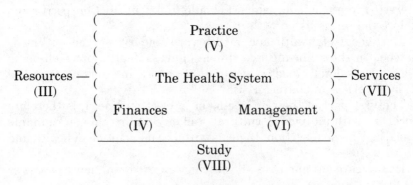

Figure 2
The Health System

CONSPECTUS OF HEALTH AND HEALTH CARE

I.   Determinants of Health and Illness
        Parker, 1987
        Uvarov, 1986
        Yule, 1985

     A.   Individual
             accident proneness
             need
             organic
             stress
             susceptibility

          1.   biology
                 abortion
                 acquired
                 acuity
                 addiction
                 adult
                 age
                     advanced age
                     Age Words, 1986
                     biologic age
                     chronological age
                     geriatric
                     Maddox, 1987
                     mental age
                     old age
                     Senior Actualization and
                         Growth Experience
                 anesthesia
                 anomaly
                 birth
                     live birth
                     natural childbirth
                     stillbirth
                 child
                     infant
                 congenital
                     Baby Doe
                 convalesce
                 death
                     fetal death
                     inquest

senile dementia
minor
    emancipated minor
morbid, morbidity
mortal, mortality
mutant, mutation
natural
natural death act
natural selection
neonate
obesity
pain
para, parity
parasite
parasitoid
pathogen
penetrance
pest
    pest control
relaxation response
reservoir
resistance
Sampson, 1975
senescence
senile dementia
Singleton, 1978
somatic
sound
standard age groups
synergy
tolerance, tolerance limit
toxin
xenograft
zygosity

2. personality
    acting out
    attitude
    behavior
        The Alameda Seven
        behavioral risk factor
        Behavioral Risk Factor
            Surveys
    behavior modification

behavior therapy
behavioral science
bond
burnout
compliance
critical incident
developmental task
differentiation of self
double-bind message
fusion
Goldenson, 1970
habituation
intelligence quotient
Jekyll-and-Hyde syndrome
life change event
living will
mental health
metacommunication
mutuality
J. Piaget
primary gain
problem of living
recidivism, recidivist
role
sanity
secondary gain
self-care
self-neglect
sick role
stressful life event
suffer
Wolman, 1973

a. diet
adulterate
Bender, 1976
deficiency disease
Delaney amendment
dietary supplement
digestion
essential
food
food additive
food irradiation

Food and Agriculture
Organization
Food and Drug
Administration
Food and Nutrition
Terminology, 1974
Food, Drug, and Cosmetic Act
Food: Multilingual Thesaurus,
1978
food chain, web
good manufacturing practice
health food
Incaparina
labeling
Lagua, 1974
La Leche League
Lapedes, 1977
mineral
natural food
nutrient
nutrition
 malnutrition
organic
pesticide
 ethylene dibromide
 herbicide
Peterson, 1978
preservative
recommended dietary
allowance
residual substance
Take Off Pounds Sensibly
tolerance
trophic
vegetarianism
vitamin
Weight Watchers
Wren, 1907

b. exercise
 aerobic
 fit

c. occupation (see *occupational safety and*
health, VII.B.2.d.)

         Aid to the Blind
         Aid to Families with
            Dependent Children
         Aid to the Permanently and
            Totally Disabled
         blue flu
         cafeteria plan
         categorically needy
         categorically related
         ergonomics
         income
               earned income
               poverty
               unearned income
         means test
         Old-Age, Survivors, Disability
            and Health Insurance
            Program
         sickout
         Supplemental Security Income
         welfare
         work capacity
         work history
         work test

    d. avocation
        scry

B. Cultural
    blaming the victim
    population
        population pyramid
    war
        biologic warfare
        chemical warfare
        yellow rain

    1. family
        abused child
        adoption
        adult-centered family
        autonomy
        battery
        blended family
        boundary

caretaker
chaotic family
child-focused family
critical incident
developmental task
differentiation of self
disengagement
dyad
dysfunctional family
emotional divorce
emotional field
engagement
enmeshment
familial
family
 active family
 attending family
 extended family
 family of origin
 family of procreation
 former family
 inactive family
 nuclear family
 registered family
Family Adaptability and Cohesion
 Scales
family constellation
family life cycle
family myth
family planning (see VII.B.3.b.)
 birth control
 planned parenthood
 Speert, 1973
 squeal rule
family system
family transference
functional family
fusion
genogram
interlocking pathology
Jekyll-and-Hyde syndrome
life change event
lover
marriage

marital schism
marital skew
metacommunication
Office of Human Development
Services, 1978
parental child, parentification
Peckham experiment
Pinney, 1982
proband, propositus
problem of living
reconstituted family
remarried family
role
role overload
safe house
scapegoat
schism
sibling position
sibling subsystem
skew
stepfamily
stressful life event
subsystems
support group, system
toxic issue
triangle
undifferentiated family ego mass

2. society
adult protective services
exploitation
anomie
boarding house
community
community psychiatry
congregate housing
day care
Encyclopedia of Sociology, 1974
Gould, 1964
herd effect, immunity
poverty area
Rinzler, 1979
rural
social problem

　　socioeconomic status
　　specific learning disability
　　suburb
　　suburban
　　support group, system
　　urban
　　welfare

3. religion

4. law (see VIII.B.3.)
　　medicine
　　reglementation

5. economics (see VIII.B.1.)
　　CPI
　　income
　　Keogh plan
　　　　individual retirement account

C. Environment
　　abatement
　　additive
　　adulterant
　　allergen
　　Ames' test
　　asepsis
　　　　J. Lister
　　C. Bernard
　　biocenose
　　biodegradation
　　biomass
　　biome
　　Brace, 1977
　　carcinogen
　　contaminate
　　control
　　diversity index
　　dump
　　Durrenberger, 1973
　　ecology
　　　　ecological community
　　　　ecological efficiency
　　　　ecological impact
　　　　ecological pyramid

ecological succession and recession
ecosystem
Energy, 1986
habitat
nutrient budget
entropy
exposure
    protective action level
Federal Insecticide, Fungicide, and
    Rodenticide Act
fomite
Hampel, 1982
Hawley, 1981
hazard
    health hazard
    safety hazard
heavy metal
    arsenic
    cadmium
    chromium
    lead
    mercury
impurity
mutagen
peril
persistence
    persistent pesticide
pest control
pesticide
    dichloro-diphenyl-trichloro-ethane
    ethylene dibromide
    organophosphate
    rebuttable presumption against
        registration
poison
pollutant, pollute, polluter, pollution
safe, safety
sanitary
sanitary code
sanitation
Sarnoff, 1971
stress
Studdard, 1973
surveillance system

system
teratogen
threshold
    threshold limit value
    zero threshold phenomenon
tolerance, tolerance limit
toxic, toxic substance
    Toxic Substances Control Act
    Toxic Substances List

1. air
    acid rain
    air pollution episode
    air quality criteria
    air quality index
    air quality standard
    Agent Orange
    beryllium
    criteria pollutant
    emission
    fluoride
    fumigant
    Glossary, 1980
    hazardous air pollutant
    nuclear winter
    occupational air
    Pollutant Standard Index
    particle, particulate
        dust
        fog
        fume
        mist
        smog
        smoke
            midstream smoke
            side-stream smoke
    radioactive fallout
        strontium
    zones

2. noise
    acoustic, acoustics
    decibel
    noise control
    occupational noise

in-plant noise
sound
sound pressure level

3. radiation
food irradiation
rad
radiation injury
radiation sickness, syndrome
radiation standard
radiation exposure
radioactive fallout
iodine
strontium
radioactive half-life
radioactive waste
radioactivity
radiography
radioisotope
radionuclide
roentgen
x-ray

4. waste
bulky waste
digestion
dioxin
discharge
food waste
hazardous waste
incombustible waste
Love Canal
Patrick, 1980
radioactive waste
sanitation
public cleansing
sanitary landfilling
sanitary sewer
septic tank
septic tank system
sewage
sewer
sanitary sewer
storm sewer
sewerage

treatment
solid waste
commercial waste
municipal waste
standard methods

5. water
acid-neutralizing capacity
acid rain
aquifer
biochemical oxygen demand
chlorinated hydrocarbon
chlorinate
coliform count
drain dumping
drinking water
erosion
fluoride
fresh water
median lethal concentration
polychlorinated biphenyl
potable
potable water standard
reservoir
sewage
Standard Methods
storm sewer
Veatch, 1966
waste water
water quality
water quality criterion

II. Description of Health and Illness
condition
case
index case
complication
defect
deformity
dementia
Alzheimer's disease
disability
developmental disability
disablement
homebound

disease
    orphan disease
disorder
handicap
    architectural barrier
    Baby Doe
    handicapped individual
    mainstream
    M-team
illness
impairment
intercurrent
International System of Units
latent
malformation
Medical Signal Code
natural history
normal
occult
pathogenesis, pathogenic
preclinical
puerperal
sickness
silent
subclinical
sylvatic
syndrome
welfare
zoonosis

A. Individual Manifestations
    pathognomic, pathognomonic
    pathosis, pl. pathoses
    organic

  1. subjective
    complaint
    Cornell Medical Index
    history
        chief complaint
        present illness
        past medical history
        family history
        social history

review of systems
primary gain
problem
    continuing problem
    diagnosis
    diagnostic criteria
    episode
    new problem
    problem of living
radiation
secondary gain
symptom, symptomatic

2. objective
    clean
    disability
        activities of daily living
        performance status
    intercurrent
    laboratory
        bioassay
        biologic monitoring
        laboratory diagnosis
    regression
    sequela
    severity
        acute disease
        Acute Physiology and Chronic
           Health Evaluation
        chronic disease
        condition
        emergency
        Medical Illness Severity
           Grouping System
  sign
  stage
  virulence

B. Diagnosis

1. type
    admitting diagnosis
    Armed Forces Institute of
        Pathology
    autopsy

diagnosis related group
　diagnosis related group creep
　outlier
　Patient Management
　　Categories
　principal diagnosis
Diagnostic and Statistical Manual
of Mental Disorders
diagnosis
discharge
International Classification of
　Disease
International Classification of
　Diseases for Oncology
International Classification of
　Health Problems in Primary
　Care
　Pri-Care
pathology
　R. Virchow
postmortem
primary diagnosis
Systematized Nomenclature of
　Medicine
　Systematized Nomenclature of
　　Dermatology
　Systematized Nomenclature of
　　Pathology
topsy

a.　etiologic
　　accident
　　agent
　　American Type Culture
　　　Collection
　　cause
　　　secondary
　　deficiency disease
　　essential
　　factitial, factitious
　　functional
　　iatrogenic

idiopathic
injury
    radiation injury
    recordable injury
malinger
nosocomial
ontologist
organic
parasitism
pathogen
psychosomatic
sexually transmitted disease
    venereal disease
toxic
trauma

b. anatomic
    lesion

2. specific illness
acute remunerative appendicitis
alcoholism
    Abel, 1985
    alcoholic
    Alcoholics Anonymous
alexithymic
Andromeda strain
attention-deficit disorder
    hyperactivity
    learning disability
    minimal brain dysfunction
    specific learning disability
Beighton, 1986
blind
blue flu
burnout
dementia
    Alzheimer's disease
cancer
    American Cancer Society
    carcinogen
    metastasis
    Reach for Recovery

tumor, metastases, nodes
child abuse
   *Office of Human Development
      Services, 1978*
   Parents Anonymous
*Current Medical Information and
   Terminology*
deaf
drug abuse, addiction, dependence,
   and habituation
   methadone program
   O'Brien, 1984
   substance abuse
   withdrawal syndrome
heart disease
hibakusha
hypochondria
Jekyll-and-Hyde syndrome
Legionnaire's disease
Lourie, 1982
Magalini, 1971
mental disorder
   WHO, 1974
mental illness
   *American Psychiatric
      Association, 1978*
   asylum
   criminally insane
   Deutsch, 1963
   Greyhound therapy
   insanity
   institution for mental disease
   maniac
   Munchhausen syndrome
   parens patriae
   police power
   psychiatric diagnosis
   recidivism, recidivist
   seasonal affective disorder
mental retardation
   phenylketonuria
   Tymchuk, 1973
obesity
pneumoconiosis

asbestosis
bagassosis
black lung
brown lung
B. Rush
silicosis
radiation sickness, syndrome
smoking
stroke
subluxation of the spine
swine flu
worried well

3. prognosis
hanging crepe
recrudescence
relapse
remission
retrospectoscope

C. Population Health Status
age-specific rate
age-specific fertility rate
birth rate
net reproduction rate
Cooperative Health Statistics System
demography
demographic data
final epidemic
gene pool
Glossary, 1984
health index
health survey
life expectancy
life table
abridged life table
cohort, generation life table
complete life table
current life table
medically underserved area
medically underserved population
Morbidity and Mortality Weekly Report
morbidity rate
mortality rate

case fatality rate
infant mortality rate
maternal mortality rate
neonatal mortality rate
perinatal mortality rate
standardized death rate
National Death Index
National Health and Nutrition
   Examination Survey
National Health Survey
parasite index, rate
physician shortage area
scarcity area
Singer, 1976
standard metropolitan statistical
   area
vital statistics
   J.S. Billings
   W. Farr
   J. Graunt
   W. Petty
Weise, 1979
zero population growth

D. Environmental Health
     Community Health and
       Environmental Surveillance System
     ecology
     monitor

III. Resources
     Donabedian, 1986
     Hogarth, 1975
     Kruzas, 1985
     provider
       direct
       health care provider
       indirect
       institutional
     vendor
     Saunders, 1984
     supplier

A. Health Manpower (People)
  area health education center
  Area Resource File
  capitation
  care giver
  certification
  chiropractor
  clerkship
  clinician
    W. Osler
  credential
  endorsement
  equivalency testing
  healer
  Health Manpower Education Initiative
    Award
  intern
  internship
  license, licensure
  National Health Service Corp.
  private corporation
  profession, professional
  professional association
  proficiency testing
  quid pro quo
  registration
  residency
    flexible residency
    residency review committee
    transitional year
  rotation
    elective
    selective
  Schedule A
  shaman
  specialist
    American Board of Medical
      Specialties, 1979
  specialty board
  staff
  steerer
  union
  witch doctor

1. medical
>Accreditation Council for
>>Continuing Medical Education
>Accreditation Council for Graduate
>>Medical Education
>Alpha Omega Alpha Medical
>>Honor Society
>>>The Pharos
>American Association of
>>Physicians and Surgeons
>American Medical Political Action
>>Committee
>American Medical Association
>>AMA Physician Masterfile
>American Medical College
>>Application Service
>Armed Forces Health Professions
>>Scholarship
>aviation medical examiner
>Bane Report
>caduceus
>consultant
>Coordinated Transfer Application
>>System
>Coordinating Council on Medical
>>Education
>coroner
>Council for Medical Affairs
>diplomat
>doctor
>Educational Commission for
>>Foreign Medical Graduates
>extern, externship
>fat doctor
>Federation Licensing Examination
>Federation of State Medical Boards
>fellow
>fifth pathway
>Flexner Report
>foreign medical graduate
>foreign medical student
>gatekeeper
>Health Professions Student Loan
>>Program

J visa
labor certification
Liaison Committee on Continuing
    Medical Education
Liaison Committee on Graduate
    Medical Education
Liaison Committee on Medical
    Education
Licentiate of the Medical Council
    of Canada
local medical doctor
locum tenens
        Project USA
Medical Activities and Manpower
    Project
Medical College Admission Test
medical examiner
Medical Sciences Knowledge
    Profile
medical staff
National Board Examination
National Board of Medical
    Examiners
National Residents Matching
    Program
physician
        admitting physician
        allopathic physician
        attending physician
        general practitioner
        hospital-based physician
        house officer
        house physician
        impaired physician
        osteopath, osteopathic
            physician
        personal physician
        *Physicians for the Twenty-First
            Century*
        private physician
        teaching physician
physician shortage area
police surgeon
pyramid system

registrar
specialist
    allergist
    anesthesiologist
    dermatologist
    dermatopathologist
    family physician
    general surgeon
    geriatrician, geriatrist
    gynecologist
    internist
        gastroenterologist
        hematologist
    neurologist
    neurosurgeon
    obstetrician
    oncologist
    ophthalmologist
    orthopedist
    otolaryngologist
    pathologist
        hematologist
    pediatrician
    physiatrist
    plastic surgeon
    proctologist
    psychiatrist
        psychoanalyst
    radiologist
    surgeon
        itinerant surgeon
        thoracic surgeon
    urologist
Study on Surgical Services for the
    U.S.
surgeon general
Visa Qualifying Examination

2. nursing
    American Nursing Association
    acuity
    associate degree program
    baccalaureate degree program
    clinical nurse specialist

diploma school
T. and F. Fliedner
graduate nurse
licensed practical, vocational nurse
F. Nightingale
nurse anesthetist
nurse midwife
nurse practitioner
nursing intensity
patient care technician
    nurse's aide
    orderly
practical nurse
private duty
private nurse
psychiatric nurse
public health nurse
registered nurse
L. Wald
visiting nurse

3. dental
    dental assistant
    dental hygienist
    dental technician
    dentist
    denturist
    endodontist
    gum farmer
    periodontist
    prosthodontist

4. allied health
    allied health personnel
    anesthetist
    apothecary
    audiologist
    barefoot doctor
    clerk
    clinical pharmacist
    Committee on Allied Health
      Education and Accreditation
    diener
    dietician
    Dox, 1985

druggist
feldsher
Frenay, 1977
health education
health educator
home health aide, homemaker
hygienist
Medex
medical assistant
medical corpsman
medical laboratory assistant
Miller, 1978
minister
nutritionist
occupational therapist
optician
optometrist
orthoptist
orthotist
paramedical personnel
paraprofessional
pedorthist
pharmacist
phlebotomy technician
physical therapist
physician assistant
physician extender
pink lady
podiatrist
prosthetist
psychologist
    clinical psychologist
    licensed psychologist
pusher
radiological technician
respiratory therapist
Schmidt, 1974
social worker
    psychiatric social worker
    social service designee
speech therapist
technician
technologist
    medical technologist

x-ray technologist
Thomas, 1977
training center
wet nurse

5. environmental
    health officer
    industrial hygienist
    safety engineer
    safety inspector
    sanitarian
    veterinarian, veterinary

6. administrative
    Frenay, 1977
    inspector
    medical record administrator
    recorder
    registrar

B. Things
    cosmetic
    Estrin, 1973
    health system
    proprietary

1. health program
    accreditation
    architectural barrier
    auxiliary
    bed
        bassinet
        bed turnover rate
        swing bed
    blood bank
    board
    capital
        amortization
        debt, debt service
        depreciation
    catchment area
    census
    channeling agency
    clinic
    collection agent, agency
    community health center

community health network
community mental health center
    consultation and education
      services
    Joint Commission on Mental
      Illness and Health
day
    day bed
dental laboratory
department
    pathology
dietary service
dispensary
emergency medical service system
episodic care center
ethics committee
experimental health service
  delivery system
extended care facility
facility
free clinic
group practice
halfway house
health maintenance organization
    basic health services
    community rating
    dual choice
    individual practice association
    medical foundation
    member
    open enrollment
    penetration
    prepaid group practice
    prepaid health plan
    qualification
    skim
    skimp
    supplemental health service
Health Policy Advisory Center
Hill-Burton
    free care
    outpatient medical facility
home health agency
hospice
hospital

affiliated hospital
administrative services only
   contract
American Medical Records
   Association, 1974
asylum
birthing center, room
Commission on Professional
   and Hospital Activities
     Medical Audit Program
     Professional Activities
      Study
Darling case
emergency room
Handbook, 1976
house staff
intensive care unit
Joint Commission on
   Accreditation of Hospitals
Joint, 1986
Kiger, 1986
lazaretto
National Residents Matching
   Program
night hospital
nosocomial
nursery
outpatient department
proprietary hospital
Quality Assurance
   Program
recovery room
sole community hospital
staff privilege
swing bed
teaching hospital
tissue committee
uncompensated care
unnumbered hospital
xenodochium
hot line
infirmary
institutional provider
intermediate care facility
joint purchasing agreement

license, licensure
    institutional licensure
laboratory
    Bennington, 1984
    clinical laboratory
    independent laboratory
    reference laboratory
life-care community
Life Safety Code
medical center
medical staff
medical trade area
modernization
National Health Law Program
National Organization to Reform
    Marijuana Laws
nurse's station
nursing home
    Beverly Enterprises
    fair rental system
    supplementation
occupancy rate
outpatient medical facility
patient mix
peer review organization
poison control center
preferred provider organization
private corporation
professional standards review
    organization
Red Cross
registry
right to treatment
Roemer's law
room
roster
Rural Health Initiative
safe house
sanitorium
school
    Bakke
scope of services
screening clinic

Senior Actualization and Growth
    Experience
shelter
sheltered workshop
skilled nursing facility
specialty board
staff
supplemental health service
surgicenter
ward
zero population growth

2. devices, equipment, and technology
    ambulance
    American National Standards
        Institute
    apheresis
    computed tomography
    Deadhead Medico
    durable medical equipment
    Graf, 1977
    health care technology
    Massachusetts General Hospital
        Utility Multi-Programming
        System
    nuclear magnetic resonance
        magnetic resonance imaging
        Subcommittee on NMR
            Nomenclature, 1983
    orphan product
    orthosis
    PaperChase
    prescription
    prosthesis
    ship's medical chest
    Sippl, 1980
    supplies
    talking book
    technology assessment
    test
    thermography

3. biologics and drugs
    acquisition cost

adequate and well-controlled
   investigations
adverse drug reaction
American Hospital Formulary
antibiotic
antibiotic certification
antisubstitution law
bioavailability
bioequivalent
biosynthesis
biotechnology
Boston Collaborative Drug
   Surveillance Program
Bowman, 1986
brand name
   proprietary name
The British Pharmacopoeia
chemical equivalents, name
chemical restraint
clinical equivalents
compassionate use
compendium
compound
controlled substance
   controlled substances analogue
   narcotic
      methadone
DEA number
DeLorenzo, 1985
designer drug
detail person
dispensing fee
dose
   critical dose
   cumulative dose
   infective dose
   lethal dose
   minimum dose
Drug Efficacy Study
   Implementation
drug monograph
Drug Products Information File
Drug Topics Red Book
P. Erlich

ethical drug
established name
The European Pharmacopoeia
Food, Drug, and Cosmetic Act
formulary
generally recognized as effective
generally recognized as safe
generic drug, equivalents, name
    nonproprietary name
genetic engineering
Griffiths, 1985
Homeopathic Pharmacopeia of the
  United States
inactive ingredient
investigational new drug
International Encyclopedia, 1973
International Nonproprietary
  Names
kiting
labeling
legend
Lingeman, 1974
litogen
Maximum Allowable Cost Program
"me too" drug
Modern Drug Encyclopedia, 1983
multisource drug
National Formulary
new drug
new drug application
not new
official
orphan product
over-the-counter drug
package insert
patient package insert
pharmacopeia
pharmacy
Physicians' Desk Reference
prescription
prescription drug
psychotropic
pusher
reaction, drug reaction

reference drug
scheduled drug
short
side effect
Sittig, 1979
substitution
tachyphylaxis
therapeutic equivalents
therapeutic index
tolerance
tranquilizer
U.S. Adopted Names Council
U.S. Pharmacopeia
unit-dose system
unofficial
vaccine
withdrawal
wonder drug

4. charities and foundations
American Cancer Society
charity
Education and Research
Foundation
foundation
Health Research Group
Howard Hughes Medical Institute
Medical Committee for Human
Rights
North American Primary Care
Research Group
Physicians for Social
Responsibility
Planned Parenthood Association
Project Hope
Robert Wood Johnson Foundation
Sex Information and Education
Council of the United States
voluntary health agency
L.F. Flick

C. Knowledge
art therapy

Association of American Medical
  Colleges
basic sciences
behavioral science
Bethesda
bioethics
biopsychosocial model
clinic
clinical
clinical medicine
clinical pharmacy
clinical psychology
clinical sciences
college
continuing medical education
      Physician's Recognition Award
      Network for Continuing Medical
        Education
dentistry
      Boucher, 1974
      dental public health
      endodontics
      Manhold, 1985
      orthodontics
      pedodontics
      periodontics
      prosthodontics
dietetics
emporiatrics
ethology
explanatory model
folk medicine
geratology, gerentology
      Gibson, 1985
graduate medical education
holistic
hygiene
medical ethics
      bioethics
      compassionate use
      ethics committee
medical literature
      Bowker, 1986
      Darnay, 1985

Family Medicine Literature Index
fugitive
Herbert Huffington Memorial
  Library
Index Medicus
    Quarterly Cumulative Index
      Medicus
Inglefinger rule
Koch, 1972
Medical Literature and Analysis
  Retrieval System
    Medline
    Medical Subject Headings
    National Library of Medicine
National Technical Information
  Service
PaperChase
reviewed literature
throw-away literature
Welch, 1985
medical model
medical physics
  McAnish, 1986
medical specialty
  algology
  allergy and immunology
  anesthesiology
  bariatrics
  behavioral medicine
  dermatology
  dermatopathology
  family medicine
    American Academy of Family
      Physicians
    American Board of Family
      Practice
    Balint group
    behavioral sciences
    Coggeshall Report
    Core Content Review of
      Family Medicine
    Essentials for Residencies in
      Family Medicine
    Family Health Foundation of
      America

blood banking
chemical pathology
dermatopathology
forensic pathology
hematology
medical microbiology
neuropathology
Sloane, 1984
R. Virchow
pediatrics
physical medicine and
rehabilitation
preventive medicine
aerospace medicine
industrial hygiene
J. Lind
occupational medicine
public health
psychiatry
Campbell, 1981
community psychiatry
deinstitutionalization
D.L. Dix
Eidelberg, 1968
A. and S. Freud
Greyhound therapy
Hinsie, 1970
Klein, 1975
Leigh, 1977
Lipton, 1978
P. Pinel
psychoanalysis
psychosurgery
psychotherapy
W. Reich
Rycroft, 1973
social psychiatry
W. Tuke
Werner, 1980
Wolman, 1973 and *1977*
WHO, 1974
radiology
diagnostic radiology
diagnostic (nuclear) radiology

Walton, 1986
midwifery
    Adams, 1983
music therapy
nursing (see III.A.2.)
    Cape, 1974
    Duncan, 1971
    Kasner, 1984
    Kolin, 1973
    Miller, 1978
    F. Nightingale
    Roper, 1973
    Thomas, 1977
    L. Wald
Omega, 1987
ontologist
optometry
    Millidot, 1986
orthoptics
orthotics
osteopathy
pearl
pedorthics
pharmacology
    Bowman, 1986
    Delorenzo, 1985
    International Encyclopedia, 1973
pharmacy (see III.B.3.)
physical therapy
play therapy
podiatry
preclinical
prosthetics
psychology
    Chaplin, 1975
    Corsini, 1987
    Drever, 1964
    Eysenck, 1972
    Goldenson, 1970
    Klein, 1975
    Krauss, 1976
    metapsychology
    J. Piaget
    B. Rush

B. F. Skinner
Zusne, 1984
recreation therapy
sanitary engineering
social work
Brieland, 1977
science
Collocott, 1972
specialty
American Board of Medical
Specialties
board certified
board eligible
Council of Medical Specialty
Societies
residency review committee
specialist
specialty board
subspecialty
certificate of special
competence
technology
health care technology
technology assessment
toxicology
undergraduate medical education
veterinary medicine
Miller, 1972
West, 1977

D. Public Systems
socialized medicine

1. Federal
Council on Environmental Quality
Department of Defense
Armed Forces Institute of
Pathology
Berry Plan
Civilian Health and Medical
Program of the Uniformed
Services
Medical Education for
National Defense

separation program number
unnumbered hospital
Department of Health and Human
Services
    Alcohol, Drug Abuse, and
    Mental Health
    Administration
    Centers for Disease Control
        Epidemiologic Intelligence
        Service
        Morbidity and Mortality
        Weekly Report
        National Institute of
        Occupational Safety and
        Health
    Child Health Assurance
    Program
    Commissioned Corps
        yellow beret
    Crippled Children's Bureau
        Crippled Children's
        Service
    Food and Drug Administration
    Health, 1984
    Health Care Financing
    Administration
    Health Resources
    Administration
        Graduate Medical
        Education National
        Advisory Committee
        Health Education
        Assistance Loan
        Program
    Health Services
    Administration
        Indian Health Service
        National Health Service
        Corporation
        Project USA
    Marine Hospital Service
    National Center for Health
    Services Research

National Center for Health
Statistics
National Center for
Toxicological Research
National Institutes of Health
Bethesda
National Library of
Medicine
Prospective Payment
Assessment Commission
Social Security Administration
U.S. Public Health Service
Department of Justice
Drug Enforcement
Administration
Department of Labor
Occupational Safety and
Health Administration
Environmental Protection Agency
Federal Register
Federal Trade Commission
Office of Technology Assessment
Veterans Administration
adjunct disability
Civilian Health and Medical
Program of the Veterans
Administration
hometown medical and dental
care
nonservice-connected disability
service-connected disability
Veterans Administration
Health Program
2. other
board of health
coroner
Food and Agriculture Organization
(FAO)
health department
Institute of Medicine
local government
medical examiner
National Health Service

North American Primary Care
  Research Group
Pan American Health
  Organization
police surgeon
United Nations International
  Children's Emergency Fund
World Health Organization (WHO)
World Organization of National
  Colleges, Academies, and
  Academic Associations of
  General Practitioners/Family
  Physicians

3. institutes and centers
Armed Forces Institute of
  Pathology
National Institute of Occupational
  Safety and Health
National Institutes of Health

IV. Financing
cost-related reimbursement
Downes, 1985
indexed
relative value scale
relative value unit

A. Direct Payment
bad debt
balance billing
factoring
Fee and Cost Index Program
fee schedule
fee for service
fee splitting
kickback
kiting
mutual benefit association
out-of-pocket cost, payment
payroll deduction
prepaid
professional courtesy
prospective reimbursement
retrospective reimbursement

sick tax
uncompensated care

B. Insurance
acquisition cost
actuary
admitted assets
administrative risk only contract
adverse selection
allocated benefit provision
antidiscrimination law
assigned risk
assurance
at risk
beneficiary
benefit
benefit period
blanket medical expense
capitation
carrier
catastrophic health insurance
certificate of insurance
claim
compulsory
conversion privilege
coordinating of benefits
cost of insurance
cost sharing
    coinsurance
    copayment
    deductible
        sliding scale deductible
    deterrent fee
cover, coverage
    first-dollar coverage
    last-dollar coverage
dual choice
dump
duplication of benefits
enroll
    enrollment period
evidence of insurability
exclusion
expense

exposure
fee screen
file
fund
grace period
group insurance
    contributory
    group
    noncontributory
health insurance
Health Insurance Institute, 1983
hold harmless provision
incur
insurance clause
insurance commissioner
insurance policy
insurance pool
insured
insurer
joint underwriting association
liability
    limit on liability
life table
    abridged life table
    cohort, generation life table
    complete life table
    current life table
loading
long-term care insurance
loss
moral hazard
major medical expense insurance
malpractice insurance
maternity benefit
    flat maternity
    swap maternity
    switch maternity
McCarran-Ferguson Act
Medical Information Bureau
member
mutual insurance company
Osler, 1972
out-of-pocket cost, payment
participation

penetration
peril
persistency
pool
portability
preexisting condition
premium
prepayment
primary payer
Rand Health Insurance Experiment
rate, rating
    community rating
    experience rating
recurring clause
reinsurance
rescission
reserve
    contingency reserve
    reinsurance reserve
    primary reserve
rider
risk
    insurable risk
risk charge
saturation
screen
secondary payer
second opinion
self-insure
Singer, 1976
skim
social insurance
stock insurance company
subrogation
subscriber
surplus
third party payer
underwrite
underwriting profit
Uniform Individual Policy Provisions
usual, customary, and reasonable plan
waiting period
waiver of premium

1. service benefits
>   ancillary expense, service
>   assignment
>   Blue Cross and Blue Shield
>   Association
>   Blue Cross discount
>   Blue Cross plan
>   Blue Shield plan
>   competitive medical plan
>   Health Service, Inc.
>   Medical Indemnity of America, Inc.
>   vendor payment

2. indemnity benefits
>   accident and health insurance
>   aggregate indemnity
>   assessment
>   bedpan mutual
>   disability income insurance
>   extra cash policy
>   fixed benefit
>   individual insurance
>   mail-order insurance
>   scheduled benefit
>   specified disease insurance
>   supplemental health insurance
>   trolley car policy
>   unscheduled benefit

C. Public Funds
>   block grant
>   bond
>   categorical grant
>   Federal Employees Health Benefits
>   Program
>   high option
>   low option
>   open season
>   formula grant
>   general revenue
>   Health Care Financing Administration
>   Maximum Allowable Cost Program

means test
ownership disclosure
project grant
prudent buyer principle
request for proposal
section 314(d)
section 1122
social security
tax
> excise tax
> marginal tax rate
> payroll tax
> progressive tax
> proportional tax
> regressive tax
> tax bracket
> tax credit
> tax deduction
> tax expenditure
> tax expenditure budget

trust fund
unemployment insurance
vendor payment
waiting period

1. Medicare
> adjusted area per capita cost
> administrative days
> assignment
> comparability provision
> competitive medical plan
> condition of participation
> diagnosis related group
> > diagnosis related group creep
> > diagnosis related group rate
> > diagnosis related group weight
> > outlier
> > Patient Management
> > > Categories
> > principal diagnosis
> > Prospective Payment
> > > Assessment Commission
> > prospective payment system
> > sole community hospital

family ganging
fiscal agent, intermediary
freedom of choice
Hyde Amendment
institution for mental disease
lock-in
Medicaid management information
   system
Medicaid mill
Medi-Cal
Medical Assistance Program
medically needy
medical review
     independent professional
       review
     professional review team
Kerr-Mills
notch
optional service
ping-ponging
prepaid health plan
prior authorization
required service
resources
Ribicoff kid
section 222
spend down
supplementation
Title XIX

D. National Health Insurance
     competition
     compulsory
     health card
     medical deduction
     medical expense
     notch
     social insurance

V. Practice
     algorithm, clinical algorithm
     alternative medicine, therapy
       acupuncture
         acupressure

moxibustion
shiatsu
Alexander technique
Bates method
biofeedback
Bricklin, 1976
chiropractic
    chiropractor
Christian Science
denturism
faith healing
    curandero
    psychic surgery
    shaman
Gerson therapy
gestalt psychology
health food
    natural
    organic
holistic medicine
homeopathy
    concordant remedies
    inimic remedies
    tissue remedies
Hulke, 1979
humanistic medicine
hypnotism
    Braidism
imagery
Ingham Reflex Method of Compression
  Massage
    foot zone therapy
    reflexology
    zone therapy
iridology
Laetrile
macrobiotics
massage therapy
    Rolfing
    structural integration
meditation
    transcendental meditation
megavitamin therapy
    orthomolecular psychiatry

naturopathy
orthopsychiatry
pelotherapy
prolotherapy
quack
Reichian therapy
 orgone
 vegetotherapy
Rinzler, 1979
Scientology
speech therapy
T'ai-chi Chu'an
Tao of Loving
vegetarianism
 lactoovovegetarian
 vegan
Walker, 1978
wholistic medicine
Wren, 1907
Yoga
bedside manner
care
 primary care
  NAPCRG, 1978
  primary health care
  (see VII.D.2.)
 secondary care
 tertiary care
chairside
cure
error
ethics
 freedom of choice
 Hippocratic oath
 medical ethics
  Duncan, 1981
  Reich, 1978
family practice
 Balint group
 biopsychosocial model
 care giver
 caretaker
 community health care
 community medicine

telephone order
verbal order
orthodontics
panel
   list
playing god
practice management
practice register
prepaid group practice
private practice
protocol
roster
round, rounds
single-handed practice
solo practice
therapy
   art therapy
   audiology
      Delk, 1973
      Nicolosis, 1978
   behavior modification, therapy
   dentistry
      denture mill
      shopper
      slicking
      wetfingered
   music therapy
   occupational therapy
   play therapy
   recreation therapy
   respiratory therapy
scut work
speech pathology
stat

A. Diagnosis
      Bloomfield, 1982
      clinicopathologic conference
      consultation
      critical incident
      diagnostic criteria
      differential diagnosis

examination, physical exam
    gundeck physical
history, history and physical
    past medical history
    family history
    social history
    review of symptoms, systems
multiphasic screening
parsimony of diagnosis
physical diagnosis
principal diagnosis
psychometrics
q-sort
rule out
second opinion
scan
serum porcelain
therapeutic test
triage
workup

B. Treatment
    acceptable risk
    accepted dental remedy
    activity level
    acuity
    adjuvant
    adverse drug reaction
    bed rest
    behavior modification
    behavior therapy
    biofeedback
    blood doping
    cardiopulmonary resuscitation
        code, code blue
        no code
    commitment
    compliance
    complication
    condition
    consent
        consent form
        informed consent
        parental consent

therapeutic privilege
conservative
contraindication
counsel
dose
detoxification
dialysis
euthanasia
follow-up
habilitation
heal
indication
International Encyclopedia, 1973
kardex
Lipton, 1978
manipulation
milieu therapy
Modern Drug Encyclopedia, 1983
Moerman, 1977
minister
nostrum
nurse
nursing intensity
panacea
palliate
partial hospitalization
pastoral counseling
patent medicine
prescribe, prescription
    paradoxical prescription
primum non nocere
psychosurgery
psychotherapy
radical
reaction
regimen
rehabilitation
remedy
respite care
sick role
side effect
staff
surgery
    ambulatory surgery

                    cosmetic surgery
                    elective surgery
                    major surgery
                    minor surgery
                    operation
                    unnecessary surgery
               tachyphylaxis
               talk down
               Take Off Pounds Sensibly
               technique
               therapeutic, therapeutics
               therapeutic community
                    token economy
               therapeutic contract
               therapy
               tomato effect
               treatment
               vegetotherapy
               Weight Watchers

C. Education (see VII.B.2.b.)
               Brace, 1983
               Drug Use Education Tips
               health education
               Health Education Information
                    Retrieval System
               health hazard appraisal
               health maintenance
               health promotion
               holistic medicine
               humanistic medicine
               patient education
               preventative
               preventive medicine
               self-care
               self-help
               Smokenders
               wholistic

D. Malpractice
               abandonment
               ad damnum clause
               against medical advice
               American Medical Assurance
                    Company

charitable immunity
claims incurred policy
claims made policy
collateral source
compensable event
contingency fee
defensive medicine
discovery rule
dump
expert witness
go bare
good samaritan law
governmental immunity
incident report
joint underwriting association
liability
    limit on liability
liability exam
locality rule
malpractice insurance
negligence
New Jersey rule
professional liability
Relman Doctrine
res ipsa loquitur
respondeat superior
screening panel
self-insure
sponsored malpractice insurance
steer
tail
warranty

VI. Management
    Bittel, 1985
    consumer participation
    Heyel, 1973
    Timmreck, 1982

    A. Policy and Planning
        appropriate
        Area Resource File
        bond
        capital expenditure review

comprehensive health planning
depreciation
    funded
goal
green screen
health planning
objective
patient origin study
provider
region
Regional Medical Program
Roemer's law
Safire, 1978
Staats, 1975
Willard Report

1. health systems agency
    annual implementation plan
    areawide comprehensive health
        planning agency
    health service area
    health system plan

2. state health planning and development agency
    certificate of need
    institutional health service
    section 1122
    state comprehensive health
        planning agency
    statewide health coordinating
        council

B. Budgeting

1. federal budget
    advance appropriation
    appropriation
    authorization, authorizing
        legislation
    backdoor authority
    budget authority
    budget mark
    concurrent resolution
    congressional budget
    continuing resolution

controllability
current services budget
deferral of budget authority
entitlement authority
forward funding
function, functional classification
impoundment
impoundment resolution
lapsed funds
mark
obligation
open-ended program
outlay
President's budget
rescission

C. Administration
affiliation
health authority
management information system
Morris, 1978
practice management
request for proposal
Slee, 1986

1. accounting
administrative services only
contract
asset
capital
human capital
working capital
chart of accounts
collection rate
cost (see VII.D.1.)
fixed cost
variable cost
cost allocation
cost apportionment
cost center
current
debt
bad debt

balloon payment debt
retirement
debt service
long-term debt
depreciation
Estes, 1981
expense
fiscal year
Kohler, 1975
prospective reimbursement
responsibility accounting
sick tax
uniform cost accounting

D. Assessment and Regulation
abuse
accountable
Anderson, 1975
claims review
criteria
cost benefit
DEA number
evaluate
Farber, 1984
fraud
monitor
norm
profile
quality
SuperPro
standard
performance standard
specification standard
utilization
variance

1. cost control
Economic Stabilization Program
state cost commission

2. medical review
admission certification
concurrent review
continued stay review

experimental medical care review
  organization
medical audit
peer review
peer review organization
professional standards review
  organization
    delegation
    medical care evaluation study
    quality review study
necessity
prior authorization
prior determination
professional review team
quality assurance
technology assessment
tissue review
tracer
utilization review
utilization review committee

VII. Services and Procedures
  basic health service
  Current Procedural Terminology
  dental health services
  encounter
    direct encounter
    indirect encounter
    problem contact
    reason for encounter
  health system
  NAPCRG Process Classification
  problem contact
  service
    diagnostic, investigative service
    preventive service
    therapeutic service
  Systematized Nomenclature of Medicine
  visit
    gang visit
    home visit
    hospital visit

inpatient visit
outpatient visit
office visit

A. Beneficiaries

1. individual
consumer
maternal and child health service
S.J. Baker
F. Kelley
Supplemental Feeding
Program for Women,
Infants, and Children
patient
activated patient
attending patient
former patient
identified patient
inactive patient
nonvisiting patient
outpatient
public patient
private patient
registered patient
service patient
staff patient
temporary patient
transient patient
visiting patient
ward patient
walk-in

2. community
community health care
community medicine
community oriented primary care

B. Purpose

1. diagnosis
categorical program
Pap smear

2. community treatment

community mental health center
monitor

a. environmental health services (see I.C.)
    abatement
    demographics
    ecology
    environment
    environmental impact
        statement
    fluoridation
    National Environmental Policy
        Act

b. health education (see V.C.)
    activated patient
    Doctors Ought to Care
    Frenay, 1977
    Health Education Information
        Retrieval System
    health fair
    health hazard appraisal
    health information
    health promotion
    Levine, 1978
    Pomeranz, 1977
    Rothenberg, 1975
    Sex Information and Education
        Council of the United States
    Thomson, 1976
    Wingate, 1976
    World Book, 1979

c. mine safety and health
    black lung
    Coal Mine Health and Safety
        Act
    Paracelsus
    unwarrantable failure

d. occupational health
    abatement, abatement period
    accident prevention
    accident proneness
    asbestos

Ashford, 1976
assumption of risk
beryllium
brown lung
carcinogen
citation
complaints about state
    program administration
contributory negligence
criteria
criteria document
Department of Labor, 1977
disability
disablement
discount
fellow-servant doctrine
Goldberg, 1981
general duty clause
industrial hygiene
industrial physician
in-plant noise
International Labor Office,
    1971 and 1972
occupational air
occupational health
occupational health service
occupational medicine
occupational noise
occupational safety and health
Occupational Safety and
    Health Information Centre,
    1976
Robens Report
standard
        national consensus
            standard
        occupational safety and
            health standard
        performance standard
        specification standard
        variance
susceptibility
workmen's compensation act,
    insurance, and program

compensable event
disability
impairment
scheduled benefit or
payment
second-injury fund

e. public health (see VIII.C.)
G.D. Baillou
E. Chadwick
Deblock, 1976
Food, Drug, and Cosmetic Act
J. Goldberger
W.H. Park
preventive medicine
multiphasic screening
screening
pratique
Public Health Service Act
quarantine
Rhazes
Rosen, 1958
T. Sydenham

3. individual treatment
checkup
community health center
community health network
personal health service

a. acute
adult protective services
exploitation
emergency medical services
categorization
emergency
first aid
operation

b. habilitation/rehabilitation
health maintenance
prospective medicine
family planning (see I.C.1.)
Adolescent Family Life
Program

National Reporting
System for Family
Planning Services
Planned Parenthood
Association
squeal rule
immunization
E. Jenner
vaccination
vaccine
physical therapy
activities of daily living
Senior Actualization and
Growth Experience
vocational rehabilitation

C. Setting
level of care

1. home
foster care
home health care
homemaker service
home visit, house call
meals-on-wheels
sick call
visiting nurse association

2. community
health care delivery system
health care system
health services system
poison control center
respite care
rural health care

3. mobile
evacuation hospital
mobile army surgical hospital

4. ambulatory
aftercare
ambulatory care
chairside
episodic care center
surgicenter

visit

5. inpatient
    admission
        outlier
        Uniform Hospital Discharge
            Data Set
    admission certification
    day
        bed day
        patient day
    discharge
        discharge abstract
        discharge planning
        discharge summary
    inpatient care
    institutional health service
    progressive patient care

    a. acute
        critical care
        emergency care
        emergency medical services
        intensive care
        special care
        turkey

    b. chronic
        alternatives to long-term care
        custodial care
        domiciliary care
        extended care services
        intermediate care
        long-term care
        milieu therapy
        minimal care
        residential care
        sick call
        skilled care
        therapeutic community
            token economy

D. Attributes
    advertising
    medical record

Computer-Stored Ambulatory
  Record
confidential
problem list
problem-oriented medical record
progress note
scope of services
use, utilization
use screen

1. price
bill
charity allowance
charge
    actual charge
    allowable charge
    customary charge
    prevailing charge
    professional component
    reasonable charge
    technical, hospital component
cost
    allowable cost
    direct cost
    external cost
    general and administrative
      cost
    indirect cost
    internal cost
    per diem cost
    overhead
    reasonable cost
dispensing fee
fee
fractionation
free care
relative value scale, schedule
replacement fee
super bill
unbundling
upgrading

2. quality
acceptability
accessibility

availability
complete
comprehensive
continuous
criteria
effective
efficacy
efficiency
input measure
intensity of service
invasive
license, licensure
    institutional licensure
    reciprocity
length of stay
    average length of stay
medical audit
medical review
norm
outcome measure
output measure
primary care
    age-sex register
    North American Primary Care
      Research Group
    practice register
    problem index
    recorder
process measure
qualification
quality assurance
secondary care
standard
    performance standard
    specification standard
    variance
tertiary care

3.   resources used
    level of care
    nursing service
    productivity screen
    shared service

VIII. The Study of Health Care

A. History
Apple, 1984
Asclepius
Borgenicht, 1981
caduceus
Erlen, 1984
Hygeia
McGrew, 1985
Morton, 1983
Panacea
Rhodes, 1985
Rosen, 1958
Wasserman, 1987

1. people
Avicenna
Guillaume de Baillou
S. Josephine Baker
Beighton, 1986
Claude Bernard
John Shaw Billings
Edward Chadwick
Aurelius Cornelius Celsus
Daniel Drake
Paul Erlich
William Farr
Lawrence F. Flick
Theodore and Friederike Fliednor
Girolamo Fracastoro
Galen
Wade H. Frost
Joseph Goldberger
William Crawford Gorgas
John Graunt
Jacob Henle
Alice Hamilton
Hippocrates of Cos
Oliver Wendell Holmes
John Howard
Kaufman, 1983
Kelly, 1978

Florence Kelley
Robert Koch
Giovanni Maria Lancisi
James Lind
Joseph Lister
Pierre-Charles-Alexandre Louis
Florence Nightingale
William Osler
Paracelsus
Ambrose Pare
William Hallock Park
Talcott Parsons
Louis Pasteur
William Petty
Jean Piaget
Philippe Pinel
Bernardino Ramazzini
Rhazes
Walter Reed
Wilhelm Conrad Roentgen
Ronald Ross
Benjamin Rush
Ignaz Philip Semmelweis
Theobald Smith
John Snow
Strauss, 1968
Thomas Sydenham
William Tuke
Andreas Vesalius
Rudolph Virchow
Lillian Wald
Weeks, 1985
Zusne, 1984

2. things
Bane Report
Bethesda
Blue Cross
Bynum, 1981
Flexner Report
Haubrich, 1984
Kelly, 1948
Skinner, 1970

B. Language
Ayers, 1972
A Manual of Style, 1969
Bishop, 1984
Bloomfield, 1982
Brace, 1983
Chabner, 1985
Dirckx, 1976
Ferguson, 1983
Gove, 1976
Haubrich, 1984
Hochberg, 1985
Hukill, 1961
Landau, 1984
Manuila, 1984
Lourie, 1982
McDavid, 1973
Merriam Webster, 1973
Mishler, 1984
operational definition
render
Research Documentation Section, 1976
Rigal, 1976
Ruiz Torres, 1982a and b
Schmidt, 1969 and 1974
Skinner, 1970
Sloane, 1982
Slee, 1986
Strauss, 1968
Tabery, 1984
use, utilization
Vaisrub, 1977
WHO, 1977

1. health economics
Baldes, 1986
capital
commodity
competition
cost (see VII.D.1.)
cost benefit
life cost
marginal cost
opportunity cost

social cost
demand
depreciation
discounting
economy of scale
efficiency
elasticity
externality
good
    economic good
    consumer good
    free good
    social good
Greenwald, 1965
incidence
inflation
Moffat, 1976
Pearce, 1985
price
profit
proprietary
resources
Sichel, 1986
Sloan, 1970
supply

2. slang and humor

  a. slang
    acute remunerative
      appendicitis
    Andromeda strain
    bedpan mutual
    crock, crick
    denture mill
    disease of the month club
    doctor shopping
    eternal care, eternal care unit
    family ganging
    fascinoma
    fat doctor
    gang visit
    gork
    gomer
    green screen

gum farmer
gundeck physical
hip-pocket hysterectomy
hired gun
local medical doctor
measure for coffin
new clear medicine
pink lady
retrospectoscope
scut work
serum porcelain
shadow gazer
shopper
shroud waving
Sienknecht, 1985
slicking
steerer
stroke clinic
topsy
to the house
troll
trolley car policy
turkey
unclear medicine
upgrading
Wernicke rounds
wetfingered
yellow beret

b. jokes
actuary
alcoholic
Bethesda
Bierce, 1911
deceased
dictionary
expert
furfuraceous
institution
medical center
Metz, 1977
psychiatric diagnosis
psychiatrist
Ryan's law

socialized medicine
zones

3. health law (see V.D.)
abandonment
abuse of process
adult
assumption of risk
Baby Doe
Bander and Wallach, 1970
battery
bill
Black, 1968
boiler plate
bond
carnal knowledge
certificate
committee report
competence
    American Law Institute
      Formulation
    Durham rule
    Freeman rule
    guardian
    irresistible impulse test
    M'Naghton rule
    ward
conference
consent
    consent form
    informed consent
    legal consent
    parental consent
    therapeutic privilege
coroner
Curran, 1975
damage, damages
Darling case
dependent
disease of the month club
dissatisfied life
doctor shopping
equity
expert witness

hired gun
exploitation
exposure
fellow-servant doctrine
Fox's laws
fiduciary
Food, Drug, and Cosmetic Act
fraud
grandfather clause, provision
hold harmless provision
inquest
insanity
legislative history
liability
lobby
mark-up
medical examiner
mens rea
Metz, 1977
Murphy's law
natural death act
neglect, negligence
    contributory negligence
Oran, 1978
O'Shea's law
parens patriae
police power
police surgeon
privilege
    physician-patient privilege
    therapeutic privilege
Public Health Service Act
public law
rape
    statutory rape
right to treatment
Roemer's law
Ryan's law
rule
    notice of proposed rulemaking
    regulation
Safire, 1978
Social Security Act
statute of limitations

Last, 1983
Michael, 1984
net reproduction rate
nomenclature
nosology
notifiable
pandemic
para, parity
plaque
population
    population pyramid
    registered population
    sample
    study population
prevalence
    period prevalence
    point prevalence
    prevalence rate in active patient
        population
problem index
rate, ratio
    age-specific rate
recorder
relative risk
reportable
reservoir
risk factor
    behavioral risk factor
Singer, 1976
J. Snow
standard age groups
vector
    G.M. Lancisi
    W. Reed
    R. Ross
    T. Smith
    R. Virchow
zoonosis

D. Research and Statistics
    applied research
    analysis of variance
    animal model
    average

bias
>   detection bias
>   experimenter bias
>   migration bias
>   susceptibility bias
>   volunteer bias

biomedical research
Chen, 1981
control
>   control group
>   subjects as their own controls

correlation
crossover experiment
datum, statistic
>   data set

demand characteristic
ecological fallacy
efficiency value
Elling, 1980
error
>   sampling error
>   systematic error

evaluate
experiment
experimental design
experimenter bias
false negative
false positive
fit
Framingham Heart Study
halo effect
Hawthorne effect
health services research
Hill, 1977
hypothesis
>   falsifiable hypothesis
>   null hypothesis

institutional review board
Jerrard, 1986
Kotz, 1985
lead-time bias
Manning, 1981
mean
>   arithmetic mean

study, trial
case-control study
cohort study
double-blind study
longitudinal study
prospective trial
retrospective study
study population
subject
subjects as their own controls
test
test of significance
Tiejten, 1986
tomato effect
true negative
true positive
University Group Diabetes Program
utilization
variable
dependent
independent
intervening variable
quantitative variable
validity
external validity
variance
volunteer bias
Weise, 1979
Will Rogers phenomenon
zero-time shift
Zupke, 1985

Abbreviations, Acronyms, and Numerology

(Alphabet Soup Expanded)[1]

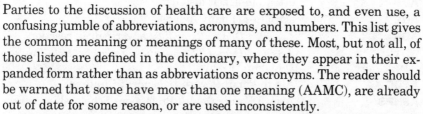

Parties to the discussion of health care are exposed to, and even use, a confusing jumble of abbreviations, acronyms, and numbers. This list gives the common meaning or meanings of many of these. Most, but not all, of those listed are defined in the dictionary, where they appear in their expanded form rather than as abbreviations or acronyms. The reader should be warned that some have more than one meaning (AAMC), are already out of date for some reason, or are used inconsistently.

Longer lists of abbreviations will be found in the works of *Crowley, 1984; Davis, 1985; Delong, 1985; Garb, 1976; Hamilton, 1984; Hughes, 1977; Kerr, 1970; Logan, 1987; Roody, 1976; Schertel, 1977;* the *Special Studies Committee, 1967; Sloane, 1985;* and *Steen, 1984*. These all have a more clinical orientation than the following list. Mnemonics, particularly common in clinical medicine, have been omitted; see *Bloomfield, 1982* and *1984*.

A

AA Alcoholics Anonymous

AAMC Association of American Medical Clinics, Association of American Medical Colleges

---

[1]This lovely phrase is taken from Florence A. Wilson and Duncan Neuhauser, *Health Services in the United States* (Cambridge, MA: Ballinger, 1974). Their book is a very useful "anatomy" of the health system.

91

AAFP	American Academy of Family Physicians
AAPCC	adjusted average per capita cost
A&H	accident and health insurance
AAPS	American Association of Physicians and Surgeons
AB	abortion, Aid to the Blind
ABFP	American Board of Family Practice
ABMS	American Board of Medical Specialties
ACA	American Chiropractic Association
ACCME	Accreditation Council for Continuing Medical Education
ACGME	Accreditation Council for Graduate Medical Education
ACS	American Cancer Society
ADA	American Dental Association
ADAMHA	Alcohol, Drug Abuse, and Mental Health Administration
ADC	Aid to Families with Dependent Children
ADD	attention-deficit disorder
ADL	activities of daily living
ADR	*Accepted Dental Remedies;* adverse drug reaction
ADT	*Accepted Dental Therapeutics;* a *placebo, as* A (any), D (damn), T (thing)
AFDC	Aid to Families with Dependent Children
AFHPS	Armed Forces Health Professions Scholarship
AFIP	Armed Forces Institute of Pathology
AFRAIDS	Afraid of AIDS, see *acquired immune deficiency syndrome*
AHA	American Heart Association, American Hospital Association, area health authority
AHCCCS	Arizona Health Care Cost Containment System
AHEC	area health education center
AHFS	American Hospital Formulary Service
AHIP	Assisted Health Insurance Plan
AIDS	acquired immune deficiency syndrome
AIP	annual implementation plan
ALI	American Law Institute
ALOS	average *length of stay*
AMA	against medical advice, American Medical Association
AMACO	American Medical Assurance Company

AMA-ERF	American Medical Association—Educational Research Foundation
AMCAS	American Medical College Application Service
AME	aviation medical examiner
AMPAC	American Medical Political Action Committee
ANA	American Nurses Association
ANC	acid-neutralizing capacity
ANOVA	analysis of variance
ANSI	American National Standards Institute
AOA	Alpha Omega Alpha Honor Medical Society
APACHE	Acute Physiology and Chronic Health Evaluation
APhA	American Pharmaceutical Association
APHA	American Protestant Hospital Association, American Public Health Association
ARC	American Red Cross; AIDS related complex, see *acquired immune deficiency syndrome*
ASFR	age-specific fertility rate
ASHD	arteriosclerotic heart disease
ASO contract	administrative services only contract
ATCC	American Type Culture Collection

B

BA	budget authority
BCA	Blue Cross Association
BC/BS	Blue Cross/Blue Shield
BCDSP	Boston Collaborative Drug Surveillance Program
BCHS	Bureau of Community Health Services
BCRR	BCHS Common Reporting Requirements
BHI	Bureau of Health Insurance
BHM	Bureau of Health Manpower
BHPRD	Bureau of Health Planning and Resources Development
Blue Sheet	*Drug Research Reports*
BNDD	Bureau of Narcotics and Dangerous Drugs
BOD	biochemical oxygent demand
BOSH	Bureau of Occupational Safety and Health
BRFS	Behavioral Risk Factor Surveys
BS	Blue Shield

C

C&Y	children and youth project of the Maternal and Child Health Program
CAHEA	Committee on Allied Health Education and Accreditation
CAP	community action program
CASPA	complaints about state program administration
CAT scanning	computed or computerized axial tomography
CBO	Congressional Budget Office
CC	chief complaint
CCME	Coordinating Council on Medical Education
CCS	Crippled Children's Service
CCU	coronary care unit, see *intensive care*
CD	communicable disease
CDC	Centers for Disease Control (formally the Communicable Disease Center)
CEQ	Council on Environmental Quality
CER	capital expenditure review
CFMA	Council for Medical Affairs
CHAMPUS	Civilian Health and Medical Program of the Uniformed Services
CHAMPVA	Civilian Health and Medical Program of the Veterans Administration
CHAP	Child Health Assurance Program
CHC	community health center
CHESS	Community Health and Environmental Surveillance System
CHN	community health network
CHP	comprehensive health planning
CHSS	Cooperative Health Statistics System
CIOMS	Council for International Organizations on Medical Sciences
CL	current liabilities
CLA	certified laboratory assistant, see *medical laboratory assistant*
CME	continuing medical education
CMHC	community mental health center
CMI	Cornell Medical Index, Medicare Case Mix Index
CMIT	Current Medical Information and Terminology
CMP	competitive medical plan
CMS	Council of Medical Staffs

CMSS	Council of Medical Specialty Societies
CMT	Current Medical Terminology
CNM	certified nurse midwife
Co	coinsurance
COB	coordination of benefits
CON	certificate of need, necessity
COPC	community oriented primary care
COSTAR	Computer-Stored Ambulatory Record
COTH	Council of Teaching Hospitals
COTRANS	Coordinated Transfer Application System
CPA	certified public accountant
CPC	clinicopathologic conference
CPHA	Commission on Professional and Hospital Activities
CPI	Consumer Price Index
CPO	certified prosthetist and orthotist
CPR	cardiopulmonary resuscitation
CPT	Current Procedural Terminology
CRV, CRVS	California Relative Value Scale
CSHO	see *compliance officer*
CT	computed or computerized axial tomography

D

D	diploma, diplomate
DC	Doctor of Chiropractic
DD	developmental disability, differential diagnosis
DDS	Doctor of Dental Surgery
DDT	dichloro-diphenyl-trichloro-ethane
DEA	Drug Enforcement Administration
DEF	Dental formula designating the number of deciduous teeth needing filling, needing extraction, and filled
DES	diethylstilbestrol
DESI	Drug Efficacy Study Implementation
DHA	district health authority
DHHS	Department of Health and Human Services
DH MEDICO	Deadhead Medico
DHSS	Department of Health and Social Security (UK)
DI	double indemnity
DMD	Doctor of Dental Medicine
DME	Director of Medical Education

DME	durable medical equipment
DMF	Dental formula representing the number of decayed, missing, and filled teeth (with reference to permanent teeth; compare DEF)
DO	Doctor of Optometry, Doctor of Osteopathy
DOA	dead on arrival
DOC	Doctors Ought to Care
DP	Doctor of Pharmacy
DPIF	Drug Products Information File
DPM	Doctor of Podiatric Medicine
DRG	diagnosis related group
DSM III	*Diagnostic and Statistical Manual of Mental Disorders,* 3d ed
D.U.E.T.	Drug Use Education Tips
DVM	Doctor of Veterinary Medicine
DVS	Doctor of Veterinary Science or Surgery

E

E book	experience book
ECF	extended care facility
ECFMG	Educational Commission for Foreign Medical Graduates
ECFMS	Educational Council for Foreign Medical Students
ECU	eternal care unit
EDB	ethylene dibromide
EE	ecological efficiency
EHIP	Employee Health Insurance Plan
EHSDS	experimental health service delivery system
EIS	Epidemiologic Intelligence Service
EMCRO	experimental medical care review organization
EMI scanning	see *computerized axial tomography*
EMS	emergency medical services
EMSS	emergency medical service system
ENT	ear, nose, and throat surgery
EOB	explanation of benefits
EPA	Environmental Protection Agency
EPSDT	early and periodic screening, diagnosis, and treatment
ER	emergency room

ERF	Educational Research Foundation
ESP	Economic Stabilization Program
ESRD	end stage renal disease
EST	Erhardt Seminars Training
EW	emergency ward

F

F	Fellow
FACES	Family Adaptability and Cohesion Evaluation Scales
FACP, FACS, etc.	Fellow of the American College of Physicians, Surgeons, or whatever; see *fellow*
FAMLI	*Family Medicine Literature Index*
FAO	Food and Agricultural Organization (of the United Nations)
FBI	flossing, brushing, and irrigation
FDA	Food and Drug Administration
FD&C Act	Federal Food, Drug, and Cosmetic Act
FDD	Food and Drugs Directorate (Canada)
FEHBP	Federal Employees Health Benefits Program
FFP	federal financial participation
FHFAN	Family Health Foundation of America
FICA	Federal Insurance Contributions Act (Social Security)
FIFRA	Federal Insecticide, Fungicide, and Rodenticide Act
FLEX	Federation Licensing Examination
FLK	funny looking kid
FMC	foundation for medical care
FMG	foreign medical graduate
FMP	Family Medicine Programme
FMS	foreign medical student
FN	false negative
FNC	family nurse clinician
FNP	family nurse practitioner
FP	family planning, false positive, family practice, family practitioner
FRCP, FRCS, etc.	Fellow of the Royal College of Physicians, Surgeons, or whatever; see *fellow*
FSA	Federal Security Administration
FSMB	Federation of State Medical Boards
FTC	Federal Trade Commission
FY	fiscal year

G

G and A	general and administrative costs
GHA	Group Health Association of Washington, D.C.
GHAA	Group Health Association of America
GMENAC	Graduate Medical Education National Advisory Committee to the Secretary, DHHS
GMP	good manufacturing practice
GN	graduate nurse
GP	general practitioner
The GPEP Report	see *Physicians for the Twenty-First Century*
GRAE	generally recognized as effective
GRAS	generally recognized as safe
GYN	gynecology

H

H&A	health and accident insurance
H&P	history and physical examination
HANES	National Health and Nutrition Examination Survey
HASP	Hospital Admission and Surveillance Program
HC	handicapped, home care, house call
HCC	health care corporation
HCFA	Health Care Financing Administration
HEAL	Health Education Assistance Loan Program
Health/PAC	Health Policy Advisory Center
HEIRS	Health Education Information Retrieval System
HEW	Department of Health, Education, and Welfare
HHS	Department of Health and Human Services
HI	Hospital Insurance Program of Medicare
HIAA	Health Insurance Association of America
HIBAC	Health Insurance Benefits Advisory Council
H-ICDA	Hospital International Classification of Disease Adapted for use in the United States
HIMA	Health Industry Manufacturers Association
HIP	Health Insurance Plan of Greater New York, Inc.
HMEIA	health manpower education initiative award
HMO	health maintenance organization
HN	head nurse

HO	house officer
Homeo(p)	homeopathy
HPSL	Health Professions Student Loan Program
HRA	Health Resources Administration
H.R. 10 plan	Keogh plan
H$_2$S	Department of Health and Human Services
HSA	health service area, Health Services Administration, health systems agency
HSI	Health Service, Inc.
HSMHA	Health Services and Mental Health Administration
HSP	health system plan
hyg	hygiene

I

IBNR	incurred but not reported
IC	intensive care
ICDA	International Classification of Diseases—Adapted
ICD-9-CM	International Classification of Diseases—Ninth Edition—Clinical Modification
ICF	intermediate care facility
ICF/MR	intermediate care facility for the mentally retarded
ICU	intensive care unit
IDB	industrial development bond, see *bond*
ID$_{50}$	median infective dose
IL	intermediary letter
IM	Index Medicus, internal medicine
IMD	institution for mental disease
IND	investigational new drug
INN	International Nonproprietary Names
ins	insurance
IOM	Institute of Medicine of the National Academy of Sciences
IPA	individual practice association
IPR	independent professional review
IQ	intelligence quotient
IRA	individual retirement account
IRB	institutional review board

ISC	International Statistical Classification
IUD	intrauterine death, intrauterine device

J

JAR	junior assistant resident
JAMA	*Journal of the American Medical Association*
JCAH	Joint Commission on Accreditation of Hospitals
JUA	joint underwriting association

K

K-P	Kaiser-Permanente

L

L	Licentiate
LCCME	Liaison Committee on Continuing Medical Education
LCGME	Liaison Committee on Graduate Medical Education
LCME	Liaison Committee on Medical Education
LC_{50}	median lethal concentration
LD	learning disability
LD_{50}	median lethal dose
LMCC	Licentiate of the Medical Council of Canada
LMD	local medical doctor
LOS	length of stay
LPN	licensed practical nurse
LTC	long-term care
LVN	licensed visiting or vocational nurse

M

M	medical, medicine, member
MAA	Medical Assistance for the Aged
MAC	maximum allowable cost
MAI	medical adversity insurance
MAMP	Medical Activities and Manpower Project

M&I	maternal and infant care project of the Maternal and Child Health Program
MAP	Medical Audit Program
MASH	Mobile Army Surgical Hospital
MBD	minimal brain dysfunction
MCAT	Medical College Admission Test
MCE	medical care evaluation
MCH	maternal and child health
MCHR	Medical Committee for Human Rights
MDC	major diagnostic category
MDR	minimum daily requirements
ME	Medical Examiner
MEDEX	*medicin extension* (F), a physician assistant, see *Medex*
MEDISGRPS	Medical Illness Severity Grouping System
MEDLARS	Medical Literature and Analysis Retrieval System
MEDLINE	Medicine On-Line, an on-line part of *MEDLARS*
MEND	Medical Education for National Defense
MERIT Project	Medical Education Requirements in Training Project
MESH	Medical Subject Headings
MFC	measure for coffin ·
MGH	Massachusetts General Hospital
MIA	Medical Indemnity of America, Inc.
MIB	Medical Information Bureau
MIMS	Monthly Index of Medical Specialties
MIS	management information system
MM	major medical
MMIS	Medicaid management information system
MMWR	*Morbidity and Mortality Weekly Report*
MO	medical officer
MODs	Schools of Medicine, Osteopathy, and Dentistry; see *health manpower*
MPH	Master of Public Health
MR	mental retardation
MRI	magnetic resonance imaging
MSA	Medical Services Administration
MSKP	Medical Sciences Knowledge Profile
MSW	Master of Social Welfare, Master of Social Work, medical social worker
MT	medical technologist
M-team	multidisciplinary team

MUA	medically underserved area
MUMPS	Massachusetts General Hospital Utility Multi-Programming System
MV	*Medicus Veterinarius* (L), veterinarian

N

N	national
NA	nurse's aide
NAIA	National Association of Insurance Agents
NAIC	National Association of Insurance Commissioners
NARC	narcotics officer, National Association for Retarded Citizens
NARD	National Association of Retail Druggists
NAPCRG	North American Primary Care Research Group
NBME	National Board of Medical Examiners
NCHS	National Center for Health Statistics
NCHSR	National Center for Health Service Research
NCI	National Cancer Institute
NCME	Network for Continuing Medical Education
NDA	new drug application, natural death act
NEJM	*New England Journal of Medicine*
NEPA	National Environmental Policy Act
NF	National Formulary
NHeLP	National Health Law Program
NHI	national health insurance
NHS	National Health Service
NHSC	National Health Service Corps
NIAAA	National Institute of Alcohol Abuse and Alcoholism
NIDA	National Institute of Drug Abuse
NIH	National Institutes of Health
NIMH	National Institute of Mental Health
NIOSH	National Institute for Occupational Safety and Health
NIRMP	National Interns and Residents Matching Program
NLM	National Library of Medicine
NLN	National League of Nursing
NMA	National Medical Association
NMR	nuclear magnetic resonance
NNR	New and Nonofficial Remedies
NORML	National Organization to Reform Marijuana Laws

NP	nurse practitioner
NPRM	notice of proposed rulemaking
NRMP	National Residents Matching Program
NRSFPS	National Reporting System for Family Planning Services
NSC	nonservice connected
NSF	National Science Foundation
NTIS	National Technical Information Service

O

OASDHI	Old-Age, Survivors, Disability and Health Insurance Program
OBG, OB-GYN	obstetrics(cian) and gynecology(gist)
OC	oral contraceptive
OD	Doctor of Optometry, Doctor of Osteopathy, officer of the day, overdose
OEO	Office of Economic Opportunity
OM	Occupational Medicine
OMF	outpatient medical facility
OPD	outpatient department or dispensary
opt	optician, optics(ical)
OR	operating room
Ortho	orthopedic surgery
OSHA	Occupational Safety and Health Act or Administration
OT	occupational therapy or therapist
OTA	Office of Technology Assessment
OTC	over-the-counter drug

P

P	pharmacopeia, private, psychiatry(ist)
PA	physician assistant, Proprietary Association
PAHO	Pan American Health Organization
P&S	physicians and surgeons
Part A	Hospital Insurance Program of Medicare
Part B	Supplementary Medical Insurance Program of Medicare
PAS	Professional Activity Study
PCB	polychlorinated biphenyl

PCMR	President's Committee on Mental Retardation
PC, p.c.	private or professional corporation
PCB	polychlorinated biphenyl
PCC	poison control center
PCOB	Permanent Central Opium Board (Geneva)
PCT	Patient Care Technician
PD	Doctor of Pharmacy
PDR	*Physicians' Desk Reference*
PE	physical examination
PET	positron emission tomography
PF	Physicians' Forum
PH	past (previous) medical history, pharmacopeia, public health
phar(m)	pharmacopeia, pharmacy, pharmaceutical
PHN	public health nurse(ing)
PHP	prepaid health plan
PHS	US Public Health Service
PHS Act	Public Health Service Act
Phys Med	physical medicine
PIP	periodic interim payment
PKU	phenylketonuria
PL, P.L.	Public law, usually with a number, as P.L. 93-641.
P.L. 15	McCarran-Ferguson Act
PM	physical medicine, preventive medicine
PMA	petition for modification of abatement, see *abatement period,* Pharmaceutical Manufacturers Association
PM&R	physical medicine and rehabilitation
PMCs	Patient Management Categories
PMH	past (previous) medical history
PMI	patient medication information
PNHA	Physicians' National Housestaff Association
PO	(tele)phone order
POMR	problem-oriented medical record
PP	private patient, physician, or practice
PPI	patient package insert
PPO	preferred provider organization
PPS	prospective payment system
PriCare	International Classification of Health Problems in Primary Care
PRO	peer review organization
PROMIS	Problem-Oriented Medical Information System

ProPAC	Prospective Payment Assessment Commission
PRRB	Provider Reimbursement Review Board
PS	plastic surgery
Ps	prescription
PSI	Pollutant Standards Index
PSR	Physicians for Social Responsibility
PSRO	professional standards review organization
Psy	psychiatry(ist)
PT	patient, physical therapy(ist)
Px	past history, physical examination, prescription

Q

QAP	Quality Assurance Program for Medical Care in the Hospital
QCIM	Quarterly Cumulative Index Medicus
QHP(S)	Honorary Physician (Surgeon) to the Queen
QRS, QRSs	Quality Review Study(ies)

R

R	radiology(ist), registered, regional, royal
rad	radiation absorbed dose
Rad(iol)	radiotherapy(ist)
RAP	Residency Assistance Program
R&D	research and development
RC	Red Cross, Royal College
RCC	ratio of *Medicare charges* to total charges applied to *allowable costs*
RCT	random controlled trial
RD	registered dietician
RDA	recommended dietary allowance
Redbook	*Drug Topics Red Book*
ref phys	referring physician
REM	remarried family
RFP	request for proposal
RHA	regional health authority
RHI	Rural Health Initiative
RMP	Regional Medical Program
RN	registered nurse

ROS	review of symptoms or systems
RPAR	rebuttable presumption against registration
RR	recovery room
RRC	residency review committee
RT	radiotherapy, recreational therapy, registered technician (American Registry of X-Ray Technicians)
RVS	relative value scale or schedule
RVU	relative value unit
RWJ	The Robert Wood Johnson Foundation
Rx	prescription, treatment, or therapy

S

S	specialty(ist), surgery(eon)
SAD	seasonal affective disorder
SAGE	Senior Actualization and Growth Experience
S&H	speech and hearing
SAR	senior assistant resident
SB	stillbirth
SC	self-care, service-connected, sick call
SCH	safe community hospital
SD	standard deviation
SES	socioeconomic status
SG	Surgeon General
SH	social history, speech and hearing
SHCC	statewide health coordinating council
SHPDA	state health planning and development agency
SI	*Systeme Internationale d'Unites,* see *International System of Units*
SIECUS	Sex Information and Education Council of the United States
SKI	Sloan Kettering Institute
SLD	specific learning disability
SMI	Supplementary Medical Insurance of Medicare
SMSA	standard metropolitan statistical area
SNDO	Standard Nomenclature of Diseases and Operations
SNF	skilled nursing facility
SNODERM	Systematized Nomenclature of Dermatology
SNOMED	Systematized Nomenclature of Medicine
SNOP	Systematized Nomenclature of Pathology

SO	standing order
SOAP	subjective, objective, assessment, and plan (see *problem-oriented medical record*)
SOII	severity of illness index
SOSSUS	Study of Surgical Services for the United States
SPL	sound pressure level
^{90}Sr	strontium 90
SRS	Social and Rehabilitation Service
SSA	Social Security Administration
SSI	supplemental security income
STD	sexually transmitted disease
SW	social worker
Sx	symptom, signs
S. 1508	McCarran-Ferguson Act

T

T	technician(ologist)
TIP	Target Industry Program
Title XVIII	Medicare
Title XIX	Medicaid
TLV	threshold limit value
TO	telephone order
TM	transcendental meditation
TN	true negative
TNM	tumor, nodes, metastases
TOPS	Take Off Pounds Sensibly
TP	true positive
Trop Med	tropical medicine
TSCA	Toxic Substances Control Act
TTH	to the house
Tx	therapy, treatment

U

UCR	usual, customary, and reasonable
UGDP	University Group Diabetes Program
UHDDS	Uniform Hospital Discharge Data Set
UNICEF	United Nations International Children's Emergency Fund

UR	utilization review
USAN	United States Adopted Names
USC-MAMP	University of Southern California *Medical Activities and Manpower Project*
USP	United States Pharmacopeia
USPHS	United States Public Health Service

V

VA	Veterans Administration
VD	venereal disease
VN	visiting or vocational nurse
VNA	visiting nurse association
VO	verbal order
VOPPS	Schools of Veterinary Medicine, Optometry, Podiatry, and Public Health, see *health manpower*
VQE	Visa Qualifying Examination
VR	voc rehab, vocational rehabilitation
VRA	Vocational Rehabilitation Administration
VS	veterinary surgeon

W

WBGH	Washington Business Group on Health
WHO	World Health Organization
WIC	Supplemental Feeding Program for Women, Infants, and Children
WONCA	World Organization of National Colleges, Academies, and Academic Associations of General Practitioners/Family Physicians
WNL	within normal limits
WRMH	Washington Report on Medicine and Health

Z

ZPG	zero population growth

abandonment. desertion of a patient by a physician or other health professional during the patient's care without giving adequate notice or making suitable arrangements for a substitute. Abandonment may be grounds for loss of *license* or suit for *malpractice*. V.D., VIII.B.3.

abatement. 1. eliminating or reducing *pollution* (in environmental health), work *hazards* (in occupational health), or other deficiencies, whether or not permanently. 2. the method by which it is done. I.C., VII.B.2.d.

abatement period. the time given an employer in a *citation* by the *Occupational Safety and Health Administration* for correction of a *hazard*.

The period must be reasonable and may be appealed by either employee or employer by contesting the citation or by *petition for modification of abatement (PMA). Failure to correct a hazard within the abatement period may cost the employer a daily civil penalty (fine) of up to $1000 until it is corrected. VII.B.2.d.

abortion (ab). 1. giving *birth* to an embryo or fetus and the other products of conception before the fetus has attained viability or has a reasonable chance of survival. 2. the product of such nonviable birth. 3. the arrest of any action or process before its normal completion.

Viability is arbitrarily legally defined, variably throughout the world, in terms of the fetus weight (more than 500–1000 grams [usually 500 in the United States]), age (20–28 weeks gestation [usually 20 in the United States] or the time since the last menses or conception [180–200 days]), or occasionally, length. Whether life begins with or before viability is at issue in the United States. Birth after viability but before full term is *premature. Use of *"miscarriage" for *spontaneous (naturally occurring) and abortion for *induced (brought on purposely) abortions is irregular but common. Abortions may be *early (less than, arbitrarily and variably, 400–500 grams or 12–20 weeks gestation) or *late, and *complete or *incomplete (leaving some products of conception in the uterus). Use of "abortion" for early abortions and "miscarriage" for late ones is obsolete. A *criminal abortion is any abortion which is illegal in the jurisdiction in which it is performed, whether because improperly done, done after viability is reached, or done for unacceptable *indications*. An *elective abortion is usually a euphemism for an abortion for purposes of birth control and sometimes refers to nonemergency therapeutic abortions and those performed to prevent birth of a defective child. A *therapeutic abortion is one induced for, or incidental to, treatment of the pregnant woman, whether to save her life, treat an illness, or because she was *raped*. Sometimes includes abortions performed to prevent birth of a defective child. I.A.1.

abstinence syndrome.   see *addiction*.

abstract.   see *discharge abstract*.

abuse.   1. improper, usually excessive, use of *benefits, resources,* or *services* by either providers or consumers. 2. see *drug abuse*. 3. for abused child or wife, see *battery*.

Abuse can occur when services are used which are excessive, unnecessary, or inappropriate for the patient's condition; when cheaper services would be as effective; or where payment does not conform to requirements. It should be distinguished from *fraud* since it may be neither intentional nor illegal. VI.D.

abuse of process.   inappropriate use of the legal system, as *commitment* of someone for reasons other than those authorized by law. VII.B.3.

acceptability.   an overall assessment of *available* health care by an individual or group.

Acceptability is influenced by such tangibles as the *efficacy, cost,* and *accessibility* of care and such intangibles as facility beauty and provider empathy. VII.D.

acceptable risk.   a chance of adverse effects from an undertaking which is trivial or has costs which are usefully less than the likely benefits. See *risk*. V.B.

***Accepted Dental Therapeutics* (ADT).**   since 1969, an official publication of the Council on Dental Therapeutics of the American Dental Association describing products which have been evaluated and found safe and effective for their indicated uses in dentistry. From 1934 through 1967 the title was *Accepted Dental Remedies* (ADR). V.B.

accessibility.   the opportunity an individual or group has to obtain health care.

Access has geographic, financial, social, and psychologic aspects and is thus difficult to measure operationally. It is a direct function of, and is sometimes defined by, the *availability* of care but is only one aspect of its *acceptability*. Many government health programs are intended to improve accessibility of certain kinds of care, access to care for specific groups, or equity of access in the whole population.

Equity of access is achieved when people make equal use of *health resources* for equal needs. VII.D.

accident.   an unexpected, unplanned event, which may involve *injury;* legally, an event whose occurrence a reasonable man would not have foreseen, because of which the law holds no one legally responsible for the harm caused. Often the basis for *disability, insurance,* or *workmen's compensation claims* but variably defined, largely by case law. II.B.1.

accident and health insurance (A&H). historically, *insurance* providing cash indemnification for loss of income in the event of illness, accidental injury, or, in some cases, accidental death, with no requirement that the money be used to purchase health care; more recently and loosely, any type of insurance involving health. IV.B.

accident prevention. keeping people from getting hurt, the *prevention* of accidents; the study and methods of such prevention.

Accident prevention is an old and essential part of *occupational health*. Principles for successful prevention include management interest and support, detailed cause analysis, proper selection and application of remedies, and enforcement of corrective practices. VII.B.2.d.

accident proneness. great *susceptibility* to accidents. Inconsistent, sometimes used whatever the cause, even youth or inexperience, sometimes limited to cases arising from personality traits or psychologic factors.

This is an important but controversial concept in *occupational health* where analyzing why people have accidents is crucial to their prevention. The concept may lead to *blaming the victim* if the worker, rather than an unsafe workplace, is fixed. I.A., VII.B.2.d.

accountable. responsible, answerable; liable; able to furnish a justification or detailed explanation of financial and other activities or responsibilities; able to furnish substantial reasons or convincing explanation.

Accountability entails an obligation to disclose in adequate detail to interested parties the purposes, procedures, results, and finances involved in an activity or program so they can be *evaluated* by responsible parties. The concept is important in health *planning, delivery,* and *regulatory* programs, as *health systems agencies,* which should be accountable to the public and those they affect for their actions. There is no specific or detailed agreement on what program accountability is or how to assure it. Federal health planning law, for example, tried to enhance accountability: agency governing boards were required to have a *consumer* majority; affected parties were to be represented on agency governing boards; data, files, and meetings were open to the public; and decisions were made according to established public procedures and *criteria*. VI.E.

accreditation. 1. the process by which an organization recognizes a program of study or an institution as meeting predetermined *standards*. 2. such recognition. Similar assessment of individuals is called *certification*.

Accrediting typically involves five basic steps: establishment of standards, self-study with respect to the standards, on-site evaluation by the accrediting agency, publication of an accredited institution or program's name in official lists, and periodic reevaluation. Standards may be applied to an institution's plant, governing body, administration, staff, and scope and organization of services. Accreditation is usually given by private nonprofit organizations created specifically for the purpose, as the *Joint Commission on Accreditation of Hospitals*. Standards and individual performance with respect to such standards are not always available to the public. In some situations governments recognize accreditation in lieu of, accept it as the basis of, or require it as a condition of *licensure*. Public and private payment programs often require accreditation as a *condition of participation*. Unlike a license, accreditation is intended as an indication of adequate quality, not as a condition of lawful operation, although it may have the latter effect where payment is conditioned on accreditation. Provisional or temporary accreditation may be available for new or inadequate organizations. In the United States, national accrediting organizations in education are in turn recognized, or "accredited," by the federal Department of Education. III.B.1., VII.D.2.

Accreditation Council for Continuing Medical Education (ACCME). an organization responsible for accrediting *continuing medical education* programs.

In 1981, the ACCME replaced and combined the functions of the Liaison Committee on Continuing Medical Education and the American Medical Association's Committee on Accreditation of Continuing Medical Education. It is comprised of and controlled by members of the establishment in U.S medicine (the American Association of Medical Colleges, American Board of Medical Specialties, American Hospital Association, American Medical Association, and the Council of Medical Specialty Societies) with representation from the Association for Hospital Medical Education and the Federation of State Medical Boards. III.A.

Accreditation Council for Graduate Medical Education (ACGME). an organization responsible for accrediting *graduate medical education* programs, particularly *residencies* in the various medical specialties.

It replaced the Liaison Committee on Graduate Medical Education in 1981. It is composed of and controlled by the same parent organizations as the Accreditation Council for Continuing Medical Education with representation from residents, the public, and the federal government. Accreditation authority is delegated to individual residency review committees (RRC) for each specialty. Costs are financed through the parent organizations and by charges to accredited programs. III.A.1.

acid-neutralizing capacity (ANC). the ability of a body of water, as a lake, to buffer or absorb acid from rain and other sources without change in pH, or acidity.

A reading of less than 200 microequivalents per liter indicates a vulnerability to acidification, although lakes with low capacities are not necessarily acidifying if they are buffered by acid-absorbing soil or vegetation. I.C.5.

acid rain. rain with an acid pH, containing particularly natural carbon dioxide and sulfuric and nitric acid resulting from atmospheric conversion of sulfur dioxide (SO_2) and nitrous oxides (NO_x) *pollutants* emitted into the atmosphere, primarily by cars and coal-burning power plants; synonym, acid precipitation.

Such rain, downwind from heavily industrialized areas, acidifies lakes, shifts the biologic balance, and sometimes eliminates all lake life. Effects on forests, crops, buildings, and bridges are all destructive but still being characterized.

Read *Acid Deposition: Long Term Trends* (Washington, D.C.: National Academy Press, 1986. 506 pp.). I.C.1., I.C.5.

acoustic. pertaining to *sound* or hearing. *acoustics. the science of sound. I.C.2.

acquired. not present at birth, developed as a reaction to environment or through use, disuse, or aging; contrast *congenital*. I.A.1.

acquired immune deficiency syndrome (AIDS). a disease caused by a virus that invades the human immune system, making the host susceptible to many, unusual, and often fatal infections; synonym, acquired immuno-deficiency syndrome. The *AIDS related complex (ARC) is a group of signs and symptoms not meeting the full definition of a case of AIDS, but suggestive of its presence. *AFRAIDS is being afraid of having AIDS.

This modern *Andromeda strain* appeared in the early 1980s in homosexuals, hemophiliacs, heroin users, and Haitians and has now begun to spread to heterosexuals. It is transmitted by unprotected sex and by blood products, and is yet without effective prevention (other than condoms and abstinence) or treatment, and incredibly virulent (promising to kill most of the hundreds of thousands of its victims). II.B.2.b.

acquisition cost. 1. the immediate cost of selling, underwriting, and issuing a new *insurance policy,* including clerical costs, agents' commissions, advertising, and medical inspection fees. 2. the cost to a pharmacist or other retailer of a supply of drugs. IV.B., III.B.3.

acting out. manifestation of feelings and impulses through behavioral acts rather than talk. I.A.2.

activated patient. in *health education* jargon, a person who has been motivated or prompted either to action which will improve and maintain his health, or to caring for his own illness. VII.B.2.a.

active placebo. see *placebo.*

activities of daily living (ADL). getting about, using the bathroom, dressing, eating, and accomplishing other ordinary necessities of life; compare *performance status.*

This is a basic concept important in *physical therapy* (where the ADLs are taught), measuring *disability* (where their description is quite standardized), determining *level of care* in nursing homes, and in designing homes for the *handicapped* and elderly (which should facilitate their accomplishment). II.A.2.c, VII.B.3.b.

activity level. the amount and kinds of physical activity in which a person can, or is allowed to, engage.

Activity levels are usually specified in a physician's *orders* for the care of an *inpatient,* and may range from strict *bed rest* to "up *ad lib.*" They may be quite specifically prescribed, many hospitals using as many as eight different levels for patients who have had heart attacks. V.B.

actual charge. the amount a physician or other practitioner actually *bills* a patient or his insurance for a medical *service* or *procedure.* The actual *charge* may differ from the *customary, prevailing,* and/or *reasonable charges* under *Medicare* and other insurance programs.
See *fractionation.* VII.D.1.

actuarial rate. synonym, *force of mortality.*

actuary. in *insurance,* the person who determines premium *rates, reserves,* and dividends by deciding what assumptions should be made with respect to each of the *risks* and other factors involved, as the occurrence of the *peril,* the *benefits* that will be payable, the rate of any investment earnings, *expenses,* and *persistency* rates; the oddsmaker in the insurance business; an accountant without personality.

Actuaries are trained in mathematics, statistics, and accounting to base their assumptions correctly on the most current and *valid* data available. IV.B., VIII.B.2.b.

acuity. 1. keenness of sensory perception, as of hearing, or perceptiveness of mind. 2. nursing jargon, requirement for nursing care; synonym, *nursing intensity*.

How much nursing time a patient needs is not the same as the acuteness or *severity* of the patient's illness. 1. I.A.1. 2. III.A.2., V.B.

acupressure. see *acupuncture*.

acupuncture. an ancient Chinese therapy for relief of pain, anesthesia, and treatment of some diseases; compare *moxibustion* and *shiatsu*.

Acupuncture uses fine needles of pure copper, gold, or silver inserted in certain points on meridians of the body for therapeutic release and control of life forces and energy. *Acupressure is an absurd (*acus* is Latin for needle) recent American invention using pressure rather than needles for the same purpose, to take advantage of popular fascination with acupuncture while avoiding the needles. Some states now regulate the practice of acupuncture, but it is rarely reimbursed by health insurance. It does sometimes work (how is unknown), but *random controlled trials* have been limited. V.

acute disease. a *disease* characterized by a single episode of fairly short duration (typically less than 30 days). Some definitions also require that the patient return to his usual state and *activity level* after the episode. Note that an acute episode of a *chronic disease* (diabetic coma in a patient with diabetes) is often treated as an acute disease. II.A.

Acute Physiology and Chronic Health Evaluation (APACHE). an index of a patient's *severity* of illness based on physiologic data and reflecting the patient's probability of death. II.A.2.

acute remunerative appendicitis. one of several facetious names for diseases leading to operations performed with more regard for the surgeon's needs than the patient's.

See *unnecessary surgery*. II.B.2., VIII.B.2.a.

ad damnum clause. in malpractice, the statement in a suit of the amount sought in damages.

Reform in some states has eliminated the *ad damnum* clause, thus not allowing the plaintiff to specify an amount sought in damages and eliminating some of the publicity arising from filing of suits. V.D.

addiction. acquired physiologic *dependence* upon a substance, as alcohol, narcotics, barbiturates, tobacco, or other drugs. *addictive. having the capacity to produce addiction in regular users; compare *drug dependence*.

Addiction ordinarily manifests itself in several ways: habituation occurs and dosage increases; physical withdrawal signs and symptoms, *the abstinence or withdrawal syndrome, occur with curtailed usage; use of the drug is compulsive and beyond voluntary control; and craving for the drug persists beyond recovery from withdrawal symptoms. I.A.1.

additive. something added, usually in small quantity to a large quantity of something else, to achieve a specific purpose, as a catalyst, preservative, colorant, or emulsifier.

Some additives are unnatural complex chemicals, and thus may present problems as wastes, pollutants, or toxins. On the other hand, many clearly make expensive processes efficient, prevent disease or spoilage, and serve other useful purposes.

See *fluoride* and *food additive*. I.C.

adequate and well-controlled investigations. the type of investigations, including clinical investigations, that must be conducted by a *new drug* sponsor to demonstrate that a new drug is *effective.*

As amended in 1962, the Federal Food, Drug, and Cosmetic Act requires that drug sponsors provide substantial evidence of effectiveness "consisting of adequate and well-controlled investigations, including clinical investigations, by experts qualified by scientific training and experience to evaluate the effectiveness of the drug involved, on the basis of which it could fairly and responsibly be concluded by such experts that the drug will have the effect it purports or is represented to have under the conditions of use *prescribed*, recommended, or suggested in the *labeling*" (section 505(d) of the Act). Food and Drug Administration *rules* further delineate the types of studies which must be conducted to satisfy this requirement, and permit waiver in certain cases. The statute and rules do not explicitly require that the *safety* of a new drug be established by adequate and well-controlled investigations; nor do they set forth explicit criteria for safety testing. III.B.3.

adjunct disability. in the Veterans Administration health program, a *nonservice-connected disability* associated with or held to be aggravating a *service-connected disability.* III.D.1.

adjusted average per capita cost (AAPCC). an estimate of annual expenditures on a Medicare beneficiary.

The AAPCC formula adjusts for age, sex, Medicaid buy-in status, institutional status, and region by dividing all beneficiaries in actuarial classes and producing different per capita amounts for the various classes. It is used to determine payments by Medicare to *health maintenance organizations* and *competitive medical plans at risk* in the program. IV.C.1.

adjusted rate. see *rate.*

adjuvant. something added to a treatment or product to increase its effectiveness, improve its characteristics, or facilitate its manufacture.

*Adjuvant chemotherapy for cancer, for example, is used with or after surgery in order to increase chances of obtaining a cure by killing any microscopic *metastases* left after surgery before they grow. V.B.

administration. the guidance of an undertaking toward the achievement of its purpose.

Administration and *management* are irregularly distinguished and may be considered synonymous. They have been differentiated by applying administration to public activities and management to private ones, or by describing one as concerned with the making of broad *policy*, and the other as concerned with the execution of that policy once formulated (use of management for the former and administration for the latter is common in the United States, while the reverse is typically British).

See *planning, goals,* and *objectives.* VI.C.

administrative day. a *day* in a hospital or other health facility which is not actually necessary for the patient's care but which is covered under *Medicare* (or other payment programs which limit coverage to *needed* days) because the stay was justifiable for reasons other than the patient's immediate needs.

Medicare recognizes various causes for administrative days (patients needing only currently unavailable *skilled nursing beds*, patients waiting extra days for a *CAT scan* while the equipment is fixed) but seeks to prevent all unnecessary days of hospitalization from becoming administrative days by limiting the total number of administrative days it will cover for each facility. IV.C.1

administrative services only (ASO) contract.   an agreement providing for an *insurance* company to administer an insurance program for an organization which chooses to *self-insure* some aspect of its *risk*, ordinarily an employer with self-insured *group insurance* providing employee health benefits. Also applied to a contract between a profit-making hospital or other health care corporation and a nonprofit one in which the latter buys management services from the former. III.B.1., VI.C.

admission.   the formal acceptance by a hospital or other *inpatient* health facility of a patient who is to be provided with room, board, and continuous *nursing* care in an area of the hospital or facility where patients generally stay at least overnight; compare *discharge*. The term is also loosely used for a *visit* to an emergency room or outpatient surgical unit.

   Admission rates, admissions per bed or unit time, and numbers are common measures of facility activity. Admissions per year times average *length of stay* equal total *patient days*. VII.C.5.

admission certification, review.   a form of *medical review* in which the medical *necessity* of an admission to a hospital or other inpatient institution is assessed to assure that only patients requiring the *level of care* provided by the institution involved are admitted, without unnecessary delay and with proper planning of the stay.

   Lengths of stay appropriate for the patient's admitting diagnosis are usually assigned and certified, and payment by any program requiring certification for the assigned stay is assured. Certification done before admission to obtain *prior authorization* is called *preadmission certification. When done shortly after admission it is sometimes called *concurrent review*. VI.E.2., VII.C.5.

admitted assets.   assets of an *insurance* company recognized and used by a state regulatory or other examining body in determining the company's financial condition. IV.B.

admitting diagnosis.   the problem requiring a patient's admission for inpatient care; compare *discharge* and *primary diagnosis*. II.B.1.

admitting order.   see *order*.

admitting physician.   the physician responsible for admission of a patient to a hospital or other inpatient health facility.

   The physician may remain responsible for the care of the patient once admitted, becoming the *attending physician,* or not, the *housestaff* often becoming responsible. Some facilities have all admitting decisions made by a single physician (typically a rotating responsibility), the *admitting officer. III.A.I.

admitting privilege.   see *staff privilege*.

adolescence.   see *child*.

Adolescent Family Life Program.   Title XX of the Public Health Service Act, created in 1981, which supports efforts to advise adolescents to abstain from sexual activity and efforts to educate in *parenting* for teenagers who are pregnant or have children. The original legislative proposal for the program was known as the *chastity bill. VII.B.3.b.

adoption. the taking of an outsider into a family, or other group, usually by legally investing him with the rights and responsibilities of a member by birth. I.B.1.

adult. 1. mature; having attained full size, strength, and reproductive ability. 2. in human society and law, having attained the ability to handle personal affairs; of full legal age or *majority.* 1. I.A.1. 2. VIII.B.3.

adulterate. mix or substitute inferior or inert ingredients in a food, chemical, or other substance, usually deceptively for gain; compare *contaminate* and *impurity.* I.A.2.a.

adult protective services. a social system for identification and care of *abused, exploited,* and *neglected* (even *self-neglected*) adults, operated by the local welfare agency in U.S. cities and counties, typically the Department of Human or Social Services.

The services include investigation of reports of adults in trouble, determination of *competence* and responsibility, and arranging for appropriate care and services. I.B.2., VII.B.3.a.

advance appropriation. in the federal budget, an *appropriation* provided by the Congress one or more years in advance of the *fiscal year* in which the *budget authority* becomes available for *obligation.*

An advance appropriation should be distinguished from forward funding, which involves an agency in obligating funds in the current year for *outlay* to programs that are to operate in subsequent fiscal years. Advance appropriations allow sufficient time to develop long-range plans with assurance of future federal funding. VI.B.

advanced age. see *age.*

adversarial model. conceptual model of the interaction between physician and patient when the patient's motive involves something other than care for an illness which only the physician is societally sanctioned to provide, as certification of disability or prescribing of narcotics for an addict. Compare *clinical* and *relational models.*

Read Cogswell, B. E., and M. B. Sussman, *Family Medicine: A New Approach to Health Care* (New York: Haworth Press, 1982). V.

adverse drug reaction (ADR), adverse reaction. an undesirable *side effect..*

The Food and Drug Administration has long-standing surveillance programs for identifying ADRs, the heart of which remains spontaneous reporting by alert physicians.

Read Faich, Gerald A., "Adverse Drug-Reaction Monitoring" (*N Engl J Med,* 314(24): 1589–92, 6/12/86). III.B.3., V.B.

adverse selection. disproportionate *insurance* of *risks* who are more prone to suffer *loss,* or otherwise make *claims,* than the average risk.

It may result from the tendency for poorer risks (sick people) to seek or continue insurance to a greater extent than do better risks (healthy people), or from the tendency for the *insured* to take advantage of favorable options in insurance contracts. Favorable, as opposed to adverse, selection, when intentional, is called *skimming.* IV.B.

advertising. calling something to the attention of the public, usually with favorable comment or endorsement, especially by means of paid printed or broadcast announcements.

Traditionally, *professionals* did not advertise because they aspired to being gentlemen who did no work with their hands, thus the gold-headed cane, and neither billed nor advertised since to do so would make them mere merchants. Advertising is regulated in the United States by the *Federal Trade Commission;* compare the regulation of *labeling* of foods and drugs by the *Food and Drug Administration.* The FTC has recently limited *professional association* barriers to advertising because they restrain trade. VII.D.

aerobic exercise, aerobics.   see *exercise.*

aerospace medicine.   the subspecialty of *preventive medicine* concerned with the medical effects of flying and space travel. III.C.

Aesculapius.   see *Asclepius.*

affiliated hospital.   one which is affiliated in some degree with another health program. Usage is often limited to hospitals with affiliations with *medical schools* and classified by degree, as a *major unit of the school's teaching program, used only to a *limited extent, or solely for *graduate training of *residents.* III.B.1.

affiliation.   an agreement, usually formal, between two or more otherwise independent programs, facilities, or individuals which defines how they will relate to each other (from the Latin *filius* for son; historically implied a senior and junior partner relationship).

   Affiliation agreements may specify procedures for *referring* or transferring patients from one to another; joint faculty and/or medical staff appointments; sharing of records or services; or provision of consultation between programs. VI.C.

aftercare.   an organized program of continued care and *rehabilitation* for patients after hospital *discharge,* typically for postpartum mothers and children, psychiatric patients, or groups with common chronic illnesses, as *Reach for Recovery.* VII.C.4.

against medical advice (AMA).   usually refers to a form a patient is asked to sign when leaving a hospital against his *attending physician's* advice. The patient is said to have *gone AMA or *eloped.

   Contrary patient behavior is common, varied in form, and probably only occasionally important. Patients are usually asked to sign AMA forms, saying they understand what they are doing, only when seeking what their physicians consider dangerously premature hospital *discharge.*

   See *commitment, compliance,* and *informed consent.* V.D.

age.   the whole, a part, or a time of life; to grow older. *chronological age, time elapsed since the birth of an individual, expressed in years and smaller units of time. *biologic age, measure of the fatigue and deterioration of tissues and organs of an individual through aging, measured by comparison with a norm of chronological age for such individuals. *mental age, degree of mental development of an individual, evaluated by reference to the norm of chronological age for each stage of development.

   The ages of man are variously divided, see *child* and *adult.* *Advanced or old age is particularly variable, beginning as young as 60 in Tennessee *adult protective services* law and as old as 85 in some *geriatric* studies. I.A.1.

age cohort, interval.   see *population composition.*

agency.   1. part of a government, with specific duties or functions, as *regulating* a profession or *administering* a funding program. 2. legal relationship in which one person, the agent, attorney in fact, or proxy, acts on behalf

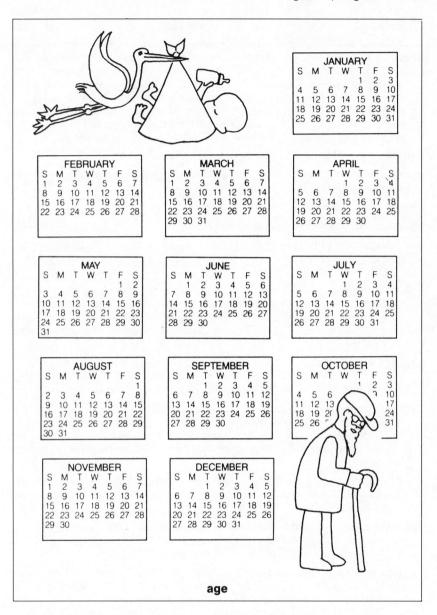

age

of another, the principal, to the extent authorized by the terms of the relationship. VIII.B.3.

agent.   a *cause;* a substance or force which, by its actions, effects change; a factor whose presence can cause a disease; compare *risk factor.*

    An agent is a necessary, but not sufficient, cause of disease when additional suitable conditions of the host or environment must also be present for the disease to develop, but the disease will not develop without the presence of the agent. II.B.1.a.

Agent Orange.   a defoliant sprayed over wide areas in Vietnam to reveal people's movements.

U.S. personnel, as well as Vietnamese, were *exposed* and now seek benefits for untoward effects, particularly from the *dioxin* with which it was *contaminated.* The code name for the spraying program in Vietnam was *Operation Ranch Hand, those who participated are *Ranch Handers, and an Air Force study of them is called the *Ranch Hand Study. I.C.1.

age-sex pyramid.   synonym, *population pyramid.*

age-sex register.   the listing by age and sex of all registered patients in a practice; compare *practice register.*

age-specific birth rate.   see *birth rate.*

age-specific death rate.   see *mortality rate.*

age-specific fertility rate (ASFR).   the number of *live births* to women in a specified age group and year, per 1000 women in that age group. II.C., VIII.C.

age-specific rate.   a *rate* of a given event for a specified age group, as 25–34 years, with specified time and population units. The numerator consists of the number of events that occur in the specified population and time; the denominator is obtained by either a census or estimate of the population. II.C., VIII.C.

aggregate indemnity.   the maximum amount payable under an *insurance policy:* either for all *coverage* under the policy, or for any specific coverage such as a specific case of malpractice, or particular services. IV.B.2.

Aid to Families with Dependent Children (ADC, AFDC).   a federally supported, state-administered *welfare* program for families with only one parent, who cannot be expected to be self-supporting because of the need to care for the children. It is authorized by Title IV of the Social Security Act. I.A.2.c.

Aid to the Blind (AB).   a federally supported, state-administered *welfare* program for the *blind* replaced in 1972 by the *Supplemental Security Income* program. I.A.2.c.

Aid to the Permanently and Totally Disabled (APTD).   a federally supported, state-administered *welfare* program for the *disabled* replaced in 1972 by the *Supplemental Security Income* program. I.A.2.c.

air pollution epidemic, episode.   occurrence of abnormally high concentrations of air *pollutants,* usually because of lack of wind and temperature inversion, with a resulting increase in illness and death.

The most serious killed 4000 people in London during a 1952 inversion. I.C.1.

air quality criteria.   a level of a *pollutant* and duration of *exposure* to air containing that level which produces adverse effects on health and welfare.

The criteria are specified by the *Environmental Protection Agency,* usually in parts per million (ppm) for a specified period, as people should not be exposed to over 50 ppm of carbon monoxide for more than 8 hours. They are based on the effects of the *criteria pollutants* on human health. I.C.1.

air quality index. a measure of air pollution published by a state or local air pollution control agency, usually on a daily basis, to inform people of the *healthfulness* of their air.

Many different specific indices have been used in different localities in the United States. These provide both a numerical measure of pollution based on the ambient concentrations of one or more of the five *criteria pollutants,* and a descriptive term indicating how hazardous the air is to health, particularly that of individuals with diseases aggravated by high levels of pollution. Because of the variability of these local indices many states and local governments have adopted the federally recommended *Pollutant Standards Index.* I.C.1

air quality standard. level of a pollutant in ambient air which may not legally be exceeded for more than a specified time in a specified geographic area.

While *air quality criteria* are related to health effects, the standards set levels for the air resource itself. Standards are specified for most recognized pollutants, including oxides of sulfur and carbon, and hydrocarbons. I.C.1.

The Alameda Seven. the seven health habits identified by the Alameda County Study as *associated* with improved health and longevity. They are: never smoking, drinking less than five drinks at a sitting, sleeping 7–8 hours each night, exercising, maintaining desirable weight for height, avoiding snacks, and eating breakfast regularly.

*The Alameda County Study was a population-based, prospective survey begun in the early 1960s in Alameda County, California, which, like the *Framingham Study,* has provided important knowledge of what behavior is, and is not, important to our health. Surprisingly, for example, sleeping either more or less than 7–8 hours was less healthful than sleeping 7–8 hours.

Read Birkman, Lisa F., and Lester Breslow, *Health and Ways of Living: The Alameda County Study* (New York: Oxford University Press, 1983. 237 pp.). I.A.2.

Al-Anon. see *Alcoholics Anonymous.*

Alateen. see *Alcoholics Anonymous.*

Alcohol, Drug Abuse, and Mental Health Administration (ADAMHA). the agency in the Department of Health and Human Services which administers federal alcohol, drug abuse, and mental health programs through their respective *national institutes.* III.D.1.

alcoholic. one who drinks more than the reader. II.B.2., VII.B.2.b.

Alcoholics Anonymous (AA). a fellowship of people who share their experience, strength, and hope that they may solve their common problem and help others recover from alcoholism.

The only membership requirement is a desire to stop drinking. There are no dues or fees, and the fellowships are self-supporting through contributions. There are over 40,000 groups in 110 countries with over 1 million members. This famous original group *self-help* approach to alcoholism has been more effective than the *medical model.* It has descendents in *Parents Anonymous,* similar groups for drug addicts, and *Weight Watchers.* There are several related organizations, *Al-Anon Family Groups for relatives of alcoholics and *Alateen, a part of Al-Anon, for the adolescent children of alcoholics. II.B.2.a.

alcoholism.   1. *addiction* to alcohol. 2. a *chronic disease* manifested by repeated drinking of alcohol in excess of the dietary and social uses and norms of the community, and to an extent that interferes with the drinker's *health,* or his social or occupational functioning.

The definition of alcoholism in both theory and practice is variable: sometimes requiring only excessive drinking, or interference with the drinker's health or functioning, rather than both; sometimes requiring, in addition to the above, physical signs of *drug dependence;* and sometimes defining it, and occasionally still viewing it, as a crime rather than a disease. There are several systems for differentiating types of alcoholism and grading its severity.

See *B. Rush.* II.B.2.

Alexander technique.   (F. Matthias Alexander, 1869–1955, Australian actor and therapist) a method of reeducating people to correct bad habits of posture, breathing, or speech, and of making people more aware of themselves and hence giving them more control of their behavior.

The technique's emphasis on the healthfulness of proper head, neck, and torso relations places it in the *chiropractic* family of therapies, although it developed independently and its practitioners have been more modest in their claims (as well as less numerous).

See Alexander, F. Matthias, *Alexander Technique* (London: Thomas and Hudson, 1974).

alexithymic.   literally, without words for moods; lacking the ability to fantasize and describe feelings verbally and reporting multiple somatic complaints.

This is not necessarily abnormal or a disease and may best be viewed as a symptom (and thus better used in the adjectival form than as a noun, alexithymia) with a *differential diagnosis* including several character disorders, depression, dementia, mental retardation, and posttraumatic stress disorder. II.B.2.

algicide.   see *pesticide.*

algology.   the branch of medicine concerned with pain and its relief.

Algology is not an established medical *specialty* but is often a particular concern of anesthesiologists and physiatrists. III.C.

algorithm.   a systematic process consisting of an ordered sequence of steps with each step depending on the outcome of the previous one, as mathematical and algebraic proofs; compare *protocol.*

Clinical algorithms for problems or symptoms lead people step by step through their diagnosis and treatment like flow sheets or guides. V.

ALI Formulation.   see *American Law Institute Formulation.*

allergen.   a substance, an antigen, like a pollen, drug, or food, which upon *exposure* induces an allergy and on subsequent reexposure elicits an allergic response in an organism. I.C.

allergist.   a physician specializing by practice or education in allergy and immunology. III.A.1.

allergy.   acquired specific alteration in biologic reactivity, *hypersensitivity; initiated by *exposure* to an allergen, and, after a latent period, characterized by evocation upon reexposure of the altered reactivity, the *allergic response.

Usually applies to hypersensitivity that harms rather than benefits an organism; *immunity* describing the same phenomenon when it is protective. II.B.1.a.

allergy and immunology. the science and medical specialty devoted to the study and care of the immune system and its disorders including allergies. III.C.

allied health personnel. all *health manpower,* other than physicians, dentists, podiatrists, and nurses, with special training and, when necessary, licensure.

The term has no constant meaning, sometimes meaning all health workers who perform tasks which must otherwise be performed by physicians; occasionally referring to health workers who do not engage in independent *practice;* and often synonymous with *paramedical personnel.* *Allied health professionals are *operationally defined* as those whose disciplines have *accredited* educational programs. Thus, *training centers* for allied health professions must provide at least one of 21 recognized curriculums: baccalaureate degree or above, dental hygienist, dietitian, medical technologist, occupational therapist, physical therapist, radiologic technologist, and sanitarian; and, associate degree or eqivalent, dental hygienist, dental assistant, dental laboratory technician, dietary technician, inhalation therapy technician, medical laboratory technician, medical record technician, occupational therapy assistant, ophthalmic assistant, optometric technician, x-ray technician, and sanitarian technician. III.A.

allocated benefit. synonym, *scheduled benefit.*

allograft. a graft of tissue between individuals of the same species but of disparate genotypes; synonyms, homograft and allogeneic graft; compare *xenograft.* This includes all grafts between two humans, except between identical (monozygotic) twins.

allopathic physician. (Gr. *allos,* other, and *pathos,* suffering or disease) a *physician* practicing a philosophy of medicine which seeks by active intervention to counteract the effects of *disease* using *treatments,* medical or surgical, which produce effects opposite to those of the disease; usually used in contrast to *osteopathic, homeopathic,* and *naturopathic* physicians. Most physicians in the United States would be considered allopathic.

See *alternative medicine* and *medical model.* III.A.1.

allowable charge. the maximum *charge* for which a *third party* will reimburse a provider for a given *service.* An allowable charge is not necessarily the same as either a *reasonable, customary, maximum allowable actual,* or *prevailing* charge as the terms are used in the Medicare program. VII.D.1.

allowable cost. an item or element of a program's *costs* that is reimbursable under a payment formula.

Some programs reimburse hospitals on the basis of certain costs, but do not allow reimbursement for all costs. Costs which are not allowable generally include those of uncovered services and luxury accommodations, costs which are not *reasonable,* expenditures which are unnecessary in the delivery of health services to persons covered under the program in question (Medicare does not allow costs of services to newborn infants), and de-

preciation on a capital expenditure which was disapproved by a health planning agency.
See *section 223* and *section 1122*. VII.D.1.

allowance.   see *Blue Cross discount* and *charity allowance.*

alpha error.   synonym, *type I error.*

Alpha Omega Alpha Honor Medical Society (AOA).   a society dedicated to the promotion of scholarship and research in medical schools, the encouragement of a high standard of character and conduct among medical students and graduates, and the recognition of high attainment in medical science, practice, and related fields.

The AOA represents the motto "Worthy to Serve the Suffering." The Phi Beta Kappa of Medicine, AOA was founded in 1902 by William Webster Root (U.S. medical student) and others and has chapters at most U.S. and Canadian Medical Schools.
See *The Pharos*. III.B.1.

alteration and renovation.   synonym, *modernization.*

alternative health care delivery system.   see *health care delivery system.*

alternative medicine.   any of many nonconventional ways of keeping people healthy and treating their illnesses. Unconventional in this context would contrast with *allopathic* medicine, based on the *medical model* and taught in accredited U.S. medical schools.

There is no single school or text of alternative medicine, but it is a useful collective term for various old (*yoga*) and new (*biofeedback*), useful (*meditation*), and suspect (*structural integration*) therapies. Some make no claim to cure disease, only increase health; as such their practice is not the practice of medicine in the eyes of the law. Some have practitioners but many are self-administered, once learned from a trainer, book, or someone selling the necessaries.

Read Hulke, Malcolm, *The Encyclopedia of Alternative Medicine and Self-Help* (New York: Schocken Books, 1979). V.

alternatives to long-term care.   the whole range of health, nutritional, housing, and social services designed to help people (particularly the aged, disabled, and retarded) live independently, rather than as inpatients in institutions like *skilled nursing* and *intermediate care facilities;* synonym, alternatives to institutionalization.

The goal is to provide all services necessary to allow the person to continue to function in the home environment. Alternatives to long-term institutional care include day-care centers, foster homes, and *homemaker services*. VII.C.2. and 4.

Alzheimer's disease.   see *dementia.*

AMA Physician Masterfile.   the primary American Medical Association file of data, and the most complete data set available, concerning U.S. physicians.

This file has made it possible to inform all state medical licensure boards when any one state identifies an *impaired physician* or otherwise disciplines a physician. Data on each physician include birthplace, age, address, medical school, residency, specialty, certification, hospital affiliation, states of licensure, and state disciplinary actions. Hospitals and government agencies routinely check credentials using the Masterfile. III.A.1.

ambulance. 1. a vehicle equipped for transporting those who are sick or injured. 2. occasionally, a temporary field hospital, organized to follow an army in its movement; hence, in civil life, an organization for rendering first aid. See *Mobile Army Surgical Hospital*. III.B.2.

ambulance service. obsolete, see *emergency medical service*.

ambulatory care. all types of medical care provided patients outside their homes without their *admission* to a health facility. Ambulatory care includes care given in physicians' offices and in *outpatient* health facilities but not to *inpatients* who are ambulatory (literally, able to walk). VII.C.4.

ambulatory surgery. *surgery* performed on a nonhospitalized patient, an outpatient; irregular synonyms, day, day-bed, day-op, in-and-out, one-day, same-day, and short-stay surgery and surgical-day care.
　　Use of this and related terms is irregular. Redefinition of levels of surgical care and standardization of terms would be helpful. V.B.

American Academy of Family Physicians (AAFP). the family physicians' professional association.
　　Its members govern the Academy, which in turn represents the interests of *family medicine* and provides educational, insurance, and other services to the members. III.C.

American Association of Physicians and Surgeons (AAPS). a nonprofit *professional association* of physicians in the United States whose purpose is the preservation of traditional ways of medical practice and life.
　　Apparently small (it has refused to reveal its membership in congressional hearings), the AAPS advocates repeal of *Medicare, Medicaid,* the rest of the Social Security Act, and the progressive income tax. III.A.

American Board of Family Practice (ABFP). family medicine's *specialty board.*
　　The board *certifies* family physicians as specialists in family medicine on the basis of their training, experience, continuing medical education, and score on the board's examination. III.C.

American Board of Medical Specialties (ABMS). the national organization of *specialty boards* in medicine, one of the parent organizations for the *Accreditation Councils for Continuing and Graduate Medical Education;* compare *Council of Medical Specialty Societies*. III.C.

American Cancer Society (ACS). a *charitable organization* founded in 1913 and dedicated to control and eradication of *cancer* through a program of research, education, and service to cancer patients. It rarely, however, provides direct support for treating people with cancer. III.B.4., II.B.2.

American Hospital Formulary Service (AHFS). a *formulary* widely used in hospitals and other health programs.
　　The AHFS is prepared and maintained by the American Society of Hospital Pharmacists. It provides subscribers with the big red book often found at *nurses' stations*, a continuously updated description of virtually all drugs used in the United States and preferred by many as an information source to the *Physicians' Desk Reference*. III.B.3.

American Law Institute Formulation. section 4.01 of the Institute's Model Penal Code, which states that "a person is not responsible for criminal conduct if at the time of such conduct as a result of mental disease or defect he lacks substantial capacity either to appreciate the wrongfulness of his conduct or to conform his conduct to the requirements of the law"; synonym, the Freeman rule.

This rule for determining competence and responsibility, known as the ALI Formulation, was adopted by the Second Circuit of the U.S. Court of Appeals in 1966 and by the U.S. Court of Appeals for the District of Columbia in 1972 (United States vs. Brawner).

See *Durham rule* and *M'Naghten rule*. VIII.B.3.

American Medical Association (AMA).   the principal *professional association* of physicians in the United States.

See *Educational Research Foundation*. III.A.1.

American Medical Assurance Company (AMACO).   an American Medical Association subsidiary that provides reinsurance for physician-owned malpractice insurance companies. V.D.

American Medical College Application Service (AMCAS).   a nonprofit, centralized, standardized application processing service for applicants for participating U.S. medical schools.

Sponsored by the *Association of American Medical Colleges* to facilitate the application process, AMCAS is supported by applicant fees. III.A.1.

American Medical Political Action Committee (AMPAC).   the (legally) independent political action committee set up by the *American Medical Association* to collect and distribute political contributions for the medical profession and engage in related political activities.

Professional associations like the AMA lose their nonprofit tax status if they engage in political activities and thus create separate organizations to handle them. Most state medical associations and some other professional associations also have such political action committees. III.A.

American National Standards Institute (ANSI).   the coordinating organization for the U.S. federated national *standards* system.

Founded in 1918, the federation consists of over a thousand companies, and trade, technical, professional, labor, and consumer organizations. It coordinates the development of standards and establishes *American National Standards, also known as *national consensus standards,* and represents the United States in international programs of standardization. Included in its over 10,000 standards are many for medical *devices* and *occupational health*. III.B.2.

American Nurses Association (ANA).   the principal *professional association* of nurses in the United States. III.A.2.

American Red Cross (ARC).   see *Red Cross*.

American Type Culture Collection (ATCC).   a nonprofit organization founded in 1925 for the collection, preservation, and distribution of authentic cultures of living microorganisms with over 28,000 strains of algae, animal and plant viruses, and antisera, bacteria, bacteriophages, chlamydiae, fungi, protozoa, and rickettsiae. II.B.1.a.

Ames test, Ames bacterial mutagen assay.   (Bruce Nathan Ames, U.S. microbiologist) a *test* of a chemical's *mutagenicity, teratogenicity,* and *carcinogenicity.*

Bacteria with similar genetic systems to humans are exposed under standard conditions to a chemical. If the bacteria mutate frequently, the chemical is considered likely to have similar effects on humans. A relatively good, rapid, and inexpensive test. Appropriate when a chemical is being considered as a possible *food additive, pesticide,* or *toxic substance.* I.C.

amortization. the act or process of extinguishing a *debt,* usually by equal payments at regular intervals over a specific period of time; see *capital.* III.B.1.

anaerobic. antonym, *aerobic.*

analysis of variance (ANOVA). a statistical procedure for determining the significance of differences or variations obtained in experimental variables, studied under two or more conditions.

Differences are commonly assigned to three aspects: the individual differences among the subjects or patients studied; group differences, however classified (e.g., by sex); and differences attributable to the various treatments which the individuals and groups have been given. The method can assess both the main effects of a variable and its interaction with other variables that have been studied simultaneously. VIII.D.

ancillary expenses. in health insurance, *costs* or *charges* for ancillary services; synonym, miscellaneous expenses. IV.B.

ancillary services. *services,* other than room and board and routine nursing care, provided by a hospital or other health facility which are separately and individually itemized and charged.

These may include anesthesia, laboratory, operating room, pharmacy, physical therapy, and x-ray services. Insurance programs may treat charges for services which a hospital calls ancillary services as part of the room and board charge when the service is given to all patients as a condition of occupancy, or every day, regardless of need. IV.B.

Andromeda strain. slang, a new, virulent, or uncontrollable infectious agent, after Michael Crichton's *The Andromeda Strain* (New York: Knopf, 1969) about such an agent imported from the Andromeda constellation and efforts to deal with it. Modern Andromeda strains include Lassa-fever virus, Marburg virus, and the agents of viral hemorrhagic fever and *acquired immune deficiency syndrome.* II.B.2., VIII.B.2.a.

anesthesia. loss of sensation, of neurogenic or psychogenic origin, induced locally in part of the body or generally by chemical, or anesthetic, agents, *hypnosis, acupuncture,* or disease. I.A.1.

anesthesiologist. a physician specializing by practice or education in *anesthesiology;* compare *anesthetist.*
Anesthesiologists are mostly *hospital-based physicians.* III.A.1.

anesthesiology. the science and specialty devoted to the study and administration of local and general anesthetics to produce the various types of anesthesia. III.C.

anesthetist. a person who administers anesthetics, not necessarily a physician; compare *anesthesiologist* and *nurse anesthetist.* III.A.

animal model. an animal disease analogous to a disease of man, the study of which aids the study of the human disease, as by preliminary testing of proposed treatment. VIII.D.

annual implementation plan (AIP). a *plan* which *health systems agencies* were required to prepare and update annually specifying, describing how to implement, and giving priority among short-run *objectives* which would achieve the long-range *goals* of the agency, detailed in its *health system plan.* VI.A.1.

anomaly.   any deviation from the usual structure or disposition of body parts, typically limited to those which are *congenital*, whether or not of any functional or aesthetic significance; any organ or part existing in an abnormal form, structure, or location. I.A.1.

anomie.   abnormal social *behavior* of an individual or group, characterized by disorientation, alienation, rejection of accepted values, and failure to conform to the norms of *society.*

Originally described by Emile Durkheim (French sociologist, 1858–1917), anomie is regarded as resulting from life in a poor, disorganized, or crowded environment, often urban and industrialized. I.B.2.

antibiotic.   a *drug* containing any quantity of any chemical substance produced by a microorganism which has the capacity, in dilute solution, to inhibit the growth of, or to destroy, bacteria and other microorganisms (or a chemically synthesized equivalent of such a substance).

Antibiotics are used in the treatment of infectious diseases. The given definition is traditional and that of the *Food, Drug, and Cosmetic Act;* in common use the term usually applies only to a drug, however made, which treats bacterial disease. III.B.3.

antibiotic certification program.   a Food and Drug Administration program in which each batch of every *antibiotic drug* manufactured for human use is certified by the FDA as possessing the identity, strength, quality, and purity needed to insure *safety* and *effectiveness* in use.

Before an antibiotic is eligible for certification, the FDA must approve it as safe and effective using procedures that are substantially equivalent to those for approving *new drugs.* Similar procedures exist for batch certification of insulin. Both antibiotic and insulin certification are supported with fees paid by the manufacturers to the FDA. There is no similar certification of the quality of other drugs. III.B.3.

antidiscrimination law.   in insurance, a state law which prohibits insurers from giving terms or rates, not *actuarially* warranted by the *risks* involved, in order to encourage or discourage enrollment of desirable or undesirable customers.

See *adverse selection* and *skimming.* IV.B.

antiduplication law.   see *duplication of benefits.*

antiseptic.   see *asepsis.*

antisubstitution law.   a state law that requires a pharmacist to "dispense as written" when filling a *prescription.* The effect is to prohibit a pharmacist from substituting for a drug prescribed by brand name a different brand name or generic equivalent drug, even if the drug to be substituted is *therapeutically equivalent* to the drug prescribed and, perhaps, less expensive.

Drug reimbursement programs such as the *Maximum Allowable Cost Program,* which limit reimbursement to the lowest cost at which a drug is generally available, are more effective if they override antisubstitution laws. Such laws have been attacked as preventing possible savings on drug expenditures, and violating antitrust statutes, and defended as assuring that patients receive exactly the drug prescribed. III.B.3.

apheresis.   removal of cells or unwanted substances from blood by various methods of filtration, followed by return of the blood to the donor.

Apheresis has been used to obtain platelets or white blood cells to give other patients and is now being used in treatment of various diseases. The latter use, therapeutic apheresis, is experimental and expensive.

Read the Office of Technology Assessment, *The Safety, Efficacy, and Cost-Effectiveness of Therapeutic Apheresis* (Washington: U.S. Government Printing Office, 1983). III.B.2.

apothecary. obsolete; synonym, *pharmacist.*

Apothecary is older and more British than "pharmacist." The English Society of Apothecaries split from the Grocers Company in 1617; prior to then drugs were not distinguished from spices. The doctors of the Middle Ages left drugs to the apothecaries and surgery to the barbers, concerning themselves with theories and fees. III.A.4.

applied research. see *research.*

appropriate. suitable for a particular person, condition, occasion, or place; proper; fitting.

Commonly used in making *policy,* usually without specific indication of which aspects of the person or thing to which the term is applied are to be judged appropriate, or how and by what standard those aspects are to be judged. For example, the Public Health Service Act requires *state health planning and development agencies* to review *institutional health services* and make findings "respecting the appropriateness of such services" (section 1523(a)(6)). No indication is given in the law or *legislative history* of what the agencies are to find either appropriate or inappropriate, as the costs or charges, necessity, quality, staffing, administration, or location of the services. VI.A.

appropriation. in the federal budget, an act of Congress that permits federal agencies to incur *obligations* and to make payments out of the treasury for specified purposes.

An appropriation usually follows enactment of *authorizing legislation* and is the most common form of *budget authority,* although in some cases authorizing legislation itself provides the budget authority. Appropriations

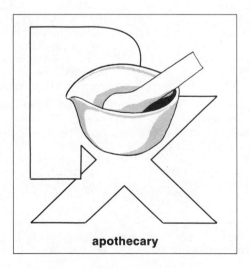

apothecary

are categorized by their period of availability (one-year, multiple-year, no-year), the timing of congressional action (current, permanent), and how the amount of the appropriation is determined (definite, indefinite). VI.B.

aquifer.   porous soil stratum capable of storing and yielding, through springs or wells, important amounts of water.

Aquifers are usually contained between impermeable layers, and located in the zone of saturation (where interstices are filled with water), below the zone of aeration (where interstices are largely filled with air and water is not under hydrostatic pressure). Aquifers can be depleted, recharged, or *polluted.* Substantial communities, particularly in the western United States, rely on aquifers for *drinking water,* as long as they are not contaminated. I.C.5.

architectural barrier.   a part of a building which limits use of the building by people with *handicaps,* as stairs rather than ramps or narrow doors.

Federal law has sought to limit architectural barriers in public buildings and those used by programs receiving federal funds. II., III.B.1.

area health authority (AHA).   see *health authority.*

area health education center (AHEC).   an organization (or organized system of health and educational institutions) whose purpose is to improve the supply, distribution, quality, use, and efficiency of *health manpower* in specific *medically underserved areas.*

The AHEC's objectives are to educate and train the health personnel specifically needed by the underserved areas and to decentralize health manpower education, thereby increasing manpower supplies and linking the health and educational institutions in scarcity areas. The policy and programs of an AHEC are usually directed by one or more medical schools. In practice, each has as its nucleus one or more hospitals, some distance away from the medical school, whose educational efforts are under the overall guidance of the AHEC and thus the medical school. The development of AHECs is assisted by the Department of Health and Human Services under the *Health Manpower Education Initiative Award* authority. III.A.

Area Resource File.   a federally maintained data set with information on the age and sex structure of the population, measures of socioeconomic and health status, and the availability of various types of health providers and facilities in virtually every county in the United States.

Read Bureau of Health Professionals, *The Area Resource File: A Health Professions Planning and Research Tool* (DHHS Publication (HRA) 81–9. Washington, D.C.: U.S. Government Printing Office, 1980). IV.A., VI.A.

areawide comprehensive health planning agency (areawide CHP 314(b) agency).   a regional, usually multicounty, health *planning* agency.

They were funded under section 314(b) of the *Public Health Service Act,* created by the Comprehensive Health Planning and Public Health Service Amendments of 1966 (P.L. 89-749), and charged with *comprehensive health planning* for the area they served, including preparation of plans for development of health services, facilities, and manpower. The agencies could review and comment upon proposals from health facilities for development of programs and expansion of facilities, but had no significant powers of enforcement. Up to three-quarters of the cost of operating the agencies was supported by federal *project grants,* the balance coming from voluntary contributions from any source, including the providers affected by the agencies' plans. Areawide CHP agencies were replaced by *health systems agencies* in 1974. VI.A.1.

arithmetic mean. synonym, *mean.*

Arizona Health Care Cost Containment System (AHCCCS). a Medicaid demonstration program established by the Arizona legislature in November 1981 to test competitive bidding by providers of indigent services; synonyms, Arizona experience or experiment, Arizona Health Care Containment Program.

Read Christianson, Jon B., and Diane G. Hillman, *Health Care for the Indigent and Competitive Contracts: The Arizona Experience* (Ann Arbor, MI: Health Administration Press, 1986. 173 pp. $18). IV.C.2.

Armed Forces Health Professions Scholarship (AFHPS). support from a program in which a student enlists as a second lieutenant or ensign and receives tuition, fees, expenses, and a stipend while attending medical school with a year-for-year obligation for active duty after completing training. III.A.1.

Armed Forces Institute of Pathology (AFIP). the U.S. Army's central *reference pathology* service located at the Walter Reed Army Hospital in Washington, D.C.

It accepts difficult pathologic specimens for interpretation from throughout the civilian, as well as military, United States. The resulting collection and experience are an important national library of pathologic knowledge. II.B.1., III.C., III.D.1.

arsenic. see *heavy metal.*

art therapy. use of art work in *therapy* of disease, particularly mental illness. III.C., V.

asbestos. a mineral fiber (calcium-magnesium silicate) with countless industrial uses.

One of the best thermal insulators, asbestos is also a *hazardous pollutant,* particularly in occupational air, since it causes cancer and a *pneumoconiosis,* *asbestosis.

Read Castleman, Barry I., *Asbestos: Medical and Legal Aspects* (2d edition. Clifton, NJ: Law and Business, 1986). II.B.2, VII.B.2.d.

Asclepius, Asklepios. in Greek mythology, the son of Apollo and god of medicine. Daughters attributed to him are *Hygeia, the goddess of health (after whom the author's practice is named), and *Panakeia (Panacea), "the all-healing," see *panacea.* *Aesculapius is the Roman name for Asclepius. *Asclepiades, of Bithynia (born circa 126 B.C.), established Greek medicine in Rome in 91 B.C. He taught a theory of disease based on the atomic theory of Democritus and rejected the humoral theory of Hippocrates. The *staff of Asclepius, a rod with only one serpent encircling it and without wings, is the correct symbol of the medical profession and the emblem of the American Medical Association, the Royal Army Medical Corps, and the Royal Canadian Medical Corps; compare *caduceus.* VIII.A.

asepsis. exclusion of microorganisms.

*Aseptic surgery is conducted in the absence of germs, everything coming in contact with the wound being sterile. Asepsis can be contrasted with *antisepsis, which limits the growth and multiplication of germs without excluding them, and cleanliness, which removes dirt rather than germs.

See *J. Lister.* I.C.

assault. see *battery*.

assessment. in *insurance,* a charge upon *carriers* to raise funds for a specific purpose such as meeting the administrative costs of a government-required program. Usually made by state government or a special organization authorized by government in law or regulation. Applied according to a formula to all carriers handling the affected lines of coverage. IV.B.2.

asset. anything of value, as money, *supplies,* or *capital.* VI.C.1.

assigned risk. a *risk* which *underwriters* do not care to *insure* (such as a person with hypertension seeking health insurance) which, because of state law or otherwise, must be insured.

Insuring assigned risks is usually handled through a group of insurers (such as all companies licensed to issue health insurance in the state) with risks assigned to the companies in turn, or in proportion to their share of the state's total health insurance business. Assignment of risks is common in casualty insurance and less common in health insurance. As an approach to providing insurance to such risks, it can be contrasted with pooling of such risks (see *insurance pool*) in which the *losses* rather than the risks are distributed among the group of insurers. IV.B.

assignment. an agreement in which a patient assigns to another party, usually a *provider,* the right to receive payment from a *third party* for *covered* services received; compare *participating.*

Assignment is an alternative to the patient paying directly for the service and then receiving reimbursement from the third party. In *Medicare,* if a physician accepts assignment from a patient, he must agree to accept the program payment as payment in full (except for specific *cost-sharing* amounts required of the patient). Assignment protects the patient against charges which Medicare will not recognize as *reasonable* and assures the provider of direct and prompt payment. In Medicare, physicians may choose assignment for some of their patients but not others, and may do so on a *claim* by claim basis for some services but not others. IV.B.1., IV.C.1.

associate degree program. a program which educates *registered nurses, technologists,* or other health manpower in a junior college, the associate degree being given upon graduation after 2 years of junior college. The student's classroom and laboratory teaching are provided in the college, and clinical teaching in an *affiliated hospital.*

See *diploma school* and *baccalaureate degree program.* III.A.2.

association. 1. in *epidemiology,* relationship between two *variables.* 2. see *professional association.*

Two related variables, as age and the incidence of diabetes, are said to be "associated." Different types of association are recognized: artifactual, causal, chance, dependent, and *spurious.* *Symmetrical associations are formulaic, noncausal, and nondirectional relationships. They may be expressed as *prevalence* equals *incidence* times disease duration. *Assymetrical associations are time and direction dependent, and may be causal; a change in a dependent variable follows a change in an independent one. *Direct associations are causal and without any intermediate variable. *Indirect ones rely on common underlying or intermediate relationships. Note that change in a dependent variable may be predicted, but is not necessarily caused, by change in an associated independent variable.

Read Hill, A. Bradford, "The Environment and Disease: Association or Causation" (*Proc R Soc Med,* 58: 295–300, 1965). VIII.C.

Association of American Medical Colleges (AAMC). a national organization representing and supporting U.S. medical schools, founded in 1890.

In addition to lobbying activities, the organization studies and aids medical education in a variety of ways, as the *American Medical College Application Service.* III.C.

association of practices. see *group.*

assuming company. see *reinsurance.*

assumption of risk. a defense in law, providing that an injured worker cannot recover damages from his employer for an injury if it arose out of *hazards* inherent in the job and the worker could be expected to know of the risk. The worker assumes the risk of injury, and his employer's liability for it, by taking the job. VIII.B.3., VII.B.2.d.

assurance. synonym, *insurance.* IV.B.

asylum. an institution for the cure, education, safekeeping, or support of those incapable of caring for themselves; compare *sanatorium.*

Deinstitutionalization has contributed to a growing population of *homeless* individuals, many of whom would benefit from humane asylum and the sanctuary it provides from worldly pressures, the *respite* it affords *caretakers,* and its *social network,* food, room, and board. II.B.2., III.B.1.

asymmetrical association. see *association.*

asymptomatic. without *symptoms.*

at risk. in danger of suffering injury, disease, loss, or other harm.

In *epidemiology,* denotes the special vulnerability of certain individuals (see *risk factors*) or groups to particular diseases or conditions: smokers are at risk for lung cancer, ghetto children for lead poisoning and rat bites, coal miners for *black lung.*

In *insurance,* refers to an individual, organization (like a Health Maintenance Organization), or insurance company assuming the chance of *loss* by taking the *risk* of having to provide or pay more for services than is gained through *premiums.* If premiums are adjusted after the fact so that no loss can occur, then there is no risk. If losses incurred in one year may be made up by increases in premiums in the next year, the "risk" is somewhat tempered. A firm at risk for losses also stands to gain from *profits* if costs are less than premiums collected. For an individual, being financially at risk usually means being without insurance or at risk for substantial *out-of-pocket* expenses. IV.B., VIII.C.

attack rate. the fraction of susceptible individuals in a *population* who acquire a disease to which the population is exposed; synonym, case rate.

Virulent diseases have high attack rates unless *herd immunity* exists. When susceptibility rates are low or unknown, attack rates may be expressed as a fraction of the whole population exposed, rather than just of the susceptibles. VIII.C.

attending, attending physician. the physician legally responsible for the care given a patient in a hospital or other health program.

This is usually a *private patient's private physician,* who is also responsible for the patient's *outpatient* care. The attending physician for a *public patient* is typically chosen by the hospital or *medical staff* upon admission from among members of the *staff,* or is one of its *teaching physicians.* *Housestaff* may take direct responsibility for an attending's patient under his supervision. III.A.1.

attention-deficit disorder (ADD). a condition of unknown cause characterized by a significantly impaired span of focused attention, which may be accompanied by a relatively high level of purposeless physical activity.

The child's inability to control this hyperactivity may produce behavioral and other problems of home and school. This new name for hyperkinetic syndrome or *minimal brain dysfunction* focuses on the probable primary problem suffered by, at most, 3 precent of children. See *learning disability.* II.B.2.

attention placebo. see *placebo.*

attitude. a stable, enduring disposition to behave or react in a given way to people, objects, institutions, issues, or other stimuli; an inferred variable operating between a stimulus and response which accounts for the nature of the response.

Attitudes come from personal, familial, and cultural sources. They may persist through generations and be so stable that they dictate an inappropriate response to a stimulus in a given situation. I.A.2.

attributable risk. the part of the *risk* of developing a *condition* or suffering a *loss* which results from a given *exposure,* where the total risk derives from multiple exposures.

The part of the rate of a disorder in an exposed population that can be attributed to the exposure, may be derived by subtracting the *incidence* or *prevalence* of the disorder in an unexposed population from the corresponding rate in the exposed population. VIII.C.

audiologist. individual trained in or practicing *audiology.*

This entails evaluating hearing and conducting *habilitative* programs which will improve the communication of individuals with impaired hearing. Licensure generally requires a master's degree in audiology. The American Speech and Hearing Association (ASHA) awards a certificate of clinical competence requiring academic training at the master's degree level, a year of experience, and passage of a national examination. Nearly half of ASHA members are employed in elementary or secondary schools, and a large majority are engaged in clinical work—either diagnostic or therapeutic. III.A.4.

audiology. the science of hearing; specifically, the study, diagnosis, and treatment of hearing defects.

Prescription of *auditory substitutional devices (hearing aids), among other forms of therapy, is a major part of audiology. It is practiced by *audiologists, otolaryngologists,* and *speech pathologists.* V.

autecology. see *ecology.*

authorization, authorizing legislation. in the federal budget, legislation which authorizes or continues the legal operation of a federal program or agency and thereby directly or indirectly authorizes spending money whether indefinitely or for a specific period of time.

Often used more narrowly to refer to annual dollar limits specified in authorizing legislation on amounts which may be appropriated for the authorized program. For many federal health programs annual authorizations are provided every 3 years in renewed authorizing legislation.

Such legislation is a prerequisite for *appropriations* or creations of other kinds of *budget authority* in appropriation acts. It may limit the amount of budget authority to be provided subsequently or may authorize the appropriation of "such sums as may be necessary." In a few instances budget authority may be provided in the authorization (see *backdoor authority*). VI.B.1.

autonomy. differentiation of self from others, allowing for self-direction and self-regulation. Compare *disengagement* and *enmeshment.*

People whose families fail to develop their autonomy often have dependent personalities and dependency diseases like alcoholism. I.B.1.

autopsy. examination of the body after death, *post mortem,* therefore also a *post or *postmortem, to determine the cause of death; synonym, necropsy.

The *autopsy rate in a hospital, the percentage of deaths followed by autopsies, is sometimes considered a measure of the quality of the hospital. *Consent* for an autopsy is required from the survivors, except when one is required by law, as with murder and sudden or unexplained death. Autopsies are done by *pathologists,* assisted by *dieners.*

See *coroner* and *medical examiner.* II.B.1.

auxiliary. an organization, traditionally of women, that assists the work of a hospital or other charitable institution, especially by donations or volunteer service.

Such auxiliaries often provide all routine patient transportation, run the snack bar and flower shop, and donate the proceeds and other funds to the hospital. The annual contribution is regular and large enough to be an important part of the budget, hence their occasional sponsorship by profit-making health programs. III.B.1.

availability. the times and places at which an individual or group may obtain health care.

Availability is often measured by the supply of health *resources* and *services* since it is largely a function of them (see *bed days*). Availability of care is in some degree independent of the *need* or *demand* for it and does not by itself make such care *accessible* or *acceptable.*

See *bioavailability.* VII.D.

average. synonym, *mean.*

average length of stay (ALOS). see *length of stay.*

Avicenna. Persian physician, 980–1037. While serving as court physician in Bagdad, he wrote the *Canon Medicinae* which codified all medical knowledge of Greek and his own time, giving him influence in medicine throughout the Middle Ages second only to Galen. He also made significant contributions to geology. VIII.A.1.

aviation medical examiner (AME). a licensed, practicing physician with a special interest in aviation who is certified, but not employed, by the Federal Aviation Administration (FAA) to perform medical examinations and use the medical standards for civilian airmen and his own judgment to decide whether an applicant for a license should receive required medical certification.

The AME's effort is guided by standards, procedures, and guidelines in the FAA's *Aviation Medical Examiners Guide.*

Read Engelberg, Alan L., et al., "A Review of the Medical Standards for Civilian Airmen: Synopsis of a Two-Year Study" (*JAMA*, 255(12): 1589–99). III.A.1.

Ayurvedic Medicine.   practice based on the Hindu sacred laws of health, the Ayurveda.

Indian medical practices of the last 3000 years stagnated during British rule but are again taught and integrated with occidental practices.

See Thakkur, Chandrashekhar G., *Introduction to Ayurveda* (New York: ASI Books, 1976). V.

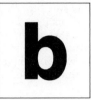

Baby Doe. pseudonym, a severely *congenitally handicapped* infant, born April 9, 1982, in Bloomington, Indiana, whose parents and physicians chose, with court approval, not to undertake therapy which might have prevented death. *Baby Jane Doe was an infant with multiple birth defects born subsequently on Long Island, New York, whose medical records were protected by the courts from federal efforts to intervene in the decision not to undertake corrective surgery.

Such cases have led to federal regulation, court action, and congressional debate to prevent either the neglect of such infants or government interference in such private matters, depending on your side. The *Baby Doe rule is the *regulation* requiring hospitals, among other things, to post notices in nurseries saying that section 504 of the Rehabilitation Act of 1973 prohibits discrimination on the basis of handicap in federally assisted programs and that therefore nourishment and medically beneficial treatment should not be withheld from handicapped infants solely on the basis of their present or anticipated mental or physical impairments. In 1986 the U.S. Supreme Court struck down the Baby Doe rule, finding that section 504 did not give the government authority to review hospital records or meddle with properly made decisions to withdraw health care.

Read Stevenson, D.K., et al., "The 'Baby Doe' Rule" (*JAMA*, 255(14): 1909–12, 4/11/86). See *quality of life*. I.A.1., II., VIII.B.3.

baccalaureate degree program. a program that educates *registered nurses* in a 4-year college or university, the bachelor of arts or bachelor of science degree being given upon graduation; compare *associate degree* and *diploma programs*.

The student's classroom and laboratory teaching are provided in the college, and clinical teaching in an *affiliated hospital*. Graduates are sometimes known as *graduate nurses,* rather than registered nurses. III.A.2.

backdoor authority.   in the federal budget, legislative *authority* for the *obligation* of funds outside the normal *appropriation* process; synonym, backdoor spending.

The most common forms of backdoor authority are borrowing authority (authority to spend debt receipts) and contract authority. In other cases, as interest on the public debt, a permanent appropriation is provided that becomes available without any current action by the Congress. *Entitlement* authority is sometimes treated as backdoor authority, since enactment of the legislation creating the entitled benefit effectively mandates subsequent appropriations to pay the statutory benefits. Backdoor authorities are found in the Social Security *trust funds*. The Congressional Budget and Impoundment Control Act of 1974 limits use of backdoor authorities. VI.B.1.

bactericide.   see *pesticide.*

bad debt.   uncollectable *debt;* income lost by a provider because of failure of patients to pay amounts owed.

Loss of revenue from bad debts is partially offset for proprietary institutions, since income tax is not payable on income not received. Such debts are usually recovered by proportionate increases in charges to paying patients, see *sick tax.* Some *cost-based reimbursement* programs reimburse certain bad debts, see *reasonable cost.*

See *uncompensated care.* IV.A., VI.C.1.

bagassosis.   *pneumoconiosis* caused by breathing moldy *bagasse, the residue of sugar cane. II.B.2.

Baillou, Guillaume de.   French physician, 1538–1616. He gave the first clinical description of whooping cough, introduced the notion of rheumatism, and was the first prominent advocate of the concept of the epidemic constitution in the sixteenth century, an idea developed by *Sydenham.* VIII.A.1., VIII.B.2.e.

Baker, S. Josephine.   U.S. physician, 1873–1945. She established child care and the protection of mothers as a health function of local government. See *maternal* and *child health.* VII.A.1., VIII.A.1.

Bakke case.   Allan Bakke v. the Regents of the University of California (U.S. Supreme Court, June 1978).

This famous court case found that affirmative action programs (favoring admission of black students to the University of California's Davis School of Medicine in this instance) may constitute illegal racial discrimination. The issue remains controversial because the court tried to steer a middle course, also saying such programs were not necessarily discriminatory. III.B.1., VIII.A.1.

balance billing.   charging a patient for the difference between an actual charge and the amount covered by insurance.

The term is irregularly used, sometimes applying to charging for *cost-sharing* amounts and sometimes to the amount by which an actual charge exceeds the covered amount plus cost-sharing. Balance billing in the latter sense is illegal for physicians who take *assignment* under Medicare. IV.A.

Balint group.   one of a series of seminars run by Michael and Enid Balint (British psychiatrist and social worker) in which general practitioners explored the effects of doctors and patients on each other and on illness.

M. Balint reported the results in a classic of family medicine, *The Doctor, His Patient, and the Illness* (Revised edition. New York: International

University Press, 1964). Similar groups are used in U.S. family medicine residencies to help learn and understand family practice. III.C.

balloon payment debt retirement. paying a debt in one payment, or a few large amounts, rather than in small regular installments.

Balloon payments may be specified or prohibited in the terms of the debt. See *debt service*. VI.C.1.

Bane Report. (Frank Bane, U.S. educator) *Physicians for a Growing America* (Report of the Surgeon General's Consultant Group on Medical Education, Publication No. 709, Bethesda, MD: U.S. Department of Health, Education, and Welfare, 10/1959).

This study of U.S. physician needs and medical education provided the analytic basis for the first federal health manpower legislation, the Health Professions Educational Assistance Act of 1963, and well represented thinking of the time on physician *supply*. III.A.1., VIII.A.2.

bare. see *go bare*.

barefoot doctor. a Chinese peasant with basic medical training who can handle medical emergencies, prescribe for simple injuries and illness, and apply treatments prescribed by qualified physicians, all without leaving productive work; Chinese transliteration, "chijiao yisheng"; compare *feldsher* and *physician assistant*.

The over 2 million barefoot doctors are the People's Republic of China's version of a venerable Chinese idea. They are chosen by communes and villages, receive several months of training, and return to their home, where they continue to be paid like other commune members.

Read Ch'ih chiao i sheng shouts'e, translator, *A Barefoot Doctor's Manual* (DHEW Publication No. (NIH) 75-695. Washington, D.C.: U.S. Government Printing Office, 1974. Reprinted, Philadelphia (PA 19103): Running Press (38 S. Nineteenth St.), 1977). III.A.4.

bariatrics. the field of medicine concerned with *obesity*. III.C.

barrier precaution. a measure taken, a *barrier technique, to prevent the spread of infection. The barrier may be erected between the patient and others, creating a *barrier patient, or at the entrance to the patient's room, a *barrier room.

There are many categories of barrier precautions, including respiratory, tuberculosis, enteric, contact, drainage/secretions, blood/body fluid, burn, and leukopenic, which protect against different modes of transmission of specified diseases.

See *nosocomial* and *quarantine*. VIII.C.

basic health services. the minimum *supply* of health *services* which should be generally and uniformly available in order to assure adequate *health status* and protection of the population from disease, or in order to satisfy some other criteria.

Given that all services cannot be supplied to everybody, it is surprising how little definition or discussion there has been of what set of services constitutes an appropriate minimum and of how to assure its availability. A beginning has been made in federal policy with the definition of *required services* for Medicaid and the basic health services required of health maintenance organizations (HMOs) for federal *qualification*. The latter includes physician services, hospital services, medically necessary emergency care, preventive health services, home health services, up to 20 visits of outpatient mental health services, medical treatment and referral services for alcoholism and drug abuse, and laboratory and radiologic services (section 1302(1) of the Public Health Service Act). Where a minimum is defined, a higher level of service also is usually defined, as *optional services* and *supplemental health services* for Medicaid required services and HMO basic health services, respectively. It is not clear in either case whether the higher level is thought of as all other, all other needed, or all other affordable services. III.B.1., VII.

basic sciences.   the disciplines which explain the normal structure and function of the body and its parts, people, families, and communities; compare *behavioral science* and *clinical sciences*.

Irregularly defined, these are the subjects taught in the first year of traditional medical education and typically include anatomy, genetics, histology, physiology, biochemistry, statistics, and psychology. III.C.

bassinet.   a baby's *bed*.

Hospital beds for infants, nursery beds, while nothing like the traditional hooded, wicker bassinet, are sometimes called bassinets. They have special design, use, and licensure. III.B.1.

Bates method.   (William H. Bates, U.S. ophthalmologist, 1860–1931). a series of techniques to improve vision by retraining the muscles which focus the lens in the eye; compare *orthoptics*.

The method sometimes provides an alternative to relying on glasses, but requires more work to succeed and is now rarely practiced. III.C., V.

battery.   in law, the use of force on a person without his *consent*, as operating on a patient without proper consent. Usually distinguished from *assault, the attempted but not successful or actual use of such force; compare *rape*.

Medicine recently, and more than law, has been concerned with violence occurring within families, recognizing first the *battered or *abused child and then his mother. This concern has led to new definitions, sometimes written into statutes, particularly at the state level, as the American Psychiatric Association's definition of an abused child as one who

has suffered repeated injuries, that may include bone fractures, neurologic and psychologic damage, and sexual abuse at the hands of a parent, parents, or parent surrogates. The abuse takes place repeatedly and is often precipitated by the child's minor and normal irritating behavior.

Assault and battery are as illegal within families as they are among them. The special problem that raising children requires the use of force without a child's consent may be solved by saying that assault and battery occur between parent and child when the threat or use of force is excessive, repeated, or damaging to the child. VIII.B.3.

bed.   a bed in a hospital or other inpatient health facility. Many definitions require that beds be maintained for continuous, 24-hour, use. A facility's *bed capacity, or *bed complement, is its number of beds, total or of a specific type, and is the principal measure of facility size.

Licenses and *certificates of need* may be granted for specific numbers of specific types of beds, as surgical, pediatric, obstetric, or extended care. Facilities may have both licensed and unlicensed beds; and active and licensed but unused beds. Beds are categorized in many other ways, as available, occupied, acute care, or observation beds.

See *bassinet, bed rest, Roemer's law,* and *swing bed.* III.B.1.

bed days. usually, the total *patient days* for a year for a health facility. *Annual available bed days for a facility is its bed capacity times 365. III.B.1., VII.C.5.

bedpan mutual. insurance slang, an insurance company selling health insurance, typically *individual, mail-order, supplemental,* or one of the other highly profitable lines, rather than group health insurance. IV.B.2, VIII.B.2.a.

bed rest. resting in bed to treat illness.
Prescribing more rest than a patient would naturally choose is much less common than previously, and useless with a child.
See *activity level.* V.B.

bedside manner. the characteristic or customary way a physician, or other health *professional,* behaves with patients.
Bedside manner may be different from the physician's manner with nonpatients, is not used just in bedside encounters, has substantial effect on the outcome of treatment, and thus is taught and studied. V.

bed turnover rate. the number of admissions per bed per year in an inpatient facility, typically a hospital. III.B.1.

behavior. a person or other organism's response to stimulation, whether internal or external.
Definitions and use sometimes limit responses recognized as behavior to ones which are conscious, expected, good, learned, observable, or social. Thus *behaviorists, adherents of a school of behavioral psychology, define only observable responses as behavior. This excludes unexpressed emotion or thought as behavior; compare *attitude.* I.A.2.

behavioral medicine. the application of scientific and technical knowledge of behavior and behavior analysis to behavior prediction and modification for the purpose of enhancing *fitness* or preventing and controlling disease. It is not a recognized medical specialty. III.C.

behavioral risk factor. the presence of a behavior known to adversely affect health, as cigarette smoking, binge drinking, heavy or chronic drinking, drunk driving, uncorrected obesity, inactivity or a sedentary lifestyle, uncontrolled hypertension, and failure to use seat belts; compare *The Alameda Seven* and *risk factor.* The *Behavioral Risk Factor Surveys (BRFS), a state population-based surveillance system for monitoring these behaviors, are sponsored by the Centers for Disease Control, Department of Health and Human Services. I.A.2., VIII.C.

behavioral science. any science concerned with understanding human or animal action, behavior, development, institutions, societies, or values, as anthropology, economics, ethology, political science, psychiatry, psychology, and sociology.
The behavioral sciences, from *family medicine's* perspective, are the disciplines which aid in caring for families. There is no standard list of the sciences included, nor much common history, function, or understanding among them.
See *basic* and *clinical sciences.* I.A.2., III.C.

behavior modification. the purpose of, and often a synonym for, *behavior therapy.* I.A.2., V.B.

behavior therapy. any specific *therapy* or therapeutic system which seeks to improve behavior.

Treatment focuses on modifying observable and, at least in principle, quantifiable behavior by means of systematic environmental and behavioral variables which determine or may affect the dysfunction or inadequate behavior being treated. Specific behavior therapies include aversion therapy, *biofeedback,* conditioning, flooding, operant shaping, systematic desensitization, and *token economy.* I.A.2., V.B.

beneficiary. someone eligible to receive, or receiving, benefits from an insurance policy (usually) or health maintenance organization (occasionally, see *member*); typically includes both people who have themselves contracted for benefits and their eligible *dependents.*

People receiving Medicare benefits are referred to as beneficiaries. Those receiving Medicaid benefits are referred to as recipients.

See *insured subscriber.* IV.B.

benefit. in insurance, a sum of money provided by the terms of an insurance policy payable for *covered losses* or *services.* The benefit may be paid to the insured or on his behalf to others. In *prepayment* programs, as health maintenance organizations, benefits are the services the program will provide a member whenever and to the extent needed.

See *allocated benefit provision, cost-benefit, indemnity benefit,* and *service benefit.* IV.B.

benefit period. the time during which payments for benefits *covered* by an *insurance policy* are available.

The availability of benefits may be limited over a specified time period, as two well-baby visits during a year. A benefit period is usually defined by a set unit of time, as a year, occasionally by other means, as a *spell of illness.* IV.B.

benign. see *cancer.*

Bernard, Claude. French physiologist, 1813–1878. His conception of homeostasis and the internal environment of the body were two profound contributions among many. I.C., VIII.A.1.

Berry plan. (George Packer Berry, U.S. physician and medical educator) a program which provided physicians with draft deferments for residency training during the Selective Service years.

Participants were obligated to as many years of military service as they had of education. The program allowed physicians to complete their training while providing the military with a planned physician supply. IV.D.1.

beryllium (Be). a divalent metallic element.

Airborne salts of beryllium cause *beryposis, which may be either an acute or chronic lung disease like *black lung.* These hazardous air pollutants are primarily discharged in machine shops, ceramic and propellant plants, and foundries. I.C.1., VII.B.2.d.

beta error. synonym, *type II error.*

Bethesda. 1. a pool described in the Bible (John 5: 2–4) and believed to have curative powers; a hallowed place. 2. the town in Maryland where the *National Institutes of Health* are located. III.D.1., VII.A.2.

Beverly Enterprises. the largest nursing home chain in the United States, with over 700 individual homes. III.B.1.

bias. inclination, prejudice, tendency, trend; in statistics, a tendency of an estimate to deviate from a true value, as by reason of nonrandom sampling; any process at any stage of inference that produces results or conclusions that differ systematically from the truth. *Biased error is nonrandom or systematic error. In controlled studies, *susceptibility bias occurs if one group is more susceptible to the disease or treatment in question than the other, *migration bias when cases are lost (or migrate) from one group faster than the other, and *detection bias when diagnostic or monitoring efforts are not equal for all groups. Bias is not necessarily just the investigator's failing, *reader bias also occurs.

    See *experimenter* and *volunteer bias.* VIII.D.

bill. 1. an itemized account of the separate charges for services provided or goods sold; a statement in gross of a creditor's claim, a statement of account: to prepare or submit such accounts. 2. a draft of a law proposed for enactment by a legislature. 3. obsolete, a medical *prescription.*

    See *super bill.* 1. VII.D.1., 2. VIII.B.3.

Billings, John Shaw. U.S. physician, 1838–1913. He planned the Johns Hopkins Hospital and Medical School and later became director of the New York Public Library. He was a leader in the development of U.S. *vital statistics* programs. It is due to Billings that since 1880 the population census has included medical data. II.C., VIII.A.1.

bioassay. an assay, or method of measuring something, which compares its effects on living organisms to standard effects of known comparable things; synonym, biologic assay.

    See *biologic monitoring.* II.A.2.b.

bioavailability. extent and rate of absorption of a dose of a given drug, measured by the time-concentration curve for appearance of the administered drug in the blood.

    Bioavailability is a major determinant of whether different *brand name* drugs, a *generic name* as opposed to a brand name drug, or different batches of the same brand name drug have *therapeutic equivalency,* since all may demonstrate differing bioavailability. Few of such differences are therapeutically significant.

    See *antisubstitution, bioequivalence,* and *Maximum Allowable Cost Program.* III.B.3.

biocenose. the various organisms or species inhabiting a particular *environment,* an *ecological community.* I.C.

biochemical oxygen demand (BOD). an index of water pollution which represents the content of biochemically degradable substances in water. I.C.5.

biodegradation. reduction in the complexity of chemical compounds in the environment by decomposition, erosion, and other natural means.

    Some modern artificial chemicals, practically without *biodegradability, have great *persistence* in the environment. I.C.

bioequivalent. biologically equal; of two or more drug preparations with indistinguishable biologic effects.

    Such drugs are also chemical equivalents (indistinguishable by chemical means), although chemically equivalent preparations are not always bioequivalent. Bioequivalence is a function of *bioavailability;* often being synonymous, or the former measured by the latter. Chemically equivalent drugs which are bioequivalent are *therapeutic equivalents* (have the same treatment effect), although therapeutically equivalent preparations need not be either chemically equivalent or bioequivalent. III.B.3.

bioethics. the study, principles, and practice of good conduct with regard to biologic matters, as *genetic engineering* and *informed consent;* compare *medical ethics.*

Read Englehardt, H. Tristram, Jr., *The Foundations of Bioethics* (New York: Oxford University Press, 1986. 398 pp. $27.95). III.C.

biofeedback. bringing bodily processes or states, of which people are not normally conscious, as temperature, blood pressure, muscle tension, or heart rate, to sensory awareness by visual readout, auditory signal, or similar sensible display.

Many people can learn to control bodily processes when thus made aware of them, and even eventually to control them without the feedback. This may help treat hypertension, headaches, and other dysfunctions of such processes. Biofeedback is practiced and studied by a few physicians and psychologists among others, usually not reimbursed by health insurance, and not yet standardized or regulated.

Read Basmajian, John V., ed., *Biofeedback: Principles and Practice for Clinicians* (2d edition. Baltimore: Williams & Wilkins Co., 1983. 390 pp.).

biologic, biological, biologic product. any virus, therapeutic serum, toxin, antitoxin, or analogous product of plant or animal origin used in the prevention, diagnosis, or treatment of disease.

Biologics, including vaccines and blood plasma products, are regulated by the Bureau of Biologics, a division of the *Food and Drug Administration.* They differ from *drugs* in that biologics are usually derived from living organisms and cannot be synthesized or readily standardized by chemical or physical means, nor can their *safety* be as easily assured. They tend to be chemically less stable and pure than drugs. III.B.3.

biologic age. see *age.*

biologic monitoring. testing for the presence or observing the effects of *hazards* by observing *exposed* living organisms; compare *bioassay.*

The classic example is the canary used by coal miners to monitor the accumulation of methane; it stops singing and falls before they do. The most important example is close medical *screening* of *cohorts* of workers exposed to known or potential hazards. II.A.2.b.

biologic warfare. 1. waging *war* by use of *biologic weapons, living organisms or their products whose harmful properties are used to destroy or debilitate an enemy. 2. the use of chemicals to destroy plant, and other, life, as defoliants like *Agent Orange;* compare *chemical warfare.*

Typically biologic weapons are infectious microorganisms introduced in a nontypical manner (as an aerosol of an organism usually ingested), or a toxin produced by a virus, bacterium, or fungus. In the broader sense, biologic warfare may include the use of higher organisms, as the bats carrying incendiary devices experimented with in World War II. I.B.

biomass. the total living matter in a specified *habitat,* expressed as weight or volume of matter per unit area or volume of habitat. *Biomass energy, or bioenergy, is energy derived from the biomass, rather than solar, nuclear, or inert sources. Brazil, for example, runs automobiles on water and alcohol from sugarcane and cassava. Other sources of bioenergy include trees, crops, manure, seaweed, algae, and urban waste. I.C.

biome. the *community* or *population* of living organisms in a given area or particular *ecological* region, ordinarily identified by characteristic vegetation. I.C.

biomedical model. synonym, *medical model.*

biomedical research. *research* concerned with human and animal biology and disease; contrast *health services research.* VIII.D.

biopsychosocial model. a *systems* approach to understanding health and illness which conceives of the person as one of a continuous hierarchy of systems, beginning with cells and organ systems and continuing through the *family, culture,* and *environment.*

Each system is complete but also an interrelated part of higher level systems. The use of this approach integrates consideration of physiologic, emotional, social, and other factors affecting health, while still permitting appropriate use of the *medical model* to understand biologic aspects of illness.

See *adversarial, explanatory,* and *relational models,* and read Engel, G.L., "The Need for a New Medical Model: A Challenge for Biomedicine" (*Science,* 196: 129–36, 77) and "The Biopsychosocial Model and Medical Education: Who Are to Be the Teachers?" (*N Engl J Med,* 306: 802–5, 82). III.C.

biosynthetic. made by biological means, as by putting human genes in bacteria so that they will make human insulin or growth hormone. III.B.3.

biotechnology. means and methods of changing biology, as recombining DNA and other forms of *genetic engineering.*

Plant genetics may be altered to produce better crops or resist disease, new organisms may be created for purposes of biosynthesis, and soon genetic illnesses will be treatable by manipulation of the genome. Appropriate regulation of this new technology is *naturally* a matter of growing public debate.

Read Olson, Steve, *Biotechnology: An Industry Comes of Age* (Washington, D.C.: National Academy Press, 1986. 120 pp.). III.B.3.

birth. the offspring's emergence from the womb of its mother; the beginning of life for *vital statistics* purposes.

See *abortion, family planning, live birth,* and *stillbirth.* I.A.1.

birth certificate. a legal *certificate* issued by the government of the state in which a birth occurs recording its date and place, the newborn's name, sex, and parents, and other pertinent information. I.A.1.

birth control. control of fertility, conception, and pregnancy; especially by *contraception,* sometimes by increasing fertility. Typically a means of *family planning,* with which it is often synonymous. I.B.1.

birthing room. a homelike room or suite in a hospital in which women labor and deliver with their families and without the encumbrance of full medical management.

With the safety of immediate help in the event of trouble, these rooms restore some of the natural family support and *bonding* found in home deliveries that is limited by inflexible, high technology labor and delivery rooms. A *birthing center is a freestanding birthing room in a facility outside a hospital, offering the best of neither world. III.B.1.

birth rate.   ratio of babies born to a *population* during a given period in a specified area; compare *mortality rate* and *rate*.

Generally expressed as the *crude, *central, or *live birth rate, the number of live births per thousand population at midyear per year. More meaningful indices of natural population growth are the *age-specific birth rate, births per thousand women of a given age group, from which can be obtained the *fertility rate, births to all women of child-bearing age; and *net reproduction rate, female births to all women of child-bearing age making allowance for the female death rate. The *total birth rate includes *stillbirths* with *live births*. Standardized birth rates eliminate in various ways the effects of differences in the age and sex structures of different populations on their birth rates. Birth rate and fertility differentials between populations are related to their composition and are due more to social (population policies) and individual (*family planning*) actions, than to physiologic reproductive capacity, *fecundity. II.C., VIII.C.

black lung.   a chronic lung disease, medically known as coal workers' *pneumoconiosis,* caused by breathing coal dust and found among coal miners; compare *brown lung.* Certain medical benefits for the victims of the disease are available under title IV of the Federal Coal Mine Health and Safety Act of 1969.

See *Mine Safety and Health Administration.* II.B.2., VII.B.2.d.

blaming the victim.   placing responsibility for suffering a condition, behavior, or disease upon the one who suffers it, as the woman for her rape, the child for his fall from a window, or the smoker for his lung cancer. Usually implies the blaming is wrong, or at least counterproductive.

Read Beauchamp, Dan E., "Public Health as Social Justice" (*Inquiry,* XIII(1): 3–14, March 1976). I.B.

blanket medical expense.   an insurance policy, or provision of one, entitling the insured to collect *benefits,* up to a specified maximum, for all hospital and medical expenses incurred, without limitations on individual types of medical expenses. Usually an added feature of a policy primarily providing some other type of coverage, as loss of income insurance. IV.B.

blind.   unable to see.

Subject to elaborate legal definition for such purposes as determining eligibility for disability: as, in Social Security, a person is blind when the remaining vision in the better eye after best correction is 20/200 or less; or peripheral visual fields in the better eye are contracted to 10° or less from the point of fixation, or have a widest diameter subtending an angle less than 20°, or have 20 percent or less visual field efficiency. II.B.2.

block grant.   a grant of federal funds to a state for a group of related purposes, as funding maternal and child health services or drug abuse control programs; compare *categorical grant.*

Recipients of block grants typically are given substantial flexibility and little supervision in their use of funds. IV.C.

blood doping.   the practice of giving athletes blood transfusions before competition to enhance their performance; synonyms, blood boosting and blood packing.

This controversial practice is apparently safe, effective, and unethical. Read Klein, Harvey G., "Blood Transfusion and Athletes: Games People Play" (*N Engl J Med*, 312(13): 854–6, 3/28/85). III.C., V.B.

blood bank.   an organization, or distinct part of a health facility, which procures and stores blood and its parts.

Blood banks usually also recruit and screen donors, bleed them, test donors and recipients for immunologic compatibility, fractionate blood into its parts (known as *blood components or products, including plasma, cells, and proteins), and, in some cases, infuse blood. Blood banking is a *subspecialty* of pathology. *Tissue, *eye, and *milk banks perform similar functions for other organs, corneas, and mother's milk. III.B.1.

Blue Cross.   1. obsolete; a branch, founded in 1912, of an English society, Our Dumb Friends' League, for the succor of horses and dogs. It was active in the Balkan and world wars. 2. also obsolete; a society, the American Blue Cross Society, formed in the United States in 1911 to further the humane treatment of animals. VIII.A.

Blue Cross allowance, discount.   the amount or percentage less than charges which Blue Cross plans using charge-based reimbursement pay hospitals or other participating providers for covered services.

Paying less than charges is rationalized by the value to hospitals of Blue Cross's large, prompt, predictable payments. In 1980 the discount in Tennessee was 2 percent. The allowance is an example of monopsony. IV.B.1.

Blue Cross and Blue Shield Association (BC/BS).   the national nonprofit organization to which the individual Blue Cross and Blue Shield plans in the United States voluntarily belong.

BC/BS administers programs of supervision for member plans, provides specific services related to the writing and administering of health care benefits across the country, and represents the plans in national affairs. Under contract with the Social Security Administration, BC/BS is *intermediary* in the Medicare program for most *participating* providers. BC/BS was formed by merger of the Blue Cross Association and the National Association of Blue Shield Plans.

See *Health Services, Inc.,* and *Medical Indemnity of America, Inc.* IV.B.1.

Blue Cross plan (BC).   a nonprofit, tax-exempt health services prepayment organization providing *coverage* for hospital and related health services.

The individual plans should be distinguished from their national association, the Blue Cross and Blue Shield Association. Historically, the plans were largely the creation of the hospital industry, and designed to provide hospitals with a stable source of revenue, although formal association between Blue Cross plans and hospital associations ended in 1972. A Blue Cross plan must be a nonprofit, community service organization with a governing body whose membership includes a majority of public representatives. Most plans are regulated by state insurance commissioners under special state enabling legislation. The plans receive special federal tax treatment, and, in most states, are exempt from state taxes (both property and premium). Unlike most private insurance companies, the plans usually provide service rather than *indemnity benefits,* and often pay hospitals on the basis of *reasonable costs* rather than charges.

See *Health Services, Inc.,* and *Blue Shield plan.* IV.B.1.

blue flu.   the illness policemen, the men in blue, are said to have when they all take *sick leave* during a *sickout, an informal or illegal strike on the part of workers without a union or the right to strike. I.A.2.c., II.B.2.

Blue Shield plan (BS).   a nonprofit, tax-exempt health service prepayment organization providing *coverage* of physicians' services.
   The individual plans should be distinguished from the national Blue Cross and Blue Shield Association. Blue Shield coverage is commonly, although not always, sold in conjunction with Blue Cross coverage. The relationship between Blue Cross and Blue Shield plans has been a cooperative one; they may have a common board, one management, and be located in the same building. Blue Shield plans were originally organized in 1939 by medical societies. They cover millions of Americans through their *group* and individual business and affect millions more through participation in government programs, including Medicare (many plans act as *carriers* under *part B*), Medicaid, and the *Civilian Health and Medical Program of the Uniformed Services.* Most states have enacted special enabling legislation for Blue Shield plans.
   See *Medical Indemnity of America, Inc.* IV.B.1.

board.   a licensure or *specialty board;* the governing body, a board of trustees or directors, of a health program. *Boards are the examination given by a specialty board or the *National Board of Medical Examiners.* III.B.1.

board certified.   a physician or other health professional who has been *certified* by a *specialty* board as a specialist in a given subject.
   This entails satisfying requirements of the specialty board for board eligibility and then passing its examination. Certification is generally permanent, only family physicians are required by their board to undergo periodic recertification. III.C.

board eligible.   a physician or other health professional who has met requirements for *specialty board* examination (including those who may have failed the examination, if they remain eligible).
   Each of the specialty boards has requirements which must be met before the examination for board certification may be taken. These typically include graduation from an approved school, training experience of specified type and length, and specified time in practice or on the job. The time needed after graduation from medical school to become board eligible may be up to 5 years. Government and other health programs which define standards for specialists occasionally still accept board eligibility as equivalent to board certification, since the only difference is usually that the board-certified professional has passed an examination. III.C.

boarding home, house.   a facility which, for a fee, provides room, board, and, sometimes, *custodial care;* synonym, board and care home irregularly limited to homes providing some care and supervision.
   Boarding homes are quite variable in size, organization, and whom they serve, but are often small, poor, and filled with old people. Medical care, social activities, and counseling are not normally included. They are not licensed as health facilities and often not subject to licensure at all, although terminology and requirements vary greatly among state and local jurisdictions.
   See *foster care, partial hospitalization,* and *shelter.* I.B.2.

board of health. an official commission responsible for maintaining *public health* in a city, county, or state, typically through *sanitation* and provision of certain laboratory and clinical services, and sometimes through *licensure, certificate of need,* and other regulatory activities.

Such boards are usually appointed by the chief executive of the area served, but are occasionally elected or may be chosen, all or in part, by the local medical society. The membership may include any mixture of *consumers* and *providers.* The board's actions may be official or advisory. VII.D.2.

boiler plate. slang, standard recurring language in health insurance or law relied on to avoid confusion in common, unchanging provisions. VIII.B.3.

bond. an attachment uniting or binding one or more parties, as the marriage bond; an engaging or connecting element or force, as of friendship or common employment.

The recent rediscovery by medicine of the maternal-infant bond is now leading to understanding of the parental, lover, and other bonds that hold people and families together. They are rooted in our biology and the basis of society. Bonding may be done by force, money, gifts, or pheromones. I.A.2.

bond. an interest-bearing document issued by a government or corporation giving evidence of a long-term debt, sometimes secured by a lien on property or other means, and usually designed to meet a particular financial need. The contract between the issuing agent and the bondholder is a *bond indenture. A *bond sinking *fund* is one in which assets are placed to pay bonds by their maturity date.

Income to the bondholder from interest on many bonds, as a federally sponsored industrial development bond (IDB), is exempt from taxation. The tax exemption enhances the value of bonds enough that they attract *capital,* typically for construction, easily and even in excess of true need or market value. IV.C., VI.A., VIII.B.3.

Boston Collaborative Drug Surveillance Program. a nonexperimental *cohort study* operating in the Boston area since 1966 in which consecutive admissions to participating hospitals are closely monitored for the effects, particularly *adverse drug reactions,* of all drugs used in the patients' care.

Read Bigby, Michael, et al., "Drug-Induced Cutaneous Reactions: A Report from the Boston Collaborative Drug Surveillance Program on 15,438 Consecutive Inpatients, 1975 to 1982" (*JAMA*, 256(24): 3358–63, 12/26/86). III.B.3.

Braidism. synonym, *hypnotism;* after James Braid (British physician, 1795–1860) who introduced its practice into medicine. V.

branded generic drug. see *drug.*

brand name. the registered trademark given a specific drug product by its manufacturer; synonyms, proprietary name and trade name.

As an example, there is a widely prescribed broad-spectrum antibiotic with the *generic* or *established name* of tetracycline hydrochloride. Its chemical name is 4-dimethylamino-1,4,4a,5,5a,6,11,13a-octahydro-3,6,10,12, 12a-pentahydroxy-6-methyl-11-dioxo-2-naphthacenecarboxamide hydrochloride. Its chemical formula is $C_{22}H_{24}N_2O_8$ HCL. Tetracycline is marketed by Lederle Laboratories using the brand name Achromycin, by Upjohn as Panmycin, by Robins as Robitet, by Squibb as Sumycin, and so on. There are no official rules governing the selection of brand names. According to the Pharmaceutical Manufacturers Association, the objective is to coin a name which is "useful, dignified, easily remembered, and individual or proprietary." Drugs are advertised to practitioners by brand name. When a physician prescribes by brand name, *antisubstitution laws* in some states forbid pharmacists from substituting either a brand or *generic equivalent* made by a different manufacturer, although either may be less expensive than the drug prescribed. III.B.3.

The British Pharmacopoeia. the official British government *pharmacopeia,* comparable to *The United States Pharmacopeia,* including in edited form all relevant monographs and methods currently contained in the *European Pharmacopoeia.*

Read the British Pharmacopoeia Commission, Sir Frank Hartley, chairman, *The British Pharmacopoeia 1980* (Two vols. London: Her Majesty's Stationary Office, 1980). III.B.3.

brown lung. popular name for byssinosis, a *pneumoconiosis* caused by breathing cotton, linen, and other plant fiber *dusts,* which is *prevalent* among textile workers, and similar to but not the same as *black lung.*

Special federal benefits, like those available for miners disabled by black lung, are not available for people with brown lung, although they may qualify for general Social Security disability benefits. Brown lung has an acute early form, known as *Monday morning fever, because its symptoms are most noticeable when workers renew their *exposure* after a weekend free of cotton dust. Exposure to cotton dust is regulated under the *Occupational Safety and Health Act.* II.B.3.

budget. a detailed plan in financial terms for carrying out a program of activities in a specified period, usually a *fiscal year.*

A budget estimates all of the program's proposed income, by source, and expenses, by purpose, as salaries and capital costs. Expenses are sometimes related to the program's *goals* and *objectives.*

See *administration, congressional* and *presidential budgets, planning,* and *policy.* VI.B.

budget authority (BA). in the federal budget, authority provided by law to enter into *obligations* which will result in immediate or future *outlays* of government funds.

The authority to insure or guarantee the repayment of indebtedness incurred by another person or government is not usually treated as budget authority. The basic forms of budget authority are *appropriations,* contract authority, and borrowing authority. Budget authority is classified by the timing of congressional action (current or permanent) and the amount available (definite or indefinite). VI.B.

budget mark. in the federal budget, the amount a federal agency is told by the Office of Management and Budget, or some other superior agency, that it may use in drawing up its budget.

The mark usually predicts income (whether or not realistically) from *appropriations* and other sources, and requires the agency to show how it will adjust expenditures to the mark. VI.B.

bulky waste. see *waste*

bundle of services. see *unbundling.*

Bureau of Narcotics and Dangerous Drugs (BNDD).   see *Drug Enforcement Administration.*

Bureau of Occupational Safety and Health (BOSH).   see *National Institute of Occupational Safety and Health.*

burnout.   loss of capacity through sustained, usually excessive, effort.
Burnout and its manifestations are common among *caretakers,* physicians and other health workers, and people with stressful jobs. Irritability, decreased productivity, and depression become more likely with increased time and stress. Rest, variety of responsibilities, and opportunity for creativity and recreation help. II.B.2.

byssinosis.   see *brown lung.*

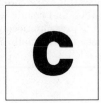

cadmium. see *heavy metal.*

caduceus, caduces. a herald's staff; a staff with two snakes curled around it and two wings at the top; one of the symbols of a physician, as the symbol of the Medical Corps of the U.S. Army; compare *Asclepius.*

A *Caduceus group or chapter is a therapeutic group for support of *impaired physicians,* comparable to *Alcoholics Anonymous.* The *Caduceus Games are a quiz contest for medical schools patterned after the "college bowl" television program and run by the East Tennessee State University Quillen-Dishner College of Medicine. VIII.A.

cafeteria plan. an employee benefit plan that allows covered employees some control over the type of benefit for which available funds are used.

Rather than simply buying employees group health insurance, an employer offers to spend a given amount on the employee's behalf on health, life, or disability insurance or other benefits, and the employee "shops" for the benefit. I.A.2.c.

cancer. an abnormal growth of cells, which usually persists and grows independently of surrounding structures and is of no use to its host. A *tumor is any mass or swelling whether or not cancerous. Cancers are, since Hippocrates, divided into the *benign (unlikely to kill the host) and *malignant (likely to do so), although the distinction is not reliable since all cancers possess a degree of malignancy determined by their propensity for growth, invasion, and distant spread.

Cancer is not one disease; the over 100 different forms have markedly different characters. However, the cancers usually are treated collectively for statistical, research, legislative, and other purposes. Cancer causes about a fifth of U.S. deaths, second only to *heart disease* as a cause.

See *American Cancer Society, carcinogen, metastasis, oncology, performance status, registry, Regional Medical Program,* and *stage.* II.B.2.

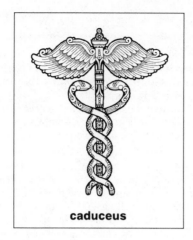

caduceus

candystriper. see *pink lady.*

capacity. see *bed.*

capacity for work. see *occupation.*

capital. 1. in economics, everything manufactured for the purpose of helping man in his productive efforts, as equipment, facilities, and roads; synonym, capital goods; the value of such *goods.* 2. commonly, liquid or spendable assets, also called capital funds, sometimes only when specifically accounted for the purchase of capital goods.

Capital goods are usually thought of as permanent and durable (when in doubt, those lasting over a year); contrast *supplies.* Capital may refer to investment in self, called *human capital, as purchase of *preventive care* for the positive effect it may have on one's future earning capacity. *Capital gains, income from the sale of a capital asset or good for a higher price than was paid for it, are usually treated differently by tax law than other types of *income.*

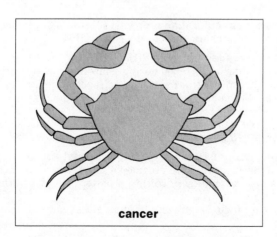

cancer

See *amortization, depreciation, working capital.* 1. VIII.B.2., III.B.1. 2. VI.C.1.

capital depreciation.   see *depreciation.*

capital expenditure review (CER).   any review of *capital* expenditures proposed by or for health facilities to determine the *need* for, and *appropriateness* of, the proposed services.

The review is usually done by a designated *regulatory* agency, as a *state health planning and development agency,* and has a sanction attached which prevents, see *certificate of need,* or discourages, see *section 1122,* unneeded expenditures. VI.A.

capitation.   1. payment fixed per person and determined by the number of people eligible for service. 2. in health services, used when a provider is paid a fixed amount for each person served, without regard to the number or nature of services each actually uses. Capitation is characteristic of *health maintenance organizations,* but unusual for physicians, see *fee for service.* 3. federal support for health professional schools in which eligible schools receive a *capitation grant for each student enrolled (Titles VII and VIII of the *Public Health Service Act*). 2. IV.B. 3. III.A.

capper.   synonym, *steerer.*

Being or dealing with a capper or steerer is expressly forbidden by at least one state medical practice act (Tennessee). I am unaware of a distinction, although both are listed in law. Might capper be from "capturing," rather than "putting on the cap," see *Gove, 1976*?

carcinogen.   a cause of *cancer,* whether by facilitation, initiation, or promotion. *Carcinogenic means cancer causing. *Carcinogenicity refers to how bad a carcinogen is. *Carcinogenesis is the causing of cancer, and the means by which it is done.

Certain viruses, chemicals (asbestos), *exposures* (coal tar), jobs (uranium mining), and behaviors (smoking) are known to be carcinogens. How these lead to cancer is not always known; in some cases the *association* may not be causal. Carcinogenesis, *mutagenesis,* and *teratogenesis* are similar at the chemical level, although not all agents have all three properties.

See *Ames' test* and *Delaney Amendment.* I.C.

cardex.   see *Kardex.*

cardiology, cardiovascular disease.   the subspecialty of internal medicine concerned with the heart and blood vessels. III.C.

cardiopulmonary resuscitation (CPR).   artificial, usually manual, breathing and/or pumping of the blood during temporary, respiratory and/or heart failure while definitive treatment can be reached and undertaken.

CPR is most often needed immediately after a heart attack that produces ineffective, irregular beating of the heart. The *Red Cross* and others have widely taught CPR to *consumers,* since the skills are easily learned and *death* occurs after only 5 minutes of respiratory or circulatory collapse. V.B.

care.   1. responsibility for, or attention to, the safety, health, and needs of a patient or other concern. 2. to provide for, or attend to the needs of, or perform necessary personal services for, a patient, child, or other dependent person.

Caring may include *curing,* although either may be done without the other. V.

care giver. usually a synonym for caretaker. The latter is better usage. One of the occasional places in English where opposites have come to the same meaning.

Care giver is more common among mental health workers. It sometimes means volunteers and community workers with some training, while caretakers are ordinarily without special training. III.A.

caretaker. one who has care or charge of a person, organization, or thing; compare *homemaker* and *nurse*. Typically, the person primarily responsible for caring for a particular sick, dependent, or aged person.

Identification, education, and support of caretakers is one of family medicine's keys to successful care of many chronic complex problems. Caretakers are chosen by circumstances and the one cared for, care givers by the health care system. I.B.1.

carnal. of the flesh, bodily. *carnal knowledge. sexual intercourse, although for legal purposes hymenal rupture or vaginal penetration may not be necessary. VIII.B.3.

carrier. 1. a commercial health *insurer,* a government agency, or a *Blue Cross/ Blue Shield* plan which *underwrites* or administers a program that pays for health services. 2. one who harbors a disease, compare *vector.*

In the Medicare *Supplementary Medical Insurance Program* and *Federal Employees Health Benefits Program* carriers are agencies and organizations with which the programs contract for administration of various functions, including payment of *claims.*

See *intermediary* and *third party.* IV.B.

case. an occurrence or episode of a *disease;* a patient with a particular disease; an *encounter* or *admission,* usually for a particular disease.

See *index case.* II.

case abstract. synonym, *discharge abstract.*

case-control study. a study, ordinarily longitudinal, in which individuals are selected because they do (cases) or, while similar, do not (controls) have the *disease* being studied.

The cases and controls are compared with respect to past, existing, or future characteristics judged likely to be relevant to the disease in question to see which of the characteristics differ, and how, in the two groups. VIII.D.

case fatality rate. see *mortality rate.*

case management. assigning one individual or institutional provider sole responsibility for furnishing *primary care* and overseeing needed referrals for an individual or family; compare *gatekeeper.*

Some *Medicaid* programs require some or all covered individuals to *lock in* to a case manager, who may or may not be at financial risk or a member of a formal primary care network, in hopes of controlling costly doctor shopping and unnecessary procedures. IV.C.2.

case mix. the disease-specific makeup of a health program's workload.

Case mix directly influences the *lengths of stays* in, and *intensity, cost,* and *scope of services* provided by, a hospital or other health program. *Case-mix severity measures how bad the cases treated are at their clinical worst; *case-mix complexity also considers their duration and other aspects of how hard they are to manage. Compare the maximum height and the area un-

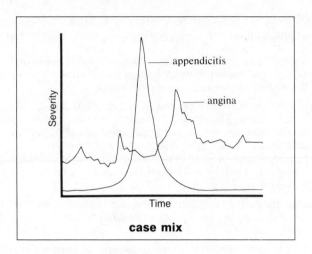

case mix

der the following curves: appendicitis may be severe but is rarely complex in this sense; angina is usually complex, sometimes also severe.

Read Cretin, S., and L.G. Worthman, *Alternative Systems for Case Mix Classification* (Palo Alto, CA: The Rand Corporation (R-3457-HCFA), 2/86). See *Acute Physiology and Chronic Health Evaluation, diagnosis related group, Medical Illness Severity Grouping System, nursing intensity,* and *Patient Management Categories.* VIII.C.

case rate. synonym, *attack rate.*

cases treated. the number of cases cared for by a health program during a year.

Inpatient discharges and *outpatient* visits may be combined into an aggregate weighted index of hospital output. VIII.C.

catastrophic health insurance. health *insurance* providing protection against the high cost of treating severe or lengthy illness or disability; the ultimate in *last dollar coverage.*

Most catastrophic policies and proposals cover all or a specified percentage of medical expenses above an amount that is the responsibility of the insured himself (or of another insurance policy up to its maximum limit of liability). Protection typically begins after an individual or family unit incurs medical expenses equal to a specified dollar amount, as $2000 within a 12-month period, or to a specified percentage of *income,* as 15 percent; or has been a hospital inpatient for a specified period, as 60 days. Individuals are liable for all costs up to specified thresholds, called *limits. There is usually no maximum amount of coverage under these plans, however, many include some *coinsurance.*

See *deductible* and *major medical.* IV.B.

catchment area. a geographic *region* defined and served by a health program, as a hospital or *community mental health center.*

Areas are delineated by use of such factors as population distribution, natural geographic boundaries, and transportation accessibility. They should be contrasted with service, medical market, or *medical trade areas.* All residents of the area needing the services of the program are usually eligible for them, although eligibility may also depend on additional criteria, as age or income. Residents of the area may or may not be limited to obtaining services from the program, known to it, or *enrolled* in it. The program may or may not be limited to providing services to residents of the area, or under any obligation to know of, *register,* or have the capacity to serve all area residents. III.B.1.

categorical grant.   a grant of federal funds for a specific purpose or program, as a *categorical program;* compare *block* and *formula grants.* IV.C.

categorically needy.   people who are both members of certain categories or groups eligible to receive public assistance, and economically needy.

As used in *Medicaid,* one who is aged, *blind, disabled,* or a member of a family with children under 18 (or 21, if in school) with one parent absent, incapacitated, or unemployed, and who also falls below state-specified *income* and *resources* limits. Most categorically needy receive cash assistance from the *Aid to Families with Dependent Children* (AFDC) or *Supplemental Security Income* (SSI) programs. A state must cover all recipients of AFDC payments under Medicaid, but is provided certain options in determining coverage for persons receiving federal SSI and/or state supplementary SSI payments. A state may cover as categorically needy additional specified groups, as foster children. Medicaid coverage may be restricted to the categorically needy or may extend to additional persons who meet the categorical requirements, as the *medically needy.* I.A.2.c., IV.C.2.

categorically related.   in the *Medicaid* program, refers to requirements, other than limits on income and *resources,* which an individual must meet to be eligible for Medicaid benefits; one who meets these requirements.

Specifically, any individual eligible for Medicaid must fall into one of the four main categories of people who are eligible for *welfare.* He must be aged, blind, or disabled (as defined by the *Supplemental Security Income Program*), or a member of a family with dependent children with one parent absent, incapacitated, or unemployed (as defined by the *Aid to Families with Dependent Children Program*). After the determination is made that an individual is categorically related, then income and resources tests are used to see if the individual is poor enough to be eligible for assistance, *categorically needy.* This means single persons; childless couples who are not aged, blind, or disabled; and male-headed families in states which do not cover such families under their AFDC programs, cannot receive Medicaid coverage no matter how poor they are because they are not categorically related. I.A.2.c., IV.C.2.

categorical program.   originally, a health program concerned with only one or a few specified, usually related, diseases, as *alcohol* treatment, or the *Regional Medical Programs;* more recently, a program concerned with only a part, instead of all, of the population or health system, as a health maintenance organization, or rate setting; often loosely and pejoratively, any existing program which the speaker opposes. VII.B.1.

categorization.   classification of health programs and other things by their differing purposes or qualities.

In *emergency medical services,* for example, hospitals are *horizontally categorized when they specialize in different emergencies, as burns or major trauma, and *vertically categorized by their sophistication, category I units caring only for simple problems and stabilizing others for transport while category III units take anything. Hospital privileges, obstetrical services, and other things are similarly, usually vertically, categorized. VII.B.3.a.

cause. that which produces or contributes to a result; a reason; a motive. In law, a basis or grounds for legal action.

May be defined negatively; something which if avoided, removed, or eliminated will prevent the occurrence of the event in question. Most things have many causes; immediate or proximate, contributory, and remote. A *necessary cause is one that must exist if a given event is to occur, but may not itself result in the event. A *sufficient cause is one which is inevitably followed by a given event.

See *agent* and *association*. II.B.1.a.

ceding company. see *reinsurance*.

ceiling limit value. see *threshold limit value*.

Celsus, Aurelius Cornelius. Roman physician, 42 B.C.–37 A.D. A noble landowner who compiled books on agriculture, veterinary medicine, and human illness. His *De re medicinae,* neglected through the middle ages, was one of the first medical books printed (1478) and subsequently very influential. VII.A.I.

census. a count, ordinarily of people served by a health program or facility at or during a given period of time. A hospital census is its number of inpatients, usually at midnight. III.B.1.

center. synonym, *institute*, but even more loosely used, as when applied to a profit-making program. III.D.3.

Centers for Disease Control (CDC). the agency within the Department of Health and Human Services principally responsible for administration of disease control, *health promotion, occupational health* (see *National Institute of Occupational Safety and Health*), and *public health* programs. Formerly the Communicable Disease Center.

The Centers provide facilities and services for the investigation, prevention, and control of disease; support *quarantine* and other activities to prevent introduction of communicable diseases from foreign countries; conduct research into the *epidemiology,* laboratory diagnosis, prevention, and treatment of infectious and other controllable diseases at the community level; conduct and support *health education* programs; provide grants for work on venereal disease, immunization against infectious diseases, and disease control programs; set *standards* for laboratories; and train state and local health workers in specific control techniques.

See *Epidemiologic Intelligence Service*. III.D.1.

central birth rate. see *birth rate*.

certificate. a document containing an official statement or signed testimony to the truth of something, as a birth certificate or death certificate. VIII.B.3.

certificate of insurance. in *group insurance*, a certificate issued to a *member* of a *group* stating that an insurance contract covering the member has been written and containing a summary of the terms applicable to that member. IV.B.

certificate of need (CON). a certificate issued by a governmental body, ordinarily a state, to an individual or organization proposing to construct or modify a *health facility*, or to offer a new or different health *service*, which determines that such facility or service when *available* will be *needed* by those for whom it is intended.

Where a certificate is required, as with proposals which will involve more than a minimum *capital* investment or will change *bed capacity,* it is required for *licensure* of the facility or service, and intended to control expansion of facilities and services in the public interest by preventing excessive or duplicative development. The National Health Planning and Resources Development Act of 1974 required states to have the *state health planning and development agency* (designated pursuant to the law) administer a certificate of need program that applied to all new *institutional health services* proposed in the state. *Health systems agencies* made recommendations to the state agencies regarding new institutional health services proposed within their areas.

See *capital expenditures review* and *section 1122.* VI.A.2.

certificate of special competence. see *subspecialty.*

certification. 1. assessment and recognition of an individual as meeting predetermined standards; the issuance of a certificate. One so recognized is said to be certified. 2. the legal process whereby a judicial authority acting on medical evidence finds a person *committable.*

Essentially synonymous with *accreditation,* except that certification is applied to individuals and accreditation to institutions. Certification programs are generally nongovernmental and do not exclude the uncertified from practice as do government *licensure* programs. In regulatory programs, certification of services sometimes means that their provision has been found necessary and payment for them is assured, see *admission certification.*

See *board certification* and *certificate of need.* III.B.

Chadwick, Edwin. British social reformer, 1800–1890. Pioneer of modern *public health,* he introduced the public to the "sanitary idea," leading to the establishment of the General Board of Health in 1848. His *Sanitary Condition of the Laboring Population of Great Britain,* published in 1842, showed the relation between poverty and ill health in the community, and provided a model for sanitary reformers in other countries. VII.B.2.e., VIII.A.1.

chairside. the dental equivalent of bedside.

See *bedside manner.* V., VII.C.4.

channeling agency. a program which serves people by finding *services* for them.

Such agencies may provide some direct services but primarily help people with multiple needs find their way through a fragmented, *categorical* system. They operate as *referral* agencies and help integrate the services people do receive. III.B.1.

charge. price assigned to a unit of medical service, as a visit to a physician, a prescription, or a day in a hospital.

Charges for services may not be related to the *actual costs* of providing the services, and when they are, the methods by which charges are related to costs vary substantially by type of service and institution. Different *third party* payers may require use of different methods of determining charges. Charges for some services provided by an institution are often used to subsidize the costs of others, while charges to one type of patient may be used to subsidize the costs of providing services to others.

See *actual, allowable, customary, prevailing, reasonable,* and *usual charges.* VII.D.1.

charitable immunity. in *malpractice,* an old legal doctrine, still in use in some states, that nonprofit, or charitable, hospitals and other health programs are not subject to suit for malpractice.

The doctrine relies on a presumed waiver of the patient's right to sue for *negligence* upon accepting the charity, the apparent unfairness of applying a doctrine such as *respondent superior,* which covers commercial pursuits, to a nonprofit enterprise, and the increased financial demands upon the assets of a charity which might result from adverse judgments. There are exceptions to the immunity: a charity may be held liable for the negligence of its agent, to a stranger who is not a beneficiary, or only to the extent of its nontrust assets. Charitable immunity has been abolished in many states, because of the illogical and conflicting bases upon which the doctrine was originally founded, the alleged unfairness of forcing the injured party to contribute indirectly to the charity by refusing him the opportunity to recover, and the availability of liability insurance.

See *governmental immunity.* V.D.

charity. 1. love, the practice of love. 2. an organization engaged in free or subsidized services to the poor, suffering, or sick. 3. in law, a program operated without *profit* and usually without *capital,* and funded publically or by private gifts, which serves the public or a part of it, indefinite as to number or individual members. Synonym, charitable organization.

Most hospitals and other health programs in the United States have historically been governmental or charities, often church operated, except in the last few decades.

See *foundation, institute,* and *voluntary health agency.* III.B.4.

charity allowance. an amount included in a health program's *charges,* or an *allowable cost* in *cost-based reimbursement,* which pays for the program's charity care to people other than the patient for whom the charge or reimbursement is made. Compare *green screen* and *sick tax.* Contrast *Blue Cross discount.* VII.D.1.

chart. synonym, *medical record;* to add information to a record.

chastity bill. see *Adolescent Family Life Program.*

checkup. informal, an *encounter* in which the patient's health and medical *problems* are assessed and treated.

A checkup usually emphasizes *health maintenance* and complete assessment, but may casually refer to any encounter for any purpose. Neither *regular nor *complete checkup has constant meaning, although the latter should include any history, physical, and laboratory investigation likely to benefit the patient. VII.B.3.

chemical equivalents. *drug* products from different sources which are chemically indistinguishable. They usually contain identical amounts of the same active ingredients in identical dosage forms and meet existing physiochemical *standards* in official *compendia.*

See *bioequivalent.* III.B.3.

chemical name. the exact description of the molecular structure of a *drug,* based on the rules of standard chemical nomenclature.

The tranquilizer with the chemical name 2-methyl-2-propyl, 3-propenediol dicarbamate will serve as an example. While long and cumbersome, this name is precise, serving as a complete identification of the compound to a trained chemist, since it is related to the drug's chemical formula, see diagram. It is sold *generically* as meprobamate, and under various *brand names* by different firms, as Miltown, Equanil, Pathibamate, and SK-Bamate. III.B.3.

$$H_2NCOO-CH_2-\underset{\underset{\displaystyle CH_2CH_2CH_3}{|}}{\overset{\overset{\displaystyle CH_3}{|}}{C}}-CH_2-OOCNH_2\ CH_2$$

chemical restraint.　a drug, as a sedative or antipsychotic, used against the recipient's will to control difficult or unwanted behavior.

Use of chemical restraint to make patients easy to care for is as unethical and destructive of their rights as tying them down. The distinction between appropriate and inappropriate use of these drugs is elusive, depending on proper diagnostic indication and patient, family, or neutral third party consent. III.B.3.

chief complaint (CC).　see *complaint.*

chijiao yisheng.　transliteration of the Chinese for *barefoot doctor.*

child.　a young person, especially between infancy and adolescence.

There are no constant divisions of childhood, although commonly used are *neonate* or newborn (the first month), *infancy (the first 2 years), *childhood (2–14), and *adolescence (15–21). For legal purposes, a child is usually any *minor,* sometimes only one under 15. Because of their special needs and dependence, and their importance to the future health of the population, children often receive special attention in health care; see *CHAP, maternal and child health,* and *Ribicoff kids.* I.A.1.

Child Health Assurance Program (CHAP).　a Carter administration proposal, first made in 1977, for expansion and revision of federal health financing and programs for children.

It would include changes in Medicaid coverage for children, the *Early and Periodic Screening, Diagnosis, and Treatment Program,* and *maternal and child health services.* III.D.1.

children and youth project (C&Y).　see *maternal and child health services.*

chiropodist, chiropody.　synonyms, *podiatrist, podiatry.*

chiropractic.　a system of mechanical therapeutics based on the principles that the nervous system largely determines the state of health and that disease results from abnormal nerve function and conformity.

Treatment consists primarily of the adjustment or manipulation of parts of the body, especially the spinal column. Some chiropractors also use physiotherapy, nutritional supplementation, and other therapeutic modalities; radiography is used for diagnosis only. Operations, drugs, and immunizations are usually rejected as violations of the human body. Chiropractic was founded in 1895 by D.D. Palmer. Its services are covered by many state Medicaid programs. Manual manipulation of the spine is covered under Medicare when *subluxation of the spine* is demonstrated on x-ray. V.

chiropractor.　a practitioner of chiropractic. Chiropractors are licensed by all states. III.A.

chirurgeon. obsolete spelling of *surgeon,* still used in such places as the names of state licensure agencies.

chloracne. see *dioxin.*

chlorinate. to treat with chlorine, as for disinfecting *sewage* or *drinking water.* I.C.5.

chlorinated hydrocarbon. any of a class of long-lasting, broad-spectrum *insecticides,* as *DDT,* first used for insect control during World War II; similar compounds include aldrin, dieldrin, heptachlor, chlordane, lindane, endrin, mirex, benzene hexachloride (BHC), and toxaphene.

Their *persistence* and effectiveness against a wide variety of insects were long felt to be desirable in agriculture, public health, and home uses. Later research showed these same qualities to represent a potential *hazard* through accumulation and concentration in the *food chain* and persistence in the environment. I.C.5.

Christian Science. a religion, and system of faith healing through prayer and the control of mind over matter, based on the teachings of the founder, Mary Baker Eddy.

The services of Christian Science *sanatoria* are covered by some health insurance programs, including Medicare and, in some states, Medicaid, sometimes with an exemption from standards applied by such programs to traditional medical providers. V.

chromium. see *heavy metal.*

chronic disease. one with long duration (more than 30 days) or frequent recurrence; contrast acute disease.

Chronic diseases often are permanent, cause *disability,* and require *rehabilitation* of the patient. II.A.

chronological age. see *age.*

citation. an official notice, and the paper embodying it, to a person or organization of a violation, as of the *Occupational Safety and Health Act of 1970* or standards under it, of a required appearance, as in court, or of some achievement, as valor.

Citations are the Occupational Safety and Health Act's principal enforcement tool. They must describe the specific violation and establish a reasonable period for its *abatement.* A copy must be posted at or near the violation. Citations must be issued promptly after a violation is found during an inspection and followed by a notice of proposed penalties. Both the citation and penalties may be contested within 15 days by the employer. VII.B.2.d.

Civilian Health and Medical Program of the Uniformed Services (CHAMPUS). a program which pays for care delivered by civilian health providers to retired members, and *dependents* of active and retired members, of the seven uniformed services of the United States (Army, Navy, Air Force, Marine Corps, *Commissioned Corps* of the Public Health Service, Coast Guard, and the National Oceanic and Atmospheric Administration).

CHAMPUS is administered by the Department of Defense. It has no *premium* but does have *cost sharing.* III.D.1.

Civilian Health and Medical Program of the Veterans Administration (CHAMPVA). a program which pays for health care provided by civilian providers to dependents of totally *disabled* veterans who are eligible for retirement pay from a uniformed service.

CHAMPVA is administered by the Department of Defense for the Veterans Administration. It has no *premium* but does have *cost sharing*. III.D.1.

claim. a request to an insurer by an insured person or, on his behalf, by the provider of a service or good, for payment of benefits under an insurance policy. IV.B.

claims-incurred policy. a *malpractice insurance* policy in which the insured, as a physician, is covered for claims arising from any injury which occurs or is alleged to have occurred during the policy period, regardless of when a claim is made. The only limiting factor is the *statute of limitations,* which varies among states.

Claims-incurred malpractice insurance was conventional until the malpractice "crisis" of the mid-seventies, at which time it was largely replaced by the claims-made approach. V.D.

claims-made policy. a *malpractice insurance* policy in which the insured is covered for any claim made, rather than any *injury* occurring, while the policy is in force.

Claims made after the insurance lapses are not covered, as they are by a *claims-incurred policy.* Administration and rate setting are easier than with the claims-incurred approach. The transition from claims-incurred to claims-made insurance is difficult because medical malpractice claims may arise years after an injury occurs, see *discovery rule.* A retired physician may be sued when not covered unless special provisions are made to continue his coverage after retirement, see *tail.* V.D.

claims review. review of claims by governments, medical foundations, peer review organizations, insurers, or others responsible for payment to determine liability and amount of payment.

This review may seek to determine eligibility of the claimant or beneficiary, eligibility of the provider of the benefit, that the benefit claimed is covered, that the benefit is not payable under another policy, see *coordination of benefits,* and that the benefit was *necessary* and of *reasonable cost* and *quality.* VI.E.

clean. free of *contagion,* as a clean patient or procedure.

Dirt and disease may be present and a patient still considered clean, as long as other patients will not be infected. Clean and *contaminated,* or "dirty," patients are ordinarily separated.

See *asepsis.* II.A.2.

clerk. 1. one who serves a clerkship, compare *extern.* 2. a secretary, as a ward clerk. III.A.4.

clerkship. an apprenticeship for a medical student, served under supervision in one of the various medical *specialties.* III.A.

clinic. 1. current, a facility, or part of one, for care of *outpatients.* Clinic is irregularly defined; sometimes excludes physicians' offices, sometimes limited to facilities for *poor* or *public patients,* and sometimes limited to ones also used for medical education. 2. older, medical instruction at the bedside or with patients. 1. III.B.1., 2. III.C.

clinical. pertaining to patients and their illnesses, as opposed to experimental, pathologic, or theoretical.

See *preclinical* and *subclinical.* III.C.

clinical equivalents. see *therapeutic equivalents.*

clinical laboratory. see *laboratory.*

clinical medicine. 1. the study of disease or instruction in medicine using living patients. 2. the *practice* of medicine. III.C.

clinical nurse specialist, clinical specialist. a professional *nurse* with highly developed knowledge and skills in the care of patients in some *specialty*, ordinarily with a master's degree in the nursing specialty.

Clinical specialists are *certified* by the American Nurses Association and include many *nurse anesthetists, nurse practitioners,* and *nurse midwives.* III.A.2.

clinical pharmacist. a *pharmacist* trained in or practicing clinical pharmacy. III.A.4.

clinical pharmacy. the division of *pharmacy* concerned with patients' use of drugs, whether prescribed or self-administered.

The discipline is concerned with drug selection and surveillance, patient response, *adverse reactions,* and drug interactions. III.C.

clinical privilege. synonym, *staff privilege.*

clinical psychologist. a *psychologist* with a graduate degree, usually a Ph.D., and clinical training who practices clinical psychology.

Clinical psychologists do a predoctoral internship year. They are licensed by most states, after additional supervised postdoctoral clinical practice, for independent professional practice, and their services are reimbursed by many health insurance programs. They do not treat physical causes of mental illness with drugs or other medical or surgical measures since they are not licensed to practice medicine. III.A.4.

clinical psychology. the branch of *psychology* that specializes in the evaluation and treatment of human mental and behavioral disorders and does research into the psychologic aspects of development, disease, and mental illness; compare *experimental psychology.* III.C.

clinical sciences. the disciplines which explain abnormal structure and function, and therapy of, the body and its parts, people and their families, communities, and environments. Compare *basic sciences* and *behavioral science.*

Irregularly defined, these are the subjects taught in the second year of traditional medical education and typically include epidemiology, infectious diseases, pathology, pharmacology, public health, and the medical specialties. III.C.

clinician. 1. one who practices medicine. 2. a physician whose knowledge is drawn from experience with live patients. 3. a *clinical* instructor, as *W. Osler.* III.A.

clinicopathological conference (CPC). a formal teaching exercise in which a patient's case is presented as an unknown to a clinician who then uses the data given to reach a *diagnosis* and comment upon the issues presented by the case. Further, usually definitive, *pathologic* information obtained at *autopsy* or operation is then presented and interpreted by a *pathologist* before further discussion. The case is typically presented by those who participated in the patient's care but is unfamiliar to the discusser.

The CPC was introduced at the turn of the century by Richard Cabot at Boston's Massachusetts General Hospital, whose weekly CPC has been published continuously by the *New England Journal of Medicine* since 1926. Always popular for the pleasure of watching someone commit himself on an interesting unknown, the CPC emphasizes careful diagnosis and the pathophysiology of disease.

Read Relman Arnold S. et al., "Are the Case Records Obsolete? Two Views" (*N Engl J Med*, 301(2): 1112–6, 11/15/79.) V.A.

closed panel. see *panel.*

closed staff. see *medical staff.*

Coal Mine Health and Safety Act of 1969. the principal federal legal authority for the coal and other mine safety and health programs administered by the *Mine Safety and Health Administration* of the Department of Labor. VII.B.

code, code blue. a cardiac or respiratory arrest requiring *cardiopulmonary resuscitation;* the coded page over a hospital paging system calling for the needed help; a patient who is to be resuscitated in the event of such arrest, compare *no code.* There are many irregular synonyms. V.B.

cohort study. a longitudinal *study* in which a group, *the cohort, is chosen for the presence of a specific characteristic at or during a specified time (the *independent variable,* as hypertension) and followed over time to discover presumably related characteristics (the *dependent variables,* as heart failure and strokes).
    Several cohorts may be treated differently in hopes of discovering differences in the results, see *prospective trial.* VIII.D.

coinsurance (Co). a *cost-sharing* requirement in a health insurance policy which provides that the insured will assume a portion or percentage of the cost of *covered* services.
    The health insurance policy provides that the insurer will reimburse a specified percentage, often 80 percent, of all or specified covered medical expenses in excess of any *deductible* amounts payable by the insured. The insured is then liable for the remaining percentage of the costs, until the maximum amount payable under the insurance policy, if any, is reached. IV.B.

coliform count, index. a measure of the purity of water based on a count of its coliform bacteria content.
    Coliform bacteria, as *Escherichia coli,* grow in the intestines of humans and animals. Their presence in water thus warns of potentially dangerous bacterial *contamination.* I.C.5.

collateral source. a source of payment for damages alternative or additional to the settlement sought from the defendant in a *malpractice* suit, as health insurance benefits for medical expenses for which the suit also seeks payment.
    In many states evidence of collateral sources cannot be introduced in malpractice trials, *the collateral source rule. Therefore, a jury disregards the availability of collateral sources in setting judgments. This contrasts with *coordination of benefits* in insurance. V.D.

collection agent, agency. an individual or organization which assists in collecting payment on accounts receivable.
    Such agencies ordinarily retain a percentage of what they collect; contrast *factoring.* III.B.1.

collection rate, ratio. percentage of charges actually collected.
    Often calculated by dividing collections in a given month or year by charges made during the same period. This is an approximation since the

collections and charges used are for services provided at somewhat different times. VI.C.

college. irregular, a school, *professional association,* or *specialty board,* as, American College of Surgeons. III.C.

colon and rectal surgery, colorectal surgery. the science and surgical specialty devoted to the study and care of the colon, rectum, and anus; synonym, proctology. III.C.

commercial waste. see *solid waste.*

Commissioned Corps of the U.S Public Health Service. the one of the seven uniformed services of the U.S. government concerned with *public health.*

The Commissioned Corps originated in 1873 as an elite career corps of government physicians. While not military service, the Corps has pay, rank, uniforms, retirement, and other characteristics in common with them, including *CHAMPUS.* Despite a great tradition, it is now essentially an employment alternative to the federal civil service for some people working for the Department of Health and Human Services. III.D.1.

Commission on Professional and Hospital Activities (CPHA). a private, nonprofit organization (Ann Arbor, Michigan; est. 1955), which collects, processes, and distributes data on hospital use for management, evaluation, and research purposes.

The two main programs of the CPHA are the *Professional Activity Study* (PAS) and the *Medical Audit Program* (MAP), which together represent a continuing study of hospital practice. More than 1800 hospitals throughout the United States, Canada, Venezuela, Saudi Arabia, and Australia participate in PAS and MAP. PAS hospitals account for almost 40 percent of all patients discharged from short-term general hospitals in the U.S. and Canada. The system abstracts and classifies information from medical records in a standard *discharge abstract.* The computer-accessible data library at CPHA contains information on over 100 million hospitalizations, the world's largest collection of such data.

See *Internation Classification of Diseases, Adapted.* III.B.1.

commitment. obligatory hospitalization of a patient in need of treatment, as for a *mental illness,* typically by *certification.*

Criteria and methods for commitment are carefully, although variably, specified in state laws. They usually require a finding by two or more physicians, or one physician and one psychologist, that the patient is dangerous to himself or others, and are subject to judicial review. *Involuntary commitment is done against the patient's will and often implied, although committal is sometimes voluntary.

See *against medical advice.* V.B.

committee. the world is full of committees, see *infection committee* and *tissue committee.*

Committee on Allied Health Education and Accreditation (CAHEA). an American Medical Association committee formed in 1977 and recognized by the Department of Education as the *accrediting* body for *allied health* education programs. III.A.5.

committee report. in Congress, a formal report by a congressional committee to the House, Senate, or both, see *conference,* on a proposed law or other matter.

The report is part of the *legislative history* and includes a summary of the proposed law, recommendations on its passage and amendments, background information, a discussion and defense of its provisions, a detailed section-by-section analysis of them, a demonstration of the changes it makes in existing law, administration views, cost estimates, and dissenting views from members of the committee. VIII.B.3.

commodity. synonym, *good.*

communicable disease (CD). a disease, usually *infectious*, transmissible from one source (either animal or person) to another, directly or indirectly (as via a *vector*). I.A.1.

Communicable Disease Center (CDC). old name for the *Centers for Disease Control.*

community. a group of organisms having common residence, organization, or interests; compare *biome*. Not consistently differentiated from *population* or *society*, usually intermediate in size between *family* and society.
  Concern for the *healthfulness* of communities, and understanding how they may affect and support families, is a growing part of family medicine. I.B.2., VII.A.2.

community health care. activities and programs intended to improve the *healthfulness* of, and general *health status* in, a specified community.
  The term is widely and irregularly used either as above, in a manner similar to *public health;* synonymously with *environmental health*; as all health services of any kind available to a given community; or synonymously with a community's *ambulatory care.* VII.A.2.

community health center (CHC). an *ambulatory* health program, usually serving a *catchment area* with scarce or nonexistent health services or a population with special health needs; synonym, neighborhood health center.
  Community health centers coordinate federal, state, and local resources in a single operation which delivers both medical care and related social services to a defined population. While such centers may not themselves provide all types of health care, they take responsibility for arranging for all medical services needed by their patients. Other ambulatory programs providing health services in areas of *medical underservice* include *family health centers* and *community health networks*. Community health centers are defined and supported by section 330 of the *Public Health Service Act*. In 1987, there were some 600 centers serving 5 million people. III.B.2., VII.B.3.

community health network (CHN). a community (state, county, or city) health system for delivering medical care to the *poor*.
  Started by the White House Office of Economic Opportunity in the early 1970s, the program was transferred to the Department of Health and Human Services and became part of the *community health center* program. A network consisted of several centrally managed community health centers with necessary hospital *affiliations.* III.B.1., VII.B.3.

community health nurse. synonym, *public health nurse* or *visiting nurse.*

community medicine. variously synonymous with *community health care, public health, preventive medicine, primary care,* or *social medicine.* VII.A.2.

community mental health center (CMHC). a program which provides comprehensive, mainly *ambulatory, mental health* services primarily to individuals residing or employed in a defined *catchment area.*

The term is defined in section 201 of the Community Mental Health Centers Act which specifies the services to be provided and requirements for the governance, organization, and operation of centers. The CMHC Act provides for federal assistance for construction, development, and initial operation of centers, and, on an ongoing basis, for the costs of their *consultation and education services.* III.B.1., VII.B.2.

community oriented primary care (COPC). an approach to *community medicine* and *primary care,* the elements of which include use of *clinical epidemiology,* a defined population, programs addressing community health problems, community involvement, the absence of barriers to care, and the integration of all kinds of services.

Read Conner, Eileen, and Mullen, Fitzhugh, editors, *Community Oriented Primary Care: New Directions for Health Services Delivery* (Washington: National Academy Press, 1983. 313 pp. $16.50, paper). VII.A.2.

community psychiatry. the branch of psychiatry concerned with the provision of a coordinated program of mental health care to residents of a designated *catchment area;* compare *social psychiatry.*

Some also extend its concern, in a manner comparable to *public health,* to identifying and changing deficient and dysfunctional *community* structure or function in hopes of creating a more mentally and socially *healthful* environment for the community's members. I.B.2., III.C.

community rating. a method of establishing or *rating premiums* for health insurance which bases the premium on the average cost of actual or anticipated health care used by all *subscribers* in a geographic area or industry and does not vary for different groups of subscribers or with such variables as individual or group claims experience, age, sex, or *health status.*

The Health Maintenance Organization Act, section 1302(8) of the *Public Health Service Act,* defines community rating as a system of fixing rates of payments for health services "which may be determined on a per person or per family basis and may vary with the number of persons in a family, but must be equivalent for all individuals and for all families with similar composition." Community rating spreads the cost of illness evenly over the subscribers (the whole community), rather than charging the sick more than the healthy for insurance. It is the exceptional means of establishing health insurance premiums in the United States today, for example the Federal Employees Health Benefits Program is *experience rated,* not community rated. IV.B., III.B.1.

comparability provision. a provision in Medicare law specifying that the *reasonable charge* for a service may not be higher than the charges payable for a comparable service insured under comparable circumstances by a *carrier* for its non-Medicare *beneficiaries,* section 1842(b)(3)(B) of the Social Security Act. IV.C.1.

compassionate use. administration of investigational or experimental drugs in circumstances or programs which violate the requirements for *adequate and well-controlled investigations* but are nonetheless acceptable because the patients receiving the drug have such grim *prognoses* that any potential benefits outweigh any conceivable risks, i.e., the patients would be better off dead. III.B.3., III.C.

compendium. a collection of information about *drugs;* synonym, *pharmacopeia.*

The Federal Food, Drug, and Cosmetic Act recognizes standards for strength, quality, and purity of drugs set forth in three official compendia: the *United States Pharmacopeia,* the *Homeopathic Pharmacopeia of the United States,* the *National Formulary,* and any supplement to any of them. See *formulary* and *Physicians' Desk Reference.* III.B.3.

compensable event, injury, or death. in *malpractice* and *worker's compensation,* a cause of, or resulting condition from, illness or death for which damages or benefits are payable. In law, the date of the event may be the date the right to compensation accrues rather than that of the actual event. V.D., VII.B.2.d.

competence, competency. in law, the possession of qualification, capacity, or soundness of mind to perform or take responsibility for an act or duty in question.

Insanity is a common basis for incompetency. Competency to stand trial applies to the defendant's state of mind at the time of trial and is present when he understands the charges and consequences of conviction, and can assist in his own defense. Responsibility for a criminal act is determined by various rules in different jurisdictions, as the *American Law Institute Formulation.*

See *guardian.* VIII.B.3.

competition. the act or action of seeking to gain what another seeks, usually at the same time and under similar circumstances.

In economics, pure competition exists when the price and quantity of a commodity or service are established by market forces of *supply* and *demand.* This requires many independent buyers and sellers, freedom for sellers to enter and leave the market, and free flow of information so buyers may compare sellers. While these conditions do not exist in health care, a competitive approach to reforming U.S. health care has attracted wide attention in the late 1970s and early 1980s. It would involve organizing physicians into competitive economic units, including *health maintenance organizations,* creating common rules regarding benefits, catastrophic expenses, and so forth, assuring people a choice among these units, and adjusting premiums and *medical deductions* so that people receive the same subsidy no matter what plan they choose. This should make differences in charges apparent, make consumers responsible for the differences, and thus lead to competition and drive charges down.

Read Ginzberg, Eli, "Competition and Cost Containment" (*N Engl J Med,* 303: 1112–5, 1980). IV.D., VIII.B.1.

competitive medical plan (CMP). a *prepaid* medical plan delivering managed care; a watered-down *health maintenance organization* (HMO).

CMPs, unlike HMOs, may have deductibles and unlimited copayments, may *experience rate,* and need not be a distinct legal entity, e.g., they may be part of a hospital or insurance company. Either CMPs or HMOs may qualify for Medicare risk contracts, although to do so CMP care need be provided only primarily (over 50 percent of the time) by CMP providers rather than exclusively (over 90 percent) as is required for HMOs. III.B.1., IV.C.1.

complaint. a *symptom, problem,* or disease which concerns a patient. The *chief or *presenting complaint is the one which causes him to seek care and regularly the initial part of the *history.* II.A.1.

Complaints About State Program Administration (CASPA). an *Occupational Safety and Health Administration (OSHA)* program for considering complaints, which may be made by any interested party, about state-operated *occupational health* programs.

Known as *CASPA,* the program is one way OSHA provides federal backup and supervision in states in which it is not active due to having approved state plans for assuming its responsibilities under the federal law. The complaints themselves are sometimes called CASPAs. VII.B.2.d.

complement. see *bed.*

complete. whole, finished, perfectly equipped or skilled. In health care a synonym for *comprehensive,* as complete *checkup.* VII.D.2.

complete history and physical. synonym, complete *checkup.*

complexity. see *case mix.*

compliance. patient cooperation with the requirements of proper care for his self and any illness.

These requirements range from demands for cooperation in diagnostic procedures despite anxiety and pain, through taking drugs on schedule and otherwise following a *prescribed regimen,* to abandonment of social and familial obligations to the needs of the health system. Discussion by providers of problems of patient compliance always focuses on failures of compliance, for which reason it is measured and manipulated. Nations vary substantially in the degree to which compliance may be enforced by law, involuntary *commitment* being an example in the United States. V.B.

compliance officer. anyone responsible for enforcing rules; synonym, *inspector.* In occupational health, known as a *compliance safety and health officer (CSHO).

complication. 1. an uncommon part of the *natural history* or an extreme manifestation of a disease, a *side effect* of its therapy, or an *intercurrent* condition. 2. an incidental circumstance, condition, or disease occurring in the course of and modifying a primary illness or process.

The second definition is traditional but is now given to "intercurrent condition" and has given way to the first definition. II., V.B.

compound. 1. in medicine, complicated or multiple. 2. something made or composed of elements, chemicals, or parts in definite proportions; to make such a compound.

In pharmacy compounding drugs refers to preparing one or more active chemicals for human use. Compounding must preserve the active ingredients, make them palatable, assure their *bioavailability,* add no *inactive ingredients* with bad *side effects,* and so forth. III.B.3.

comprehensive. including much, having a wide scope.

One of the clichés of medicine; comprehensive care, like *continuity,* is often promised and rarely defined or delivered. Comprehensive health care seeks to provide all the health services eligible or enrolled people need. Since no health insurance program can cover, nor any individual practitioner or program provide, complete care, comprehensive care usually refers to direct provision of any reasonably broad set of services, as health maintenance organizations *basic* and *supplemental* services together, coupled with responsibility on the part of the provider for assisting people with obtaining rare services which are not directly available. The Royal Australian College of General Practitioners defines comprehensive care as meaning "the ability to make decisions about health problems in all age groups." VII.D.2.

comprehensive health planning (CHP). health *planning* which encompasses all factors and programs which impact on people's *health;* planning *health care.*

Federally assisted CHP was done on a *regional* basis by *areawide* and *state CHP agencies,* which had authority to concern themselves with *environmental* and *occupational health, health education,* and personal health behavior, as well as medical resources and services. CHP was initiated by the Comprehensive Health Planning and Public Health Services Amendments of 1966, P.L. 89-749, and replaced by the National Health Planning and Resources Development Act of 1974, P.L. 93-941. CHP also was noteworthy for the fact that the planning was guided by a council, a majority of the membership of which were health services *consumers.* VI.A.

compulsory. in health insurance, insurance which requires that *coverage* be offered or taken.

A plan may be compulsory only for an employer, as coverage must be offered to employees and a specified portion of the *premium* paid if they opt to take it, or for individuals as well. Any universal public plan of *social insurance* is necessarily compulsory in that the payment of taxes to support the plan is not optional. IV.B.

Computer-Stored Ambulatory Record (COSTAR). a medical information and communication system which includes computer-stored medical records and management information.

COSTAR was developed in the 1970s by the Massachusetts General Hospital Laboratory of Computer Services for the Harvard Community Health Plan, a large early *health maintenance organization.* The system is fully operational and, in addition to replacing the paper medical record, assists with claims, appointments, enrollment, and quality assurance. Its ability to make complete legible information readily available, acceptable to providers, at a comparative cost, and protection of *confidentiality* have proved satisfactory in use. Transferability to other locations and types of practices is now at issue. VII.D.

computer tomography, computerized tomography, computerized axial tomography (CT, CAT, EMI scanning). a method of imaging in which a computer is used to reconstruct the anatomic features registered by x-rays of plane cross sections of the body. Parallel sections, a centimeter apart, are usually recorded along several perpendicular axes, as front-to-front, side-to-side, and vertical. Multiple colors may represent different tissue densities (not the true colors of the tissue). Sometimes known as EMI scanning, after English Music Inc., an early manufacturer.

CT, introduced in the 1970s, is very powerful as a diagnostic tool, very expensive, and usually safe. As such, it has spread widely and been much used and debated.

See *nuclear magnetic resonance.* III.B.2.

concordant remedies. in homeopathy, remedies of similar action but dissimilar origin. V.

concurrent resolution on the budget. in the federal budget, a resolution passed by both houses of Congress, but not requiring the signature of the president, setting forth, reaffirming, or revising the *congressional budget* for the U.S. government for a *fiscal year*. VI.B.1.

concurrent review.   review of the medical *necessity* of *admissions,* upon or within a working day of an admission, and periodic review of services provided during the admission.

Initial review assigns an appropriate *length of stay* to the admission (using *diagnosis* specific *criteria*), and may also reassess the stay periodically. Where concurrent review is required, third party payment for unneeded days of care or services may be denied. Review is typically conducted by a physician member, or by a qualified nonphysician member, of the institution's *utilization review* committee. Concurrent review contrasts with retrospective *medical audit,* done for quality assurance purposes and unrelated to payment, and *claims review,* done after discharge. VI.D.2.

condition.   1. something that limits or modifies the existence or character of something else, as a *disease* or *deformity.* 2. the physical or mental status of the body as a whole, or of one of its parts; *fitness;* compare *severity.* 3. necessary, established, or agreed upon requisite to something else, as a condition for funding a grant.

There is no standard approach to reporting a sick person's condition, although gradations like critical, serious, fair, and good are common. Condition, a description of the present, is often confused with *prognosis.* 1. II. 2. IA.2.c.

condition.   1. to establish, by training or repeated exposure, a specific response to a particular stimulus. 2. to put into proper or desired condition, as training an athlete. 3. to set a condition, as contractually, upon awarding a grant. V.B.

conditions of participation.   the various conditions which a provider, as a *home health agency, hospital, skilled nursing facility,* or *supplier* of services, must meet to participate in the *Medicare* program.

These conditions, specified in law and *regulations,* include compliance with civil rights requirements; signing an agreement to participate acceptable to the secretary of DHHS; meeting the law's definition of the particular institution or facility, as a hospital must be a hospital within the meaning of section 1861(3) of the Social Security Act; conforming with state and local laws; and having an acceptable *utilization review* plan. Determining whether a facility meets conditions of participation is done by a state health agency, which certifies that the conditions have been met and the provider or supplier is eligible to participate. IV.C.II.

conference.   in Congress, a formal meeting of representatives of the House and Senate at which the differences between House and Senate versions of proposed legislation or *policy* are resolved.

See *consensus conference.* VIII.B.3.

confidential.   private or secret, as of information, practices, or procedures; characterized or marked by trust, intimacy, or willingness to confide.

Confidentiality, as of a *medical record,* refers to the degree and circumstances in which the record's content is private, or secret. Confidential information may include medical, financial, or other information about patients obtained in the course of medical practice, and information about the cost, quality, and nature of the practice of individual and institutional providers obtained through payment and regulatory programs. Confidentiality in reality is hard to protect. Detailed efforts to do so have already been written into health law, as section 333 of the Comprehensive Alcohol Abuse and Alcoholism Prevention, Treatment, and Rehabilitation Act of 1970, and part B of title XI of the Social Security Act. Confidentiality is difficult because it may keep secret inappropriate acts by patients or providers, but its absence may limit the freedom and confidence with which medicine is practiced, or expose people to unnecessary embarrassment.

See *Hippocrates of Cos, physician-patient privilege,* and *separation program number.* VII.D.

congenital. arising before or during birth, though not necessarily recognized at that time. Compare *familial, genetic, heredity;* contrast *acquired.*

The World Health Organization has distinguished *congenital malformations, structural deformity present at birth, and *congenital anomalies, all biochemical, functional, structural, and other disorders present at birth. Such anomalies are primarily genetic but include intrauterine infections, effects of toxins on the embryo, and results of birth trauma. I.A.1.

congregate housing. designed or devoted to housing a usually undifferentiated and unrelated group of individuals, although they may have something in common.

Boarding homes, communes, and missions are congregate housing. Sometimes applied to prisons, mental institutions, and their facilities. Congregate housing creates special public health and sanitation problems and is therefore sometimes subject to special regulation. Financial assistance for construction of congregate housing for the elderly is available from the Department of Housing and Urban Development. I.B.2.

congressional budget. in the federal budget, the budget set forth by Congress in a *concurrent resolution.* VI.B.1.

conjoint family therapy. therapy in which the whole family is the therapeutic unit for treatment, meeting as a group with the therapist in order to change family interaction.

The objective is to change family processes that contribute to disorder in family members. Conjoint therapy is increasingly replacing *collaborative, *combined, and *concurrent approaches, in which family members are seen respectively by separate therapists, in individual and group therapy simultaneously, or separately by the same therapist. V.A.

consensus conference, consensus development conference. one of a series of formal meetings sponsored by the *National Institutes of Health* at which new, or otherwise important, medical technologies are assessed for the purpose of developing and disseminating a group statement on appropriate use of the technology and other issues concerning it.

Read Mullan, Fitzhugh, and Itzhak Jacoby, "The Town Meeting of Technology: The Maturation of Consensus Conferences" (*JAMA,* 254(8): 1068–72, 8/23/85). III.B.2., VIII.D.

consensus standard. see *national consensus standard.*

consent. accept, approve, or permit implicitly or explicitly what is done or proposed by another, as agreement by a patient, or one who can legally bind him, with a proposed course of medical action.

In emergencies, consent is implied by law. Consent is valid and legal when deliberately and voluntarily given by one *competent* to do so. It thus implies free will and mental power. To submit, as to rape, is not necessarily to consent.

See *informed consent, parental consent, physician-patient privilege,* and *therapeutic privilege.* V.B., VIII.B.3.

consent form. a document, usually standardized, which a person signs to attest to his consent to something.

Use of such forms prior to surgery or other medical treatment is common and helps establish *informed consent.* However, even if specific to the procedure in question and readily understood by the person signing, they do not always establish after the fact that consent was properly obtained, nor are they legally required to do so. V.B., VIII.B.3.

conservative. of treatment by expectant observation, by preservation and restoration of injured parts, or by limited, well-established means without unnecessary or risky interference; contrast *radical.* V.B.

consultant. a physician or other *professional* asked by an *attending physician* to give counsel on a *problem;* "a physician having in-depth knowledge of a particular area of medicine who provides services related to this area on the request of another health care provider" (*NAPCRG, 1977*). III.A.1.

consultation. in health care, deliberation among physicians or other health professionals concerning the proper *management* of a *problem.* Occasionally, synonym, *encounter* or *visit.*

A consultant, often a *specialist,* reviews the history, examines the patient, and gives his written or oral opinion to the requesting practitioner. Consultation should be distinguished from *referral* since responsibility for patient care is not usually transferred to a consultant, although how care is shared is a highly variable art. V.A.

consultation and education services. *community mental health center* services consisting of consultation with, and education for, the staffs of programs in the community mental health center's community concerned with people with *mental illness,* as schools, prisons, bars, and courts.

These services are required of CMHCs by section 201, and specially subsidized by section 204 of the CMHC Act, because they are high priority *preventive care,* not usually reimbursed by the recipient institutions, and not covered under health insurance (which rarely covers services not directly delivered to insured individuals). III.B.1.

consumer. one who may receive or is receiving health *services.*

While anyone may use health services, "consumer" as used in health legislation and programs is usually someone who is never a *provider,* and is not associated in any direct or indirect way with the provision of health services. The distinction has become important in programs in which a consumer majority on a governing or advisory body is required, as is the case with federally assisted *community health centers* and *health systems agencies.*

See *food chain* and *patient.* VII.A.1.

consumer good. see *good.*

consumer participation. involvement of users of a program's services in its policy making or management in either an advisory or controlling capacity.

Many efforts, as *comprehensive health planning* and *community health centers,* were made in the late 1960s and early 1970s to require and give *operational definition* to consumer participation, principally in hopes of assuring program responsiveness to people's needs. VI.

Consumer Price Index (CPI). an economic *index* prepared by the Bureau of Statistics of the U.S. Department of Labor. It measures the change in average prices of the goods and services purchased by urban wage earners and clerical workers and their families.

The CPI is widely used as an indicator of changes in the cost of living, as a measure of inflation, and as a means of studying price trends. It is made up of several components which measure prices in different sectors of the economy. One of these, the medical care component, reflects trends in medical care *charges* based on specific indicators of hospital, medical, dental, and drug prices. The medical care component of the CPI often rises faster than the CPI itself, as do some other service components. However, since the CPI measures charges, which are not always closely related to *costs,* it may fail to accurately reflect changes in medical care costs.

See *indexed.* I.B.5.

contagion. the process whereby *disease* or its causative agent spreads from person to person; the organism which spreads.

Contagion causes *infection.* I.A.1.

contaminant. something that contaminates. Occasionally limited to, and frequently refers to, infectious agents or radiation, but may be chemical, noise, or other harmful agent. I.C.

contaminate. soil, stain, corrupt, or *infect* by contact or association; render unfit for use by the introduction of harmful agents.

Living organisms may be contaminated. When used of inanimate objects the meaning is often that they have become dangerous to living organisms; compare *fomite* and *pollute.* I.C.

contamination. the act or process of contaminating; the state of being contaminated.

The distinction between contamination and *pollution* is irregular: pollution often connotes a completed process of contamination. Pollution is sometimes limited to contamination caused by man; contamination usually refers to pollution which is actually dangerous to life, rather than just ugly or unnatural. I.C.

contextual family therapy. "a family treatment developed by Ivan Boszormenyi-Nagy which focuses not only on the individual's gratification of needs from others (the 'centripetal' criteria of relationships, as described in Freudian motivational theory), but also on fulfilling the partner's emotional needs (the 'centrifugal' aspect of relational reality which maintains the relationship)" (*Pinney and Slipp, 1982*). V.A.

contingency fee. a charge based or conditioned on future occurrences or conclusions, or on the results of services to be performed.

Contingency fees are used by lawyers representing patients as plaintiffs in malpractice cases, and are usually a set fraction of damages, as a third of any settlement. If no settlement is awarded, the lawyer is not paid. Such fees are said to give the lawyer incentives to try the case with full vigor, to choose only cases which are likely to succeed or will have large settlements, and to increase the settlements sought.

See *New Jersey rule.* V.D.

contingency reserve. in insurance, a reserve set aside by an insurance company for unforeseen or *unplannable* circumstances and expenses other than the normal *losses* incurred by the *risks* insured. IV.B.

continued stay review. review during a patient's hospitalization to determine the medical necessity and appropriateness of the patient's continued stay at a hospital level of care.

Such review may also include assessment of the quality of care being provided. It is occasionally applied to similar review of patients in other health facilities, see *medical review*. In the peer review organization and Medicare programs it is sometimes called *extended duration review. See *concurrent review*. VI.D.2.

continuing medical education (CME). formal education obtained by a health professional after completing his degree and full-time postgraduate training. The American Medical Association (AMA) has defined CME as "any education or training which serves to develop, maintain, or increase the knowledge, interpretive or reasoning proficiencies, applicable technical skills, professional performance standards or ability for interpersonal relationships."

For physicians, some states require CME for continued licensure, as do some specialty boards for certification, usually 50 hours a year. This has led to registration programs, see *Physician's Recognition Award, accreditation*, and a variety of categorizations and definitions of subtypes. These are as yet inconsistent; the AMA's is representative. CME is tax deductible, often subsidized by drug manufacturers, and of largely unproven efficacy. III.C.

continuing problem. "a previously assessed problem which requires ongoing care.

"It includes follow-up for a problem, or initial presentation to the provider of a problem previously assessed by another provider, and may be subdivided into old problem and follow-up for a problem" (*NAPCRG, 1977*). II.

continuing resolution. in the federal *budget,* legislation enacted by the Congress to provide *budget authority* for specific ongoing activities during a *fiscal year* in which the regular *appropriation* for such activities has not been enacted by the beginning of the fiscal year.

The continuing resolution usually specifies a maximum rate at which the administering agency may *obligate* funds, based on the rate of the prior year, the *President's budget* request, or an appropriation bill previously passed by either House of the Congress. VI.B.1.

continuous. without interruption, as in continuity of care; always available and consistent with the past.

One of medicine's clichés, continuity of care is traditionally and best achieved through a *personal physician* delivering all care, but also through good medical records, and effective team practice. *Consultation*, a controlled discontinuity, may correct continuous error while making continuity a possibility in the face of any one physician's limitations. VII.D.2.

contract. see *therapeutic contract*.

contraindication. 1. a reason not to do something, usually not to give a particular drug in a given situation, as many ordinarily safe drugs are contraindicated during pregnancy; antonym, *indication*. 2. the particular symptom, sign, or condition which makes a treatment inadvisable or improper. V.B.

contributory insurance. *group insurance* in which all or part of the *premium* is paid by an employee, the remainder, if any, being paid by an employer or union.

In this context, *noncontributory insurance is insurance for which the employer pays all of the premium. So-called because the *risk*, or employee, contributes to the cost of the insurance as well as the *insured*, the employer. See *enrollment period*. IV.B.

contributory negligence. *negligence* on the part of an injured party which, together with negligence on the part of another, resulted in the injury, or without which the injury would not have occurred.

The legal doctrine of contributory negligence in many circumstances, as occupational injury, provides that a negligent party cannot be sued for damages if the injured party contributed to his injury through his own negligence. VIII.B.3.

contributory tax. see *payroll tax*.

control. in *research*, a member of a *control group*; a standard for checking observations and insuring *validity*. VIII.D.

control. 1. to regulate, guide, monitor, keep constant; to have skill in the use of something; a means of control. 2. to keep the relevant conditions of an experiment constant; to cause a *variable* to change in a specified and known manner; to use a spontaneously occurring and discoverable fact as a check or standard of comparison to evaluate the results of changing a variable. 3. in biology and *demography,* to regulate the *population* of an organism by *environmental* conditions, as by disease, predators, shortage of resources, and even war and automobiles. Usage sometimes limits this meaning to active efforts to control an organism by manipulation of the environment, as by introduction of sterile insects to control an insect population. I.C.

control group. a portion of a population under study, set aside and not subjected to the *independent variable* being studied, used to compare with another portion which is subjected to the independent variable, *the experimental group.

Change in the control group allows separation of naturally occurring change from that caused by the *experiment* in the experimental group. The control group may be selected at random, see *random controlled trial*, by matching its members to those of the experimental group, see *case-controlled study*, or by finding a comparable population at another place in time or space; see *adequate and well-controlled investigations* for controls allowed by the Food and Drug Administration. VIII.D.

controllability. in the federal *budget*, the ability under existing law of the Congress or the president to control *outlays* during a given *fiscal year*.

Uncontrollable outlays cannot be increased or decreased without changes in existing substantive law. Such spending is usually the result of *entitlements,* as *Medicare* and *Medicaid,* fixed costs, and *obligations* incurred or commitments made during prior years. VI.B.1.

controlled substance. in the United States, a substance, as a drug, identified as having potential for *abuse* and subject to the special manufacturing, *prescribing,* and other controls required by the Controlled Substances Act of 1970 and administered by the *Drug Enforcement Administration.*

These controls are graded according to the drugs' varying potentials for abuse in *schedules,* with the narcotics most stringently controlled and the mild sleeping pills least so. III.B.3.

controlled substances analogue.   synonym, *designer drug.*

convalesce.   get well; recover health and strength gradually after an illness. I.A.1.

convalescent home.   synonym, *nursing home.*

convenience medicine.   the services of an *episodic care center.*

conversion privilege.   in group health insurance, the right given an insured to change his *group insurance* to some form of individual insurance, without medical examination, upon termination of the group insurance, as upon termination of employment or membership in the group.

Group insurance does not always offer a conversion privilege and, when it does, the available individual insurance is often not of a comparable scope of benefits or price, typically being more expensive. IV.A.

Cooperative Health Statistics System (CHSS).   a National Center for Health Statistics program in which federal, state, and local governments cooperate in collecting health and *vital statistics,* so that standard data are collected by the governmental level best equipped to collect and distribute it to all levels.

When in full operation CHSS will collect data in seven subject areas: health manpower, health facilities, hospital care, household interviews, ambulatory care, long-term care, and vital statistics. Legislative authority for the CHSS is found in section 306(e) of the PHS Act.

See *CHESS.* II.C.

Coordinated Transfer Application System (COTRANS).   a system begun in 1970 by the American Association of Medical Colleges in cooperation with the National Board of Medical Examiners for evaluating U.S. citizens receiving undergraduate medical education outside the United States. COTRANS determines eligibility and sponsors those it deems qualified for Part I of the *National Board Examination.*

Students who take and pass the board with this sponsorship may then apply to a U.S. medical school for completion of their training with advanced standing. Some students obtain sponsorship for the boards from an individual school without using COTRANS. III.A.1.

Coordinating Council on Medical Education (CCME).   a supervisory body, established in 1972, and replaced in 1980 by the *Council for Medical Affairs,* to coordinate *policy* matters and *accreditation* at all levels of medical education. III.A.1.

coordination of benefits (COB).   provisions and procedures used by insurers to avoid duplicate payment for *losses* insured under more than one *insurance policy.*

Some people have a *duplication of benefits,* as for medical costs arising from an automobile accident, in their automobile and health insurance policies. A coordination of benefits, or *antiduplication, clause in either policy prevents double payment by making one insurer the primary payer, and assuring that no more than 100 percent of the cost is covered. Standard rules determine which of two or more plans, each having COB provisions, pays its benefits in full and which pays a sufficiently reduced benefit to prevent the claimant from making a *profit*. IV.B.

copayment.   a *cost-sharing* requirement in a health insurance policy which provides that the insured pay a specified constant amount per unit of covered service, as $2 per visit or $10 per inpatient hospital day, the insurer then paying the rest.

The copayment is incurred at the time the service is used. Unlike *coinsurance*, the amount paid does not vary with the cost of the service. IV.B.

Core Content Review of Family Medicine.   a self-testing *continuing medical education* program for family physicians.

Endorsed by the American Academy of Family Physicians and prepared by the Connecticut and Ohio Academies of Family Physicians, the Review provides 32 hours of Category 1 credit toward the American Medical Association *Physician's Recognition Award* or American Board of Family Practice recertification. It consists of eight sets of 75 questions with educational answers and references each year. III.C.

Cornell Medical Index (CMI).   a medical history form that can be self-administered by clerks or patients. II.A.1.

coroner.   a legal officer, now often but not always a physician, of a city or county whose principal duty is investigating sudden, violent, or unexplained deaths; compare *medical examiner*.

Many coroners are elected, some are political appointees. Only in large jurisdictions is it a full-time job. III.D.2., VIII.B.3.

correlation (r^2).   the extent to which two measures vary together; a measure of the strength of the relationship between two *variables*.

It is usually expressed by a coefficient, the r^2, which varies between $+1.0$, perfect agreement, and -1.0, a perfect inverse relationship. A correlation coefficient of 0.0 means a *random* or no relationship. The correlation coefficient shows the degree to which a measure of one variable can predict a measure of the other. A high correlation between two variables does not necessarily indicate a *causal* relationship between them; the correlation may follow because each of the variables is highly related to a third, yet unmeasured, factor. VIII.D.

corridor deductible.   see *deductible*.

cosmetic.   1. serving or intended to improve appearance. 2. a preparation applied to the body, especially the skin or hair, to protect, beautify, or cover blemishes.

Labeling of cosmetics is regulated by the Food and Drug Administration under the authorities of the Food, Drug, and Cosmetic Act, although somewhat less stringently than of food and drugs. III.B.

cosmetic surgery.   an *operation* done to improve appearance, except when required for the prompt repair of injury or to improve functioning of a malformed body member; compare *plastic surgery*.

The term does not apply to surgery for treatment of severe burns or repair of the face following an automobile accident, or to surgery for some therapeutic purpose which coincidentally serves a cosmetic purpose, but does include reshaping an ugly nose. Most health insurance plans do not cover cosmetic surgery. V.B.

cost.   1. outlay or expenditure made to achieve an object, as the provision of services or goods. 2. unfortunate synonym, *charge* or *price*.

Many different costs are recognized, see *actual* and *allowable, direct* and *indirect, fixed* and *variable, general and administrative, internal* and *external, marginal* and *opportunity,* and *private* and *social cost.* Charges may or may not be the same as, or based on, costs (one man's charge is another's cost). Hospitals, for example, often *cross-subsidize by charging more for a given service than it actually costs in order to recoup losses from providing other services whose costs exceed feasible or collectible charges. Despite their name, cost control programs often seek to control increases in charges rather than in real costs. IV.C.1., VII.D.1., VIII.B.1.

cost allocation.   the distribution of *overhead* costs among *revenue*-producing cost centers. VI.C.1.

cost apportionment.   the distribution of costs associated with a revenue-producing cost center among the payers of the revenue. VI.C.1.

cost-based reimbursement.   synonym, *cost-related reimbursement.*

cost benefit.   the ratio of costs of an activity to its benefits, whether known or projected.

Cost-benefit analysis helps determine the relative merits of alternative proposed actions by identifying all potential *social, external,* and other costs and benefits associated with each and assigning monetary values to them. This allows development of comparable cost-benefit ratios. *Cost-effectiveness analysis limits itself to consideration of known *direct* costs and effects, usually with established *prices* or otherwise known values, in comparing alternatives. Cost-benefit and cost-effectiveness analyses are powerful tools, limited by the difficulty of forecasting and valuing all possible costs and benefits.

See *life cost.* VI.D., VIII.B.1.

cost center.   in responsibility accounting, an activity, product, or service within a program to which costs of whatever type are attributed as having been incurred by that center or function.

Contrasts with segregating costs of different types, as nursing, drugs, or laundry costs, regardless of why they were incurred or who pays them. Cost centers are usually revenue producing. Such accounting is used in developing charges for the various centers' services. VI.C.1.

cost-effectiveness.   see *cost benefit.*

cost of insurance.   the amount a policyholder pays an *insurer* minus what he gets back from it, usually in the aggregate or on the average; distinguish *expenses,* and the *rate* for a given unit of insurance.

Such costs, difficult to obtain and rarely compared, are approximated by the *loading,* or the ratio of amounts paid in benefits to income produced from premiums. IV.B.

cost-push inflation.   see *inflation.*

cost-related reimbursement.   payment of medical care programs by *third parties,* typically *Blue Cross* plans or government agencies, in which the amount of payment is based on the *cost* to the provider of delivering the service.

The actual payment may be based on any of several different formulas, as full cost, a percentage of full cost, or *allowable costs.* Other reimbursement methods use *charges* for the services delivered, or budgeted or anticipated cost for a future time period, see *prospective reimbursement.* Historically, *Medicare, Medicaid,* and some Blue Cross plans reimbursed hospitals on the basis of cost; most private insurance plans pay charges. IV.

cost sharing. a provision of a health insurance policy which requires the insured, or otherwise covered individual, to pay some portion of covered expenses or services. Several forms of cost sharing are used, particularly *deductibles, coinsurance,* and *copayments.*

Cost sharing does not refer to or include the amounts paid in premiums for the coverage. The premium amount relates to both the benefits provided and the cost sharing required. For a given set of benefits, premiums increase as cost-sharing requirements decrease. In addition to being used to reduce premiums, cost sharing is used to control *utilization* of covered services, as by requiring a large copayment for a service which is likely to be overused. IV.B.

Council for Medical Affairs (CFMA). an organization founded in 1980 by five member organizations to provide a forum for the members to consider issues related to medical education and other matters of mutual concern.

The CFMA replaced the Coordinating Council on Medical Education in its eighth year of existence, without in the process continuing the CCME supervisory role over the accrediting bodies for medical education. The member organizations include the American Association of Medical Colleges, American Board of Medical Specialties, American Hospital Association, American Medical Association, and Council of Medical Specialty Societies (the interlocking directorate of U.S. medicine). III.A.1.

Council of Medical Specialty Societies (CMSS). the national organization of *trade associations* representing the medical specialties, one of the parent organizations of the *Accreditation Councils for Continuing and Graduate Medical Education;* compare *American Board of Medical Specialties.* III.C.

Council on Environmental Quality (CEQ). a three-member national advisory council required by the *National Environmental Policy Act.*

It is appointed by and advises the president on the quality of the U.S. *environment,* is responsible for *rules* on *environmental impact statements,* and writes an annual public report on the environment. III.D.1.

counsel. advice or instruction, sometimes mutual; especially that given as the result of *consultation.* *counsellor. one who gives counsel.

Giving counsel is a skill which many practice, some with special training, some for a fee, and some with some success. V.B.

cover. insure, afford protection or security. IV.B.

coverage. the guarantee against specific *losses* provided under the terms of an insurance policy; the extent of insurance afforded by a policy; synonyms, *benefits, insurance,* and *insurance contract.*

A covered benefit, individual, or risk is one for which a policy provides insurance.

See *first-* and *last-dollar coverage.* IV.B.

creaming. see *skimming.*

credential. something which recognizes or attests to *professional* or technical competence, as a *registration, certificate, license,* professional association membership, or educational degree.

Credentials affect the supply of health manpower by controlling entrance into practice, influence the geographic distribution, mobility, and retention of workers, and help determine quality by providing *standards* for evaluating people's competence and defining the scope of their functions. III.A.

crick. a sick *crock*.

criminal abortion. see *abortion*.

criminally insane. an individual with mental illness who has committed a crime and been committed to a mental hospital for treatment of his insanity, whether not competent to stand trial or not guilty because of the insanity.

   In some jurisdictions, the criminally insane are hospitalized separately from others with mental disorders, whether the others have been committed or admitted voluntarily. They may also be subject to separate, sometimes vague, rules for release. II.B.2.

Crippled Children's Services (CCS). a state-operated, *formula grant* program of medical and *habilitative* services for children with *congenital* or other permanent *handicaps*. Federal funding is provided by the maternal and child health block grant program authorized in 1981.

   See *maternal and child health*. III.D.1.

criteria document. a report of research on a *safety* or *health hazard* by the *National Institute of Occupational Safety and Health*, in which it recommends to the OSHA criteria for standards intended to protect workers from the hazard.

   Most documents have dealt with health hazards, including *asbestos*, *carcinogens*, and vinyl chloride. VII.B.2.d.

criteria pollutant. one of the five *pollutants*, among the hundreds that may *contaminate* the air, which are monitored and controlled by air pollution control programs.

   They are measurable, common, and either have significant health effects or represent and correlate with important groups of pollutants. They include carbon monoxide, sulfur dioxide, total suspended particulates, ozone or other chemical oxidants, and nitrogen dioxide.

   See *air quality standard* and *pollutant standards index*. I.C.1.

criterion. a quantity or quality of something, as of an environment, workplace, or health care; particularly one used as a reference for testing *necessity*, *appropriateness*, or *quality*, suitability to a certain purpose, or conformity to a *standard*. Typically plural, *criteria. Synonym, *guideline*.

   In the *peer review organization* program, criteria thus are elements of care which, with *norms*, may be the basis for standards. Criteria for appropriate diagnosis of a urinary tract infection may be a urinalysis and urine culture. VI.D., VII.D.2.

critical. see *condition*.

critical care. synonym, *intensive* or *special care*.

   This is becoming the preferred generic term; *certification* is now available for nurses in critical care nursing, and the NIH has had a consensus conference on "Critical Care Medicine" (*JAMA,* 250: 798–804, 1983). VII.C.5.a.

critical incident. an event, as a crisis, illness, or sudden growth spurt, which permits, catalyzes, or causes change in stable individual and family illnesses and patterns.

A family physician may use such incidents to free and improve family structures and function. Without such support, these events may stress coping skills, thus receiving an inadequate response and producing symptoms in family members. I.B.1.

crock. deprecating *house staff* slang, a patient whose illness the house staff (but not the patient) feels is unreal, nonphysical, or insignificant. Use of the term should be discouraged since it often blinds the user to real patient needs, whether or not correctly perceived by the patient. VIII.B.2.a.

crossover experiment. a study in which subjects are divided, usually randomly, into as many groups as there are treatments to be tried, and the groups then interchanged until each subject has received each treatment.

This allows each subject to serve as his own *control* and compensates for spontaneous time trends. VIII.D.

cross-subsidize. see *cost.*

crude birthrate. see *birthrate.*

crude death rate. see *mortality rate.*

culture. in anthropology, the whole learned way of life of a *society.* I.B.1.

culture. to grow or cultivate, as microorganisms or cells, ordinarily in artificial medium; a group of such microorganisms or cells. V.A.

curandero. Spanish, *shaman* or *healer.*

cure. 1. recovery from an illness, or correction of a defect, as a result of treatment. 2. a course or program of related therapeutic measures. 3. a remedy. 4. to restore to health, bring about recovery or correct a defect.

People may recover without cure, although they may need *care* to do so. Cure is more technological, predominantly a physician's responsibility. V.

current. in accounting and economics, assets, liabilities, and other things available or occurring within the present accounting or fiscal year; contrast *long-term debt.* VI.C.1.

current liabilities (CL). see *liability.*

Current Medical Information and Terminology (CMIT). a system for naming, identifying, and describing disease.

CMIT is published by the American Medical Association. The fifth edition, January 1981, provides quick reference to the preferred names, causes, characteristics, course, and pathologic findings of diseases with codes for each. II.B.2.

Current Procedural Terminology (CPT). a systematic listing and coding of *procedures* and *services* performed by physicians.

Services are each identified by five digit codes which are used in reporting them for insurance, epidemiologic, and other purposes. *CPT-4, as the fourth edition is known, is authored and annually updated by the American Medical Association. The annual updates are known by year, as CPT-1987.

Read Fanta, Charlotte M. et al., eds., *Physicians' Current Procedural Terminology* (4th ed. Chicago: American Medical Association, 1987). VII.

current services budget. in the federal *budget,* a budget that estimates *budget authority* and *outlays* for the upcoming *fiscal year,* assuming continuation at the same levels of service as in the fiscal year in progress.

The Congressional Budget and Impoundment Control Act of 1974 requires that the president submit a current services budget to the Congress by November 10 of each year. The budget estimates take into account anticipated changes in economic conditions, as unemployment and inflation, and legally mandated changes in such things as eligibility and benefits. VI.B.1.

custodial care.   *care,* other than medical care, which assists people in the *activities of daily living.*

Custodial care may include room, board, and personal care, as assistance with walking, preparing food, and using the bathroom. It is usually provided on a long-term basis in informal settings, as *boarding homes.* Because it does not require trained medical personnel, custodial care is not usually covered by health insurance or Medicaid, except when given in conjunction with medical care in a hospital or nursing home. Consequently, whether a person's care, including his room and board, is covered by health insurance depends on whether it includes medical care, rather than on *competence,* diagnosis, or rehabilitation potential. VII.C.5.b.

customary charge.   the amount which a physician or other professional or program normally or usually *charges* the majority of patients for a given service or procedure. In *Medicare,* the median charge used by a particular physician for a specified service during the calendar year preceding the fiscal year in which a *claim* is processsed.

There is therefore an average delay of a year and a half in recognizing any increase in *actual charges.* Customary, actual, and *prevailing charges* are all used by Medicare in determining *reasonable charges.* VII.D.1.

cytology.   the part of biology dealing with cells.

*Cytologic services involve study by pathologists and trained cytologists or cytology technicians of cells gathered by *Pap smears,* needle aspiration, washing the bronchi at bronchoscopy, or other methods, sometimes after subsequent cell culture. Changes in the cells may be diagnostic of various diseases, particularly cancers and genetic defects. III.C.

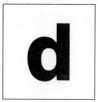

damage. in law, *loss,* injury, or deterioration of one person, his property, or his reputation caused by *negligence,* design, or accident on the part of another person. *Damages are the estimated, demanded, or otherwise established reparation in money for the damage sustained; the compensation imposed by law for a tort. VIII.B.3.

Darling case. the principal precedent for a health facility's, particularly a hospital's, responsibility for the care of patients admitted to it, and for *medical staff accountability* to the hospital for the care provided by staff members.
Read *Darling v. Charleston Community Memorial Hospital* (33 Ill. 2d. 326, 211 N.E.2d 253 (1965), *cert. denied,* 383 U.S. 946(1966)). III.B.1., VIII.B.3.

data. plural of datum.

data set. a standard group of uniformly defined and classified facts that describe an element, episode, or aspect of health care, whether a hospital *admission,* see *discharge abstract,* ambulatory *encounter,* or *physician* or *hospital.* Data sets are used for evaluation and research. VIII.D.

datum. something given, either by experience or assumption, for a purpose; a fact or principle presented for inference or argument. Usually plural, *data, a set of similar such facts; the subject of *statistics.* VIII.D.

day. a day (and/or night, since the daily count is often taken at midnight) spent by a patient in a health facility or program. Usually refers to inpatients, but may speak of people using day care programs.
Various types of days are counted as measures of institutional use, see *administrative day, bed days,* and *patient days.* III.B.1., VII.C.5.

day care. a program of personal care for *dependent* people, whether children, elderly, or mentally incompetent; compare *custodial care, nursery,* and *partial hospitalization.*

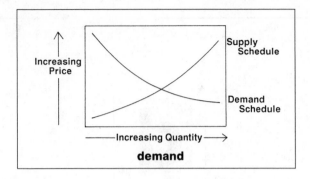

↑
Increasing
Price

Supply
Schedule

Demand
Schedule

──── Increasing Quantity ──→
demand

Day care frees the dependent's *caretaker*. It does not ordinarily provide medical care, education, or other services. I.B.2.

day hospital.   a facility, usually part of a hospital, for day hospitalization, see *partial hospitalization*.

day surgery.   see *ambulatory surgery* and *surgicenter*.

Deadhead Medico (DH Medico).   a service that furnishes medical advice by radio to ships at sea.
    Since 1921, officers of the U.S. Public Health Service have received and answered requests for advice through Coast Guard, Navy, and commercial radio stations. The service is free, a "deadhead" being railroad slang for a free rider, and now international in scope.
    See *Medical Signal Code* and *ship's medicine chest*. III.B.2.

deaf.   unable to hear normally, because of a defect or disease of the ear, brain, or connecting nerves.
    Hearing is measured by the abilities to hear sound and to distinguish speech. For purposes of granting disability, the Social Security Administration, DHHS, requires that the *impairment,* after maximum correction by hearing aid, be worse for air conduction than an average hearing threshold of 90 *decibels* in the better ear (determined as an average of the threshold hearing levels at 500, 1000, and 2000 hertz), or produce speech discrimination scores less than 40 percent in the better ear. II.B.2.

death.   the ceasing of all vital functions beyond possibility of recovery; the last of life's tasks; the act, process, or fact of dying; compare *mortality*.
    A simple thing whose actual occurrence medicine has made difficult to define. *The Uniform Determination of Death Act, adopted in some form in all states, provides that, "an individual who has sustained either (1) irreversible cessation of circulatory and respiratory function or (2) irreversible cessation of all function of the entire brain, including the brain stem, is dead. A determination of death must be made in accordance with accepted medical standards." The first proviso is the traditional common law definition of death, the second, *brain death, allows removal of surviving organs from the dead and ending support of other bodily functions. *Time of death is either the time some authorized government official puts on the forms or a misnomer, since death is not momentary but occurs during a

period of time during which irreversible loss of the functional organization regarded as life occurs.

See *eternal care, euthanasia, hospice,* and *quality of life.* I.A.1.

death benefit. a *benefit* payable or contingent upon someone's death; synonym, survivor benefit.

The beneficiary, a survivor, is not the *risk.* V.

death rate. see *mortality rate.*

debt. something owed, a *liability.*

Many specific debts are important in health care; a hospital may have both a *debt service* and *bad debts* for which to account.

See *amortization, balloon payment, capital, current,* and *long-term.* VI.C.1.

debt service. the payment of matured interest on and principal of debts; the amount needed, supplied, or accrued for meeting such payments during any given accounting period; a budget or operating statement heading for such items.

See *amortization* and *capital.* III.B.1., VI.C.1.

decay. decline in health or vigor; waste away, rot; decrease gradually in some respect, as number, size, or power.

Decay may (tooth decay in children) or may not (aging) be *disease,* depending on its rate, necessity, and *naturalness.*

See *radioactive half-life.* I.A.1.

deceased. the future tense of diseased. VIII.B.2.b.

decibel (dB, DB). one-tenth of a bel, the unit of measurement of the relative loudness or power of *sounds;* expressed as 20 times the common logarithm of the ratio of the sound measured to a reference sound.

A decibel is approximately the smallest degree of difference in loudness detectable by the human ear, which normally can distinguish sounds ranging from 1 dB (barely audible) to 130 dB (jets taking off). I.C.2.

deductible. the amount of *loss* or expense that must be incurred by an insured, or otherwise covered individual, before an insurer will assume any liability for all or part of the remaining cost of covered benefits, a form of *cost sharing.*

Deductibles may be either fixed dollar amounts or the value of specified services, as two days of hospital care or one physician visit. Deductibles are usually tied to some reference period over which they must be incurred, as $100 per calendar year, *benefit period,* or *spell of illness.* They may be either *static deductibles, which are fixed dollar amounts, or *dynamic deductibles, which are adjusted from time to time to reflect increasing medical prices. In a *sliding scale deductible the deductible would increase as income increases. *Corridor deductibles lie between two amounts, as covering the first $1000 in expenses and resuming coverage at a *catastrophic* level like $5000. IV.B.

deem. determine, as by law.

Deeming is more common; the process, or result, of deciding, as for determining Medicaid eligibility, what *income* and *resources* are available to an applicant. *Deeming of income rules exist for social security, disability, and welfare programs, ordinarily at least deeming one spouse's income as available to pay for another's care and that a parent's is available to a minor child. IV.C.2.

defect.   a deficiency, fault, or flaw in structure or function, ordinarily of such severity that appearance or performance is compromised; compare *disability, handicap,* and *impairment.* I.A.1., II.

defensive medicine.   medical *practice* induced by the threat of liability for bad results, rather than patients' needs, and intended to prevent *malpractice* suits by patients and provide adequate legal defense in the event of such suits.

A majority of physicians say they practice defensive medicine, producing unknown increases in the cost of care and the incidence of *iatrogenic* illness. V.D.

deferral of budget authority.   in the federal *budget,* any action or inaction of the executive branch which temporarily withholds, delays, or effectively precludes *obligation* or *outlay* of *budget authority;* compare *rescission.*

The Congressional Budget and Impoundment Control Act of 1974 requires the president to report each proposed deferral to the Congress. Deferrals may not extend beyond the end of a *fiscal year* and may be overturned by the passage of an *impoundment* resolution by either House of Congress. VI.B.1.

deficiency disease.   a disease, or pathologic state with characteristic clinical signs, due to an insufficient intake of energy or essential *nutrients.*

When of dietary cause, rather than such causes as malabsorption and *parasites,* deficiency disease can be prevented or cured by bringing the intake up to an adequate level or otherwise changing the *diet.* I.A.2.a, II.B.1.a.

deformity.   1. the state of being misshapen. 2. marked deviation from the normal size or shape of the body or of a part; disfigurement; *malformation.*

Deformity may or may not be a *disability* or *handicap.* II.

deinstitutionalization.   change in the locus of mental health care, particularly for schizophrenics and the mentally retarded, from traditional, residential settings to community-based services; ugly occasional synonym, *transinstitutionalization.

Spurred by development of effective antipsychotic drugs and the rising costs of institutional care, deinstitutionalization has often amounted to little more than transferring state mental hospital patients to *intermediate care facilities, boarding homes,* or *halfway houses* or making them *homeless.*

Read Gudeman, Jon E., and Miles F. Shore, "Beyond Deinstitutionalization: A New Class of Facilities for the Mentally Retarded" (*N Engl J Med,* 311(13): 832–6, 9/27/84). See *asylum* and *outpatient commitment.* III.C.

Delaney amendment, clause.   (James Delaney, U.S. Congressman) a provision of section 409(c)(3) of the Federal Food, Drug, and Cosmetic Act added by Rep. Delaney which deems any *food additive* unsafe "if it is found to induce cancer when ingested by man or animal..."

The amendment has the effect of making the addition of any *carcinogen* to food illegal. It also forbids giving carcinogens to animals if they are dangerous to the animals or if detectable residues remain in human food prepared from them. The amendment has become increasingly important as tests for carcinogenicity, like the *Ames test,* have improved, methods of detecting residues have become sensitive to the molecular level, and food additives have become more common. I.A.2.a.

delegation. in the Professional Standards Review Organization (PSRO) program, the formal process by which a PSRO, after an assessment of the willingness and capability of a hospital or other health program to effectively perform PSRO review functions, assigned the performance of some, *partial delegation, or all, *full delegation, review functions to the program.

Delegation is done by a written memorandum of understanding signed by both the PSRO and the program. The PSRO monitors the program's performance of the delegated functions without itself conducting them and retains responsibility for the effectiveness of reviews. VI.D.2.

demand. in economics, the quantity of *goods* or *services* sought at varying *prices,* given constant *income* and other factors.

Demand must be distinguished from *use* (the amount of services actually used), and *need* (for various reasons services are often sought which either the *consumer* or *provider* feel are unneeded). Demand is not always translated into use, particularly when queues develop. Either demand or *supply* may be shown as a schedule or graph. Their schedules together specify price and quantity sold in a *competitive* market and the effect that shifting either will have on the price and quantity sold, assuming other market factors are constant. VIII.B.1.

demand characteristic. in research, a cue that communicates the purpose of an experiment and the nature of the behavior expected of the subject; compare *Hawthorne effect* and *placebo.*

Demand characteristics may be derived from the manner in which the subject is solicited and treated, scuttlebutt about the experiment, the instructions, or the experimental procedure itself. Subjects may confirm the investigator's hypothesis in an effort to behave appropriately, rather than responding directly to the *independent variables* under investigation. By extension, in nonexperimental settings, the tendency of individuals to do what is implicitly expected of them, a tendency that may play a major role in the outcome of treatment. VIII.D.

demand-pull inflation. see *inflation.*

dementia. global *impairment* of thinking that usually is gradually progressive and that interferes with normal social and occupational activities.

*Primary dementia is an unexplained process with early onset compared to the different signs of *advanced age.* *Alzheimer's disease, as it is known (A. Alzheimer, German physician and neuropathologist, 1864–1915), is characterized by preserved alertness and unclouded consciousness with gradual global deterioration of memory, judgment, and intellectual performance. *Secondary dementias are those known to be caused by some other process.

Read the Council on Scientific Affairs, "Dementia" (*JAMA,* 256(16): 2234–8, 10/24/86). II., II.B.2.

demographic data. information about a population.

Basic demographic data include unique identification for each individual, date of birth, residence, sex, race and ethnic information, marriage and family information, and occupational and social information. II.C.

demography. the science and study of *populations,* especially the statistical study of human populations with reference to their *control,* density, distribution, growth, and *vital statistics.* II.C.

denominator problem. the trouble knowing who is in the denominator of many *incidence, prevalence,* and other *rates* or ratios, as when the number of people in the denominator is unknown or the denominator is defined differently in different countries. VIII.C.

dental assistant. an individual who assists a *dentist* at the *chairside* in a dental operatory, and may perform reception and clerical functions, dental radiography, and selected *dental laboratory* work.

Most dentists train and employ dental assistants who are neither *certified* nor *registered* as members of an official organization. Dental assistants who have completed *accredited* educational programs are eligible for national certification examinations conducted by the Dental Assisting National Board, Inc. III.A.3.

dental health. complete normality and functional efficiency of the teeth and supporting structures, the surrounding parts of the oral cavity, and the various structures related to chewing and the maxillofacial complex; mouth *health.* I.A.1.

dental health services. all services designed or intended to promote, maintain, or restore dental health, including educational, preventive, and therapeutic services. VII.

dental hygienist. a specially trained and licensed individual who works under the supervision of a dentist in providing dental health services: performing complete oral prophylaxis, applying medication, performing dental radiography, and providing dental education services both for *chairside* patients and in community health projects.

Dental hygiene programs are either 2- or 4-year programs at the college level. III.A.3.

dental laboratory. an organization where *dental technicians* make complete and partial dentures, *orthodontic* appliances, bridgework, crowns, and other dental restorations and appliances, as *prescribed* by dentists. A *commercial dental laboratory is independent of and separate from the dentist's office. III.B.1.

dental laboratory technician. synonym, *dental technician.*

dental public health. the *specialty* of *dentistry* concerned with dental health in the community, and the prevention and control of dental disease. III.C.

dental technician. an individual who makes complete and partial dentures, *orthodontic* appliances, bridgework, crowns, and other dental restorations and appliances, as prescribed by dentists.

Most dental technicians work in commercial *dental laboratories.* However, increasing numbers are employed by dentists, and by government and private programs. Traditionally, dental technicians have been trained on the job, but the predominant method of training is now formal programs offered by 2-year postsecondary educational institutions. Upon completion of an aggregate of 5 years of dental technology training and experience, technicians are eligible to apply for examination and *certification* by the National Board for Certification in Dental Laboratory Technology.

See *dental hygienist* and *denturist.* III.A.3.

dentist. a *professional* person qualified by education and authorized by law, usually by having obtained a *license,* to *practice* dentistry.

There are eight dental *specialties,* including *dental public health, endodontics,* oral and maxillofacial surgery, oral pathology, *orthodontics, pe-*

dodontics, periodontics, and *prosthodontics.* A Doctor of Dental Surgery (DDS), or one of the corresponding doctorates, requires 4 years of postcollege education in an accredited school of dentistry. III.A.3.

dentistry. the promotion, maintenance, and restoration of individual *dental health,* and treatment of diseases of the teeth and mouth. V.

denture mill. a dental practice specializing in low price, high volume, often rapid production of dentures.

These might provide one day service, motel room included.

See *Medicaid mill.* V., VIII.B.2.a.

denturist. a *dental technician* who provides dentures or other dental appliances for patients without benefit of a dentist's professional services or *prescription.*

Denturists are rarely found in the United States, and their practice is illegal in all states but Oregon. Independent practice of dental technology is known as *denturism. III.A.3.

department. a *functional* or *administrative* division or *service* of a health program or other agency.

A department within a hospital or medical school is typically headed by a chairman or director, has its own *budget,* and admits it own patients, but is not a separate legal entity. They are frequently organized by medical specialty, as a surgery department. There is no standard departmental organization for health programs. III.B.1.

Department of Health and Human Service (DHHS, HHS, H₂S). the cabinet agency of the U.S. government which administers most federal health programs.

Originally created as the *Federal Security Administration (FSA), it was known for many years as the *Department of Health, Education, and Welfare (DHEW, HEW) before acquiring its current name and responsibilities in 1980. III.D.2.

Department of Health, Education, and Welfare (DHEW, HEW). see *Department of Health and Human Service.*

dependence. see *drug dependence.*

dependent. 1. one who relies on another for significant or essential support. 2. determined or controlled by something else, thus one studies the effects of *independent variables* on dependent ones.

In addition to a requirement for financial support, legal definitions may require a blood relationship. The Internal Revenue Code defines dependents confusingly as:

> any of the following over half of whose support for the calendar year was received from the taxpayer: children (biologic or adopted), grandchildren, etc.; stepchildren; brothers and sisters; stepbrothers and stepsisters; half brothers and half sisters; parents, grandparents, etc.; stepparents; nephews and nieces; uncles and aunts; in-laws (father, mother, son, daughter, brother, or sister); non-relatives living as members of the taxpayer's household; and a descendent of a brother or sister of the father or mother of the taxpayer who is receiving institutional care and who, before receiving such care, was a member of the taxpayer's household.

In insurance and other programs such specific definitions are quite variable, often being limited to the individual's spouse and children. Other dependents of the kinds recognized by the IRS are sometimes known as *sponsored dependents. 1. VIII.B.3. 2. VIII.D.

dependent variable. see *variable*.

depreciation. the decline in value of *capital* goods over time with use, decay, increasing obsolescence, or the effects of the elements.

The rate and amount of depreciation is calculated by a variety of different methods, as straight line, sum of the digits, and declining balance, often with quite different results. Reimbursement of health services usually includes an amount intended to be equivalent to the capital depreciation experienced by the provider of the services in conjunction with their provision.

See *amortization, debt, funded,* and *section 1122*. III.B.1., VI.A., VIII.B.1.

dermatologist. a physician specializing by practice or education in dermatology. III.A.1.

dermatology. the science and specialty devoted to the study and care of the skin. III.C.

dermatopathologist. a physician specializing by practice or education in dermatopathology. IV.A.1.

dermatopathology. the science and subspecialty of *pathology* devoted to the study of skin structure and abnormalities produced by diseases of the skin. III.C.

designer drug. a synthetic chemical, usually designed in a makeshift laboratory, to elicit specific psychic responses and then sold on the street to drug abusers, as a chemical cousin of the amphetamines with the same effects but chemically different enough that it is not a *controlled substance;* synonym, *controlled substance analogue*. Originally and more generally, any synthetic chemical designed to meet particular consumer specifications.

The demand for these drugs is a disease of society. They are potent (3-methyl fentanyl, a narcotic, is 2000 times as potent as morphine), cheap, and easy to make, often contaminated or inaccurately dosed, and legally probably uncontrollable.

Read Ziporyn, Terra, "A Growing Industry and Menace: Makeshift Laboratory's Designer Drugs" (*JAMA*, 256(22): 3061–3, 12/12/86). III.B.3.

detail person. a sales representative of a manufacturer of drugs, devices, or medical supplies.

Detail people call on physicians, dentists, pharmacists, and others with personal presentations, advertising, and drug samples and educational materials. Many are now pharmacists. III.B.3.

detection bias. see *bias*.

deterrent fee. British synonym, *copayment*. IV.B.

detoxification. treatment to restore physiologic functioning after it has been disturbed by an overdose or habitual use of alcohol, benzodiazepines, or other addictive drugs; treatment of poisoning. IV.B.

developmental disability (DD). a *disability* which originates before age 18; can be expected to continue indefinitely; constitutes a substantial *handicap* to the disabled's ability to function normally in society; and is attributable to *mental retardation,* cerebral palsy, epilepsy, autism, or another condition closely related to mental retardation because it results in similar *impairment* of general intellectual functioning or adaptive behavior or requires similar treatment and services, or dyslexia resulting from one of the conditions listed.

The term was thus badly defined in 1977 in section 102(7) of the Developmental Services and Facilities Construction Act, which authorizes federal assistance for services and facilities for the developmentally disabled. II.

developmental task. a task, conflict, or problem to be mastered at one of the various stages of the *life cycle* of an individual or family, as weaning or leaving the family.

The distinction between individual and family tasks is elusive and their number and nature are still incompletely and variably described. A family's task is quite different from the tasks for the various individual members. I.A.2., I.B.1.

device. an item or piece of equipment used in the healing arts that is not a *drug*.

As defined in the Federal Food, Drug, and Cosmetic Act, devices include instruments, apparatus, and contrivances, including their components, parts, and accessories, intended for use in the diagnosis, cure, mitigation, treatment, or prevention of disease in man or other animals or to affect the structure or any function of the body of man or other animals. Devices are crutches, bandages, wheelchairs, artificial heart valves, cardiac pacemakers, intrauterine devices, eye glasses, hearing aids, and other *orthoses* and *prostheses*. A device is distinguished from a drug by not achieving any of its principal intended purposes through chemical action within or on the body. Devices are regulated by the Food and Drug Administration using *standards* and *premarket approval* to assure that they are *safe* and *effective*. III.B.2.

diagnosis. the art or act of determining the nature and *cause* of a problem or differentiating among diseases; a conclusion or label respecting the nature or cause of a problem; "a formal statement of the provider's understanding of the patient's problem" (*NAPCRG, 1978*).

Diagnosis, one of the basic clinical skills, is accomplished by *history, physical examination*, laboratory study, and thinking, and is a necessary condition of effective treatment.

See *clinicopathological conference, differential diagnosis*, and *parsimony of diagnosis*. V.A.

diagnosis related group (DRG). a set of *cases* with a common primary diagnosis, each of which can be expected to require similar *services*.

The groups are defined by using cases with common characteristics, as diagnosis, age, and treatment. The services a DRG receives may be measured approximately by *length of stay*, cost of treatment, or nursing requirements. Comparing services which different hospitals provide the same DRG controls for differences in *case mix*.

See *outlier* and *Patient Management Categories*. II.B.1., IV.C.1.

diagnosis related group creep (DRG creep). fudging the diagnosis for an admission or case so it is assigned to a diagnosis related group with greater reimbursement or longer length of stay than is actually appropriate.

DRG creep in the aggregate is the part of increases in the *Medicare Case Mix Index* attributable to change in documentation and coding practice, after controlling for changes in the Medicare inpatient population and in medical practice. II.B.1., IV.C.1.

diagnosis related group rate (DRG rate). the basic amount paid a hospital for an admission by the Medicare *prospective payment system.*
DRG rates vary by region of the country and location, urban or rural. The actual payment for an episode of care is the DRG rate times the DRG weight for the DRG that includes the *principal diagnosis.* IV.C.1.

diagnosis related group weight (DRG weight). the multiplier assigned to a particular DRG which reflects its relative cost and *complexity.* IV.C.1.

***Diagnostic and Statistical Manual of Mental Disorders* (DSM).** the American Psychiatric Association's official classification of *mental disorders;* usually known as *DSM-III after the third edition, published in 1980.
DSM-III is compatible with and nearly identical to the *International Classification of Diseases* but goes far beyond it and most *nosologies* in specifying criteria for making diagnoses. II.B.1.

diagnostic criteria. "those facts and observations that lead to a diagnosis" *(NAPCRG, 1978).* V.A.

diagnostic index. synonym, *problem index (NAPCRG, 1978).*

diagnostic profile. see *profile.*

dialysis. separation of substances in solution by using their differing diffusibility through porous membranes; often short for hemodialysis.
*Hemodialysis, in which one of the solutions is blood, is the principal way human and artificial kidneys remove wastes from the body. Hemodialysis is paid for by special provisions of the Medicare program through the *End Stage Renal Disease Program.* V.B.

dichloro-diphenyl-trichloro-ethane (DDT). the first *chlorinated hydrocarbon* insecticide; synonyms, chlorophenothane and dicophane.
Registration and sale of DDT have been banned since 1972 because of its 15-year *half-life* and its accumulation and concentration through the *food chain* in fatty tissues of such organisms as fish. I.C.

dictionary. "a malevolent literary device for cramping the growth of a language and making it hard and inelastic. This dictionary, however, is a most useful work" (Bierce, Ambrose, *The Devil's Dictionary.* New York: Neale Publishing Company, 1911). VIII.B.2.b.

diener. a laboratory worker, especially one who assists a *pathologist* at *autopsy.*
Dieners are trained on the job and suffer no educational requirements, although some are former medical corpsmen. They often acquire remarkable proficiency in human anatomy and its dissection. III.A.4.

diet. 1. nutrition, food and drink, ordinarily or actually consumed; eating *habit.*
2. food prescribed in kind or amount for therapeutic, religious, or other purposes, see *macrobiotics* and *vegetarian.* 3. to follow such a prescription, commonly a caloric restriction for purposes of weight loss, see *Weight Watchers.*
Diet is an important source of *exposure* to *contagion* and *carcinogens.* Excesses and deficiencies both produce disease, the latter being *deficiency diseases.* Major therapeutic diets include the salt restricted, diabetic, soft for the toothless, liquid for sick or weak intestines, and bland for sensitive intestines. I.A.2.a.

dietary service. a hospital or other institutional *department* responsible for feeding and teaching patients proper and prescribed diets. III.B.1.

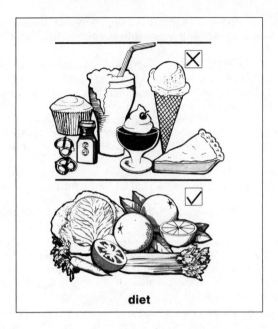

diet

dietary supplement. anything advertised or *labeled* as useful for improving or completing regular diets.

These supplements include vitamin and mineral pills, some protein preparations, and many *health foods*. They are subject to special regulation by the Food and Drug Administration because they are more expensive and rarely more *effective* than an extra meal. I.A.2.a.

dietetic. pertaining to diet, suitable for a prescribed diet.

dietetics. the science concerned with the principles of *nutrition* and their application, aiming at satisfying human nutritive needs under various social, economic, age, and health conditions. III.C.

dietician. a professional trained in or practicing dietetics.

Many dieticians are responsible for hospital and other institutional dietary services, some assist individuals in understanding and following proper or special diets. A *registered* dietician (RD) is one who has successfully participated in the American Dietary Association's registration program. III.A.4.

differential diagnosis. the various *diagnoses* which could explain a given *problem;* the act of distinguishing the correct diagnosis among the often quite similar ones in the differential. V.A.

differentiation of self. the process by, and degree to which, one's individual self is separated from the larger selves of one's family and society.

Whether part of ourself is actually part of a common self of other members of our family, or is simply similar to and easily affected by them, poses a nice theoretical issue. Successful differentiation of self, the development of individual autonomy, comes with maturity in happy, functional families. I.A.2., I.B.1.

digestion. the biochemical decomposition of organic matter, as in making absorbable *food* and rotting *waste* into usable or disposable form. I.A.2.a., I.C.4.

dioxin. any or several of about 75 chlorinated dioxins, the most notorious being 2,3,7,8-tetrachlorodibenzo-*p*-dioxin (TCDD).

TCDD and other dioxins are chemically very stable, practically insoluble in water, and *persist* for years in soil. They enter the environment as *contaminants* of pesticides or defoliants, as *Agent Orange,* and as products of incomplete burning of wood and wastes. Human *exposure* produces transient *chloracne, a skin irritation resembling common acne. *Exposure* has been said, but not shown, to cause cancer, birth defects, and psychiatric effects. The enormous, perhaps unnecessary, fuss about dioxin contamination has helped improve waste control law and practices in the United States.

Read Abelson, Philip H., "Chlorinated Dioxins" (*Science,* 220(4604): 6/24/83). I.C.4.

diploma school. a program which educates *registered nurses* in a hospital; compare *associate degree* and *baccalaureate programs.*

Classroom and laboratory teaching may be obtained from a college, but are the responsibility of the hospital. It awards a diploma, but no college degree is given. III.A.2.

diplomate (D). one who has a diploma. Sometimes describes a *board certified* physician because a diploma is given with certification. III.A.1.

direct association. see *association.*

direct cost. a *cost* which is identifiable directly with a particular activity, service, or product of the program experiencing the cost; compare *cost center, indirect cost,* and *overhead.* VII.D.1.

direct encounter. an *encounter* in which there is a face-to-face meeting of the patient and professional. A direct encounter is the same as a *visit.*

A direct encounter may be classified as (1) an office visit—a direct encounter occurring in the provider's office; (2) a home visit—a direct encounter occurring at the patient's residential location (this includes home of friend where a patient is visiting, hotel room, etc); (3) a hospital visit—a direct encounter in the hospital setting. Count one encounter for each patient visited: (a) hospital inpatient visit—a direct encounter with an inpatient; (b) outpatient visit—a direct encounter with an outpatient in either the emergency room or the outpatient clinic; (4) other direct encounters—

dioxin

these include accident scene, extended-care facility, and professional visits in a social setting, etc. Note: When more than one person is seen for problems of a single patient, the encounter is counted as one visit. When more than one person is seen for a shared problem, the encounter is counted as one visit (from *NAPCRG, 1977*). VII.

direct provider. see *provider.*

dirty. see *clean.*

disability. a "restriction or lack (resulting from an *impairment*) of ability to perform an activity in the manner or within the range considered normal for a human being" (*International Classification of Impairments, Disabilities, and Handicaps.* Geneva: World Health Organization, 1980); a physical or mental *condition, disease,* or impairment which prevents a person from engaging in his ordinary activities or normal life, or from doing a job, i.e., results in a loss of functional ability.

Disability may refer only to limitation of major activities, most commonly vocational. There are varying types (functional, vocational, or learning), degrees (partial or total), and durations (temporary or permanent) of disability. Benefits for disability may be available only for specified disabilities, as permanent and total disability, required for Social Security.

See *developmental disability, handicap, rehabilitation, specific learning disability,* and *workmen's compensation.* II., VII.B.2.d.

disability income insurance. health insurance that provides periodic payments to replace income when the insured is unable to work as a result of injury or disease.

See *workmen's compensation.* IV.B.2.

disablement. synonym, *disability.*

Theoretically distinguishable; disability being a *condition,* disablement being the state of a person with that condition. II., VII.B.2.d.

discharge. 1. emit, evacuate, release, relieve of, secrete, send forth, unload. 2. anything so discharged. 3. in medicine, release from an inpatient facility, discharges plus deaths equal admissions plus births. 4. in environmental health, gaseous discharges are *emissions,* liquid ones are *effluents,* and *solid wastes* are discharges. 3. VII.C.5., 4. II.C.4.

discharge abstract. a standardized brief description of an *admission* prepared upon a patient's discharge from a hospital or other health facility; compare *discharge summary.*

The abstract records selected data about the hospital stay including *diagnoses, services* received, *length of stay,* source of payment, and demographic information. The information is obtained from the patient's medical record and abstracted in standard coded form without interpretation or judgment.

See *Uniform Hospital Discharge Data Set.* VII.C.5.

discharge diagnosis. the problem primarily treated during an *admission;* compare *primary diagnosis.*

The discharge diagnosis is sometimes defined synonymously with *admitting diagnosis* and increasingly likely to be the most expensive problem treated, see *diagnosis related group.* It is correct to list all problems cared for during the admission as discharge diagnoses. II.B.1.

discharge planning. planning and preparing for a patient's care after discharge.

Physicians may be assisted in discharge planning by a nurse or social worker, a *discharge planner, who will obtain needed special equipment, arrange *home health services,* and teach the patient and family the post-discharge *regimen.* VIII.C.5.

discharge summary.   a review of an episode of inpatient care or *admission.* The discharge summary is prepared by the attending physician and becomes part of both the inpatient record and the physician's office record. It is more complete and less standardized than a *discharge abstract,* which may be obtained from it. The summary ordinarily describes the patient upon admission, records all laboratory results, reviews the hospital course, and lists major procedures performed, and discharge diagnoses, medications, and diet. VII.C.5.

discount.   a reduction in the price, significance, or value of something; to make such a reduction.

In economics and accounting, future costs, benefits, or earnings may be discounted in making present decisions because their occurrence is irrelevant to the decision maker, uncertain, or remote. Discounting should be, and sometimes is, done consciously, usually at a constant rate per year. Thus, in occupational health the substantial costs of chronic occupational disease, manifest years after the causative *exposure,* are discounted (perhaps excessively) when weighing the present costs of preventing the exposure.

See *Blue Cross discount.* VIII.B.1.

discovery rule.   in malpractice, a rule in some jurisdictions providing that the *statute of limitations* does not begin to run until a wrongful act is discovered, or, with reasonable diligence, should have been discovered.

Use of the discovery rule is sometimes limited to cases involving a foreign object left in the body of a patient. Some states have statutory rules for malpractice specifying time limits within which an action must be brought, both after discovery and after the *negligent* act occurred. V.D.

disease.   literally, "without ease"; any *condition* that limits life in its powers, enjoyment, or duration; in biology, a failure of the adaptive mechanisms of an organism to counteract adequately, normally, or appropriately the stimuli and stresses to which it is subject, resulting in a disturbance in the function or structure of some part of the organism.

The last definition emphasizes that disease is multifactorial and may be prevented or treated by changing any of the factors. Disease is an elusive concept, difficult to define, being variably defined by different societies. Thus, crime and *drug dependence* presently tend to be seen as diseases, when previously considered moral or legal problems.

See *acute, chronic, communicable, health, illness, impairment,* and *sickness.* II.

disease index.   synonym, *problem index (NAPCRG, 1977).*

disease of the month club.   facetious name, from the journal, *Disease of the Month,* for the people advocating and legislating special, often trivial, programs for victims of specified diseases, rather than programs that benefit all people or that improve the whole health system.

Such *categorical* legislation is easy to pass, politically popular, and basically unimportant. VIII.B.2.a., VIII.D.

disengagement. development in a family of "overly rigid boundaries around subsystems.

"Members of disengaged subsystems may function autonomously, lack feelings of loyalty and belonging, and the ability to function interdependently or request support when needed" (*Pinney and Slipp, 1982*).
See *enmeshment*. I.B.1.

disorder. a disturbance of normal physical or mental function; synonym, *disease*. II.

dispensary. a place where medicines or medical care is given, typically free or at low cost to *ambulatory* patients; compare *infirmary*.
Dispensaries, common in the military, businesses, and schools, do not usually serve the general public. III.B.1.

dispensing fee. a fee charged by a pharmacist for filling a *prescription*.
Pharmacists charge for filling a prescription with a dispensing fee or percentage markup on the *acquisition cost* of the drug involved. A dispensing fee is the same for all prescriptions, and thus a larger markup on an inexpensive drug or small prescription than an expensive drug or large prescription. It reflects the fact that a pharmacist's service is the same whatever the cost of the drug. Some pharmacists use both a percentage markup and a minimum fee.
See *maximum allowable cost program*. III.B.3., VII.D.3.

dissatisfied life. see *wrongful life*.

district health authority (DHA). see *health authority*.

diversity index. a measure of the number and variety of species living in a given *environment* and thus of the quality of the environment.
The index reflects the ecological principal that deterioration in the *healthfulness* of an environment produces a decrease in the number of species that can survive in that environment. I.C.

Dix, Dorothea Lynde. U.S. author of children's books, 1802–1887. An early crusader for improvement of institutional care for the mentally ill. III.C.

doc-in-a-box. condescending slang, *episodic care center*.

doctor. from Latin, *docere,* to teach. 1. synonym, *physician*. 2. anyone with a doctoral degree. 3. to practice medicine, to be treated by a physician. 4. to tamper with or falsify. 1. III.A.1.

doctor shopping. police slang, obtaining *controlled substances* by *fraud* from multiple physicians using fictitious complaints, a felony in most states.
Physicians use the term more generically when a patient sees multiple providers, often for the same complaint, without telling each physician about the others. VIII.B.2.a., VIII.B.3.

Doctors Ought to Care (DOC). a program of anti*smoking* advertising and related *health maintenance* and public health activities sponsored by family physicians. VII.B.2.b.

domiciliary care. provision of room and board, ordinarily without medical care, for people incapable of independent living; compare *boarding home, custodial care,* and *residential care*.
Some U.S. veterans hospitals, for instance, house incompetent but not sick veterans in facilities known as *domiciliaries or *doms. VII.C.5.b.

dose. 1. a measured quantity of anything *prescribed,* given, or received for beneficial effect; to give such a quantity; compare *exposure.* 2. in radiology, the quantity of energy or *radiation* absorbed. *dosage. the proper dose for a given situation. *dose-effect or *dose-response curve. any graph relating varying doses to their varying effects, see *threshold.* *dosimetry. the measurement of doses, usually with *dosimeters.

Many specific doses are defined, including the *critical dose, one sufficient to produce nonbeneficial, toxic effects; *cumulative dose, total dose over time; *infective dose, one sufficient to cause infection; *lethal dose, one sufficient to kill (the LD_0 is the maximum dose that kills no one; the LD_{50}, or median lethal dose, kills half; and the LD_{100} kills all); and *minimum dose, the smallest that produces an effect. III.B.3., V.3.

double bind. an "interaction in which one person demands a response to a message containing mutually contradictory signals while the other person is unable either to comment on the incongruity or to escape the situation.

"The term...describes a type of communication initially considered to be pathogenic of schizophrenia. Now it is recognized as not necessarily pathogenic but, if so, not only of schizophrenia. Double binds involve two conflicting and usually negative injunctions that are expressed at different levels (verbal and nonverbal) and come from a person who has survival significance, ordinarily a parent, who threatens punishment for not complying with either contradictory message. Further injunctions prevent the victim escaping the field or commenting (metacommunicating) on this no-win dilemma. Damage occurs when a child or person is exposed to these double-bind messages repeatedly over a long period" (after *Pinney and Slipp, 1982*). I.A.2.

double blind study. a *study* in which both subjects and investigators are unaware of (blind to) who is actually receiving the drug, procedure, or treatment being tested.

The method eliminates *bias,* conscious or unconscious, in both subjects and investigators. Classically, in drug studies a look-alike *placebo* is given to those not receiving the experimental drug. In *single blind studies either the subjects or the investigators, usually, know which treatment is being used in each case. In *triple blind trials people analyzing the data also are unaware of the treatment used. VIII.D.

drain dumping. disposal of liquid *waste* by pouring it down the drain into the public *sewer* system.

Drain dumping of *hazardous,* particularly radioactive, waste is often illegal but hard to prevent. I.C.5.

Drake, Daniel. American physician, 1785–1852. He studied the problems of health and *sanitation* connected with the settling of the West. The results were published in his classic, *On the Principal Diseases of the Interior Valley of North America* (1850–1854). VIII.A.1.

dread disease insurance. synonym, *specific disease insurance.*

drinking water. water that is *safe* and acceptable for human consumption.

Drinking water must be free of both *pathogens* and ugly odor, color, and taste. *Water quality standards,* based on criteria such as clarity and *coliform counts,* are of necessity incomplete since they fail to measure *contamination* by viruses and chemicals.

See *aquifer* and *chlorinate.* I.C.5.

drug. 1. a chemical used to change a person, animal, or other organism. 2. in the Food, Drug, and Cosmetic Act, any substance, other than food and water, intended for use in the diagnosis, cure, mitigation, treatment, or prevention of disease, or intended to affect the structure or function of the body, or components of these substances. Substances recognized in the *U.S. Pharmacopeia,* the *Homeopathic Pharmacopeia of the U.S.,* and the *National Formulary* are drugs. 3. to administer such a substance.

See *antibiotic, biologic, brand name, compendium, controlled, device, effective, established, ethical, formulary, generic, investigational new drug, label, maximum allowable cost, new drug application, new, not new, over-the-counter, package insert, prescription, safe,* and *scheduled.* IV.B.3.

drug abuse. persistent or sporadic drug use inconsistent with or unrelated to accepted medical or cultural practice; compare *alcoholism.*

Specific definitions are variable, sometimes also requiring excessive use of a drug, unnecessary use (thus incorporating recreational use), *drug dependence,* or that the use be illegal. II.B.2.

drug addiction. usually synonymous with *drug dependence;* sometimes limited to drug dependence with physical *addiction.* Not synonymous with *drug abuse* and irregular in meaning. II.B.2.

drug compendium. see *compendium.*

drug dependence. *habituation* or *addiction* to a drug or other chemical substance.

It is usually characterized by a psychologic compulsion to take the drug on a continuous or periodic basis to experience its psychic effects; the cretin's use of thyroid hormone is thus not thought of as drug dependence. Tolerance for the drug may or may not be present. A person may be dependent on more than one drug. The nature of the dependency varies with the agent involved, which requires designating the type of dependency in each case, as in drug dependence of *narcotic,* cannabis, barbiturate, or amphetamine type, *alcoholism,* or tobacco dependence. Drug dependence may or may not be dangerous, severe, or illegal. Psychic and physical dependence are sometimes separated as *drug habituation* and *drug addiction,* but usage is irregular and the distinction difficult. II.B.2.

Drug Efficacy Study Implementation (DESI). the Food and Drug Administration program implementing the evaluations and recommendations of the Drug Efficacy Study Group of the National Academy of Science—National Research Council respecting the *effectiveness* of drugs marketed prior to 1962 under approved *new drug applications.*

The Drug Efficacy Study was undertaken in 1966 to evaluate the efficacy of drugs the FDA had approved as safe prior to 1962 when Congress first required that drugs also be proved effective before marketing. The Drug Efficacy Study Group evaluated nearly 4000 individual drug products, finding many of them ineffective or of only possible or probable effectiveness. The FDA is still slowly removing some of the drugs from the market, and some efforts have been made to limit their coverage by Medicaid and other health insurance programs. III.B.3.

Drug Enforcement Administration (DEA). the agency within the Department of Justice which administers federal programs to control the use of dangerous, *scheduled,* drugs under the *Controlled Substances* Act of 1970.

The DEA was previously called the *Bureau of Narcotics and Dangerous Drugs (BNDD). III.D.1.

Drug Enforcement Administration number (DEA number). the registration number assigned people and programs *registering* with the federal government for use of *scheduled* drugs.

Physicians, hospitals, and others are required by the Controlled Substances Act of 1970 to register and obtain a number before they can obtain, *prescribe*, sell, use, or do research using scheduled drugs. III.B.3., VI.E.

druggist. one who sells drugs or operates a drugstore; compare *apothecary*.

Druggist is not synonymous with *pharmacist* since it is not limited to people with a pharmacy degree and is used only of pharmacists who operate or work in drugstores. III.A.4.

drug habituation. usually synonymous, *drug dependence;* sometimes limited to psychic drug dependence, without *addiction*. Not synonymous with *drug abuse* and irregular in meaning; compare *habituation*. II.B.2.

drug monograph. a Food and Drug Administration *rule* which specifies for a drug or class of related drugs the kinds and amounts of ingredients which it may contain, the conditions for which it may be offered, and directions for use, warnings, and other information which its *labeling* must bear.

Drug monographs state conditions under which drugs may be marketed as *safe* and *effective* without an approved *new drug application*. The FDA has established monographs for some *over-the-counter* drugs. Special statutory provisions already authorize use of monographs for antibiotic drugs. Once a monograph is promulgated, anyone who meets its requirements may market the product without seeking approval of a new drug application. III.B.3.

Drug Products Information File (DPIF). a computer processible data base on commercially available drug products developed and maintained by the American Society of Hospital Pharmacists.

The file contains for each listed product the *generic* and *brand names,* manufacturer, dosage form and size, and *labeling*. All are coded for various sorting purposes. The DPIF is leased by hospitals and others for inventory control, purchasing, and *utilization review*. III.B.3.

drug reaction. see *reaction*.

Drug Topics Red Book (The Redbook). an annual publication, principally for pharmacists, providing prices and descriptions of products distributed through retail and hospital pharmacies.

This book, known by its cover color, provides wholesale and retail prices for over 170,000 drug products (supplied by manufacturers), pictures of drugs, and tables on drug interactions, manufacturers' return policies, and pharmacy math.

Published by Medical Economics Company (Oradell, NJ 07649), which also publishes the *Physicians' Desk Reference*. III.B.3.

Drug Use Education Tips (D.U.E.T.). a cooperative effort of the American Academy of Family Physicians and the United States Pharmacopeial Convention (USP) intended to help family physicians provide patients with information on prescribed drugs.

Consisting of 300 monographs abstracted from the 1984 USP *Advice for the Patient*, it is printed in looseleaf form to facilitate photocopying for patient distribution. V.C.

dry-fingered. see *wet fingered*.

dual choice.   giving people a choice of more than one health insurance program to pay for or provide their health services.

Dual choice occurs when employers offer employees more than one group health insurance program, or a health insurance program and a prepaid group practice to choose from as a benefit of their employment. It is characteristic of the *Federal Employees Health Benefits Program*. The Health Maintenance Organization Act requires employers to offer a choice of *qualified* HMOs in addition to whatever health insurance they offer (section 1310 of the Public Health Service Act). III.B.1., IV.B.

dummy.   British, *placebo*.

dump.   to unload, throw away, or get rid of, as of unwanted patients or wastes.

Dumping often implies inappropriate or irresponsible action, as when toxic wastes are dumped by the roadside to avoid the costs of proper disposal or when uninsured sick people are transferred from private to public hospitals, see *Relman Doctrine*. Patients should be transferred with *informed consent* for medical or humanitarian, not financial, reasons.

See *drain dumping*. I.C., IV.B., V.D.

duplication of benefits.   occurs when a person covered under more than one health or other insurance policy collects, or may collect, for the same medical expenses or other loss from more than one insurer; compare *coordination of benefits*.

Individual health insurance policies sometimes include *antiduplication clauses* against overinsurance due to two similar policies issued by the same insurer, loss-of-time coverage in excess of the insured's monthly earnings, and duplicate coverage with other insurers. *Group insurance* usually contains such clauses, especially in *major medical* policies. However, most states will not allow group policies to apply such clauses to individual insurance. Where duplication exists the insurer responsible for paying its benefits first is the *primary payer*. IV.B.

durable medical equipment (DME).   equipment which ordinarily can remain in use for over a year without unusual maintenance or calibration.

Medicare, Medicaid, and some private health insurance companies limit coverage for rental or purchase of such equipment. DME includes such items as beds and respirators. III.B.2.

Durham Rule.   a ruling by the U.S. Court of Appeals for the District of Columbia in 1954 that held that "an accused is not criminally responsible if his unlawful act was the product of mental disease or mental defect."

The rule has since been replaced in the District of Columbia by the *American Law Institute Formulation;* compare the earlier *M'Naghten Rule*. VIII.B.3.

dust.   particulate matter, usually dry, derived from larger masses by grinding, crushing, or other physical force and capable of suspension in air.

Inhalation of dust causes *pneumoconioses* and other damage to lungs. Its control is thus important in environmental and occupational health. The damage done depends on the size and density of the *particles,* their concentration in the air, the composition of the dust itself, the length of *exposure,* the rate and depth of breathing during exposure, the dust's solubility, and the rate of elimination from the body. I.C.1.

dyad.   a liaison, temporary or permanent, between two people.

See *triangle*. I.B.1.

dynamic deductible. see *deductible.*

dyscalculia, dysgraphia, and dyslexia. see *learning disability.*

dysfunctional family. "a family that cannot accommodate to and cope with stresses, as those arising from changes in the life cycle of the family, usually involving addition or loss of a member.

"Boundaries between individual members are too loose, rigid, or distant, so that cooperation and support cannot occur. The family is not responsive to the developmental needs of its members. Homeostasis often (but not always) is sustained by one member being induced into being the *identified patient,* who overtly manifests symptoms" (*Pinney and Slipp, 1982*). I.B.1.

dysfunctional marriage. "a marital relationship lacking role complementarity, which may result in a dominant-submissive power relationship, coercion of one member, or the isolation of each member.

"Each strives for his or her own needs. There is poor conflict resolution, i.e., role induction or manipulation of others, avoidance of conflict or differences, *triangulation* of another member to form a coalition with, or expression of conflict through a scapegoat" (*Pinney and Slipp, 1982*). I.B.1.

Early and Periodic Screening, Diagnosis, and Treatment Program (EPSDT). a part of the *Medicaid* program requiring states to have a program for eligible children under 21 "to ascertain their physical or mental defects, and such health care, treatment, and other measures to correct or ameliorate defects and chronic conditions discovered thereby" (section 1905(a)(4)(B) of the Social Security Act).

Eligible children must include at least all children in families receiving *AFDC* payments. State programs are not just to pay for services but also to have an active outreach component to inform eligible persons of available benefits, actively bring them into care so they can be screened, and, if necessary, assist them in obtaining appropriate treatment. EPSDT should properly refer only to programs which have all of these elements. IV.C.2.

ear, nose, and throat surgery (ENT). see *otolaryngology*.

E-book. synonym, *experience book*.

ecdemic. brought into a region from without, not *endemic* or *epidemic*.

Ecdemic diseases are often unusually virulent, as was measles when it first reached the Fiji Islands and killed much of the population of all ages. VII.C.

ecological community. the organisms of all types sharing a specified *environment*.

Some of the many interdependent relationships, among communities as among members of a *food chain*, may be represented by *ecological pyramids*. I.C.

ecological efficiency (EE). a measure of the energy an organism uses to produce protoplasm.

Expressed in common units to allow comparison among organisms, ecological efficiencies are functions of the organisms' absorption, assimilation, growth, and increase ratios. Pollution and other environmental changes can reduce the ecological efficiency of living things, to the detriment of all life on earth. I.C.

ecological fallacy. variously used, the erroneous assumption that because two things are *associated* or *correlated*, one must be caused by the other; the erroneous attribution of *average* conditions for a group to a subset of the group; compare *halo* and *Hawthorne effects.* VIII.D.

ecological impact. the total effect of an environmental change, either natural or man-made, on the ecology of an area. I.C.

ecological pyramid. a graphic representation of the trophic levels in a food chain, shown as stacked horizontal bands, as below, with the producers at the base, under consumers of the first, second, third, and further orders. Consumption and transfers at each trophic level may be expressed in terms of the numbers of organisms, a *number pyramid; amounts of energy, an *energy pyramid; or quantity of biomass, a *biomass pyramid.

ecological succession. ecology's rule that, as a young ecological community grows and matures, there is an accompanying increase in species diversity, which creates a growing degree of complexity and gradually changing character.

This tends to change an unstable and simple community into a stable and complex one. Overgrowth or the introduction of *pollution* can produce *ecological recession, the counterpart of ecological succession in that during recession a complex community loses its diversity of species and becomes simple again. I.C.

ecological validity. see *validity.*

ecology. the relationships of living things to one another and their *environment;* the science and study of such relations. *Autecology studies a single species. *Synecology studies a group of organisms, as a *biocenose.* I.C., II.D.

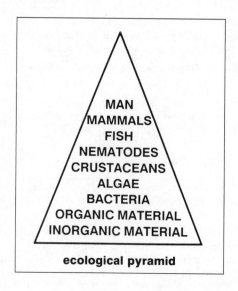

ecological pyramid

economic good.   see *good.*

Economic Stabilization Program (ESP).   a federal program established to control wages and prices from August 1971 until April 1974.

The time the controls were in effect remains one of the few periods since the enactment of Medicare and Medicaid in which medical care price increases slowed markedly, increases in prices being limited to 4.3 percent per annum. VI.D.1.

economy.   1. a system, usually largely monetary, by which *resources* are allocated; a type, stage, or part of such a system, as a barter, underdeveloped, or farm economy. 2. thrift and efficiency in resource allocation. 3. household management. VIII.B.1.

economy of scale.   any reduction in unit cost a producer achieves as larger quantities are produced; decrease in average cost when all factors of production are expanded proportionately.

Hospital costs per day are often less in 300-bed than 30-bed hospitals, an economy of scale, and sometimes more in 1000-bed than 300-bed hospitals, a diseconomy of scale. The term is often used less accurately, for savings achieved when underused resources are used more efficiently, as when health programs share the costs and use of expensive underused personnel or equipment. Economy of scale occurs when *marginal costs* are decreasing. VIII.B.3.

ecosystem.   the combination and interaction of a biologic community or *biocenose* and its nonliving *environment;* a contraction of ecological *system.* See *nutrient budget.* I.C.

educable.   see *mental retardation.*

Educational Commission for Foreign Medical Graduates (ECFMG).   an organization which operates a program for educating, testing, and evalu-

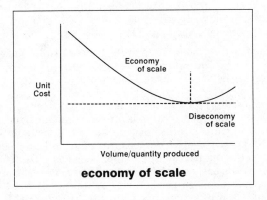

economy of scale

ating foreign medical graduates who seek internships and residencies in the United States.

The ECFMG was formed in 1974 by merger of the Educational Council for Foreign Medical Graduates, incorporated in 1956, and the Commission for Foreign Medical Graduates. It is sponsored by the American Medical Association, American Hospital Association, Association of American Medical Colleges, Association for Hospital Medical Education, and Federation of State Medical Boards of the U.S. *Certification* of FMGs is granted by the ECFMG after receiving documentation of their education, and passage of examinations of their medical competence and English comprehension. Such certification is needed for full licensure of FMGs in most states. The clinical exam uses National Board of Medical Examiners questions and would be passed by over 90 percent of U.S. graduates if they took it; over the years a fifth to a third of foreign graduates have passed.

See *Federation Licensure Examination* and *fifth pathway.* III.A.1.

Education and Research Foundation (ERF).   an American Medical Association sponsored foundation (AMA-ERF) which guarantees private loans to medical students and makes grants to support medical education and health services research.

It is funded largely with contributions from individual physicians. III.B.4.

effective.   able to cause a useful intended *outcome* or result in actual use. *effectiveness. the degree or amount of power to be effective, the state of being effective; compare *efficacious* and *efficient.*

Effectiveness requires consideration of outcomes but not costs to measure; compare *cost-benefit analysis.* The Federal Food, Drug, and Cosmetic Act requires prior demonstration of effectiveness for most drugs marketed for human use. No similar requirement exists for most other medical action paid for or regulated under federal or state law.

See *DESI, quality,* and *safety.* VII.D.2.

efficacious.   having the capability to cause a useful intended outcome, whether or not realized. *efficacy. the power to produce a result.

Use of effectiveness, efficacy, and efficiency is irregular, often synonymous. However, they may be distinguished by using efficacy for results of actions undertaken under ideal circumstances, using effectiveness for results under usual or normal circumstances, and reserving efficiency as a synonym for *cost-effectiveness.* Actions can thus be efficacious and effective, or efficacious and ineffective, but not the reverse, and can be either without being very efficient about it. VII.D.2.

efficiency.   capacity to produce maximum desired results with minimum use of energy or other resources; measured as a ratio of an *output* to an *input* where increasing efficiency increases the ratio, as encounters per physician hour.

In economics, efficiency varies with three components: input productivity, or *technical efficiency; input mix, or *economic efficiency; and the scale of operation. Colloquially, efficiency measures the "bang for the buck," but is difficult to quantify since its measures often fail to account for all its dimensions, as the relative quality of inputs and outputs. Efficiency should be measured by the costs of achieving health *outcomes* of comparable quality. Defining it in terms of productivity assumes that what is produced is *efficacious* and used in an *effective* manner. VII.D.2., VIII.B.1.

efficiency value. a measure of a test's yield of correct results; the number of *true positive* plus true negative results as a percentage of the total number of results obtained.
See *predictive value, sensitivity,* and *specificity.* VIII.D.

efficient. competent, productive, marked by the ability to choose and use the most *effective* and least wasteful means of doing a task. VII.D.2.

effluent. liquid *discharge.* II.C.5.

Ehrlich, Paul. German physician, 1854–1915. He developed chemotherapy as an effective part of medicine. In public health, his greatest achievements were the extraordinarily fruitful side-chain theory of immunity and the synthesis of arsphenamine, the first specific treatment of syphilis. III.B.3., VIII.A.1.

eidetic. of vivid lifelike imagery which is projected into the external world and not merely "in one's head"; a halfway house to hallucination; of the ability or disposition to project images, frequent in children; pertaining to forms or images, especially those voluntarily reproducible; intuitive. I.A.1.

eidetic image. an image, usually visual, so clear as to seem like an external or perceptual experience, but ordinarily recognized as subjective. May be a fantasy, dream, or memory.

eidos. something seen or envisioned; a form or essence; a logical structure used by a culture in thinking and acting. I.B.

elasticity. in economics, a measure of the degree to which a change in the quantity of a product or service demanded or supplied is dependent on changes in its price, known as *price elasticity, or the income of consumers, *income elasticity. Price *elasticity of demand, or *coefficient of elasticity, is the ratio of the resulting percentage change in demand to a given percentage change in price.
Necessities usually have inelastic demand while luxuries or items with close substitutes have elastic demand schedules. Knowing the elasticity of demand for health services allows prediction of the effects of different *cost sharing* in insurance programs and thus the potential effects of changes. VIII.B.1.

elective. in medical education, a rotation or experience chosen by, but not specifically required of, a physician in training; compare *selective.* III.A.

elective abortion. see *abortion.*

elective surgery. surgery which need not be performed on an emergency basis because reasonable delay will not affect the *outcome* unfavorably. Such surgery is usually necessary and may be *major.* V.B.

elephant policy. see *trolley car policy.*

emancipated minor. a *minor* considered to have the rights of an adult because he exercises control over his own life, usually by living alone. I.A.1.

emergency. a disease or condition which requires immediate attention.
Many emergencies are neither life threatening nor serious, as cuts, although their proper care should be immediate. Since emergency rooms rarely refuse anyone care, emergencies may be defined operationally as problems which a patient perceives as an emergency or for which, for whatever reason, he is willing to pay emergency room charges. II.B.2.c., VII.B.3.a.

emergency care. care for patients with emergency conditions. VII.C.5.a.

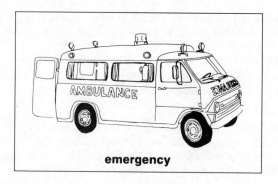

emergency

emergency room (ER). a hospital department or area with personnel and equipment for the care of acute illness, trauma, or other conditions needing immediate medical attention. III.B.1.

emergency medical services (EMS). services intended for the care of emergencies, including those of ambulances, emergency rooms, and emergency telephone numbers and hotlines. VII.C.5.a.

emergency medical services system (EMSS). an integrated system of appropriate health manpower, facilities, and equipment which provides all necessary emergency care in a defined geographic area.

The development of such systems was federally assisted under the Emergency Medical Service Systems Act of 1973, P.L. 93-154, which amended the Public Health Service (PHS) Act by creating a new Title XII. The term is defined, and the necessary components of the system listed in sections 1201 and 1206 of the PHS Act. Characteristic of such a system are a central communications facility using the universal emergency telephone number, 911, direct communications with all parts of the system, and dispatching of cases to properly *categorized* facilities. The EMSS was folded into the Preventive Health and Services Block Grant, created in 1981. III.B.1.

emergency temporary standard. see *occupational health and safety standard.*

emission. *discharge* of gases, radiation, or energy. II.C.1.

emporiatrics. the science of the health of travelers.

Read Mann, I.M., "Emporiatric Policy and Practice: Protecting the Health of Americans Abroad" (*JAMA*, 249(24): 3323–5, 6/24/83). III.C.

encounter. any contact between a patient and health professional in which care is given. Some definitions exclude either telephone contacts or home *visits.*

An *encounter form records selected information describing an encounter, including, at least, identification and description of the patient and provider involved, the diagnoses or *problems* treated, see *ICD-9-CM*, the *services* or *procedures* performed, see *CPT*, the *charges*, and sometimes the *outcomes* of the treatment.

See *experience book, indirect encounter,* and *superbill.* VII.

endemic. occurring more or less constantly in a certain region or people, whether of a disease in medicine or a particular species in ecology; compare *ecdemic* and *epidemic.* VIII.C.

endocrinology. the study of the endocrine glands and their function in control of bodily metabolism.

The endocrine glands are those which secrete hormones directly into the bloodstream without ducts and thus control a great variety of bodily functions. They include the pituitary or hypophysis, pineal, thyroid, parathyroid, pancreatic islets, adrenals, and ovaries or testicles. III.C.

endocrinology and metabolism. the subspecialty of internal medicine concerned with, and commonly known as, endocrinology. III.C.

endodontics, endodontia. the *specialty* of dentistry concerned with diagnosis and treatment of oral conditions which arise as a result of *pathoses* (sic) of the dental pulp, supporting structures, and periradicular tissues. III.C.

endodontist. a specialist in endodontics. III.A.3.

endodontology, endodontia. in dentistry, the study of the dental pulp and its diseases. III.C.

endorsement. recognition by a state of a license given by another state when the qualifications and standards required by the original licensing state are equivalent to or higher than those of the endorsing state.

The licensee is relieved by endorsement of the full burden of obtaining a license in the endorsing state. There is not necessarily any *reciprocity* between the two states. III.A.

End-Stage Renal Disease (ESRD) Program. a part of the Medicare program which pays for the treatment of patients disabled by chronic renal failure, i.e., end-stage renal diseases (having kidneys which no longer work, for whatever reason).

This special part of Medicare was enacted in 1972 and in 1987 covered 103,997 patients. It only pays for dialysis (use of artificial kidney machines) provided by specifically regulated facilities. IV.C.1.

enmeshment. entanglement, excessive intermingling, as the members of a family or vines grown so together that they choke each other.

An enmeshed family, as the one whose members were never allowed to close their doors, has trouble with growth, change, and freeing members to form new families. Some connection or engagement among family members is obviously necessary, and *disengagement* or dysfunctional connection may be as bad as enmeshment. I.B.1.

enroll. agree to participate in a contract for benefits from an insurance company or health maintenance organization (HMO). One who enrolls is an *enrollee. The number of people and their dependents enrolled with an insurance company or HMO is its *enrollment.

See *beneficiary, member, open enrollment,* and *subscriber.* IV.B.

enrollment period. a period during which individuals may enroll for insurance or health maintenance organization benefits.

There are two enrollment periods, for example, for supplementary medical insurance of Medicare: the initial enrollment period, the 7 months beginning 3 months before and ending 3 months after the month a person first becomes eligible, usually by turning 65, and the general enrollment period, the first 3 months of each year. Most *contributory group insurance* has an annual enrollment period when members of the group may elect to begin contributing and become covered. IV.B.

entitlement authority.   in the federal budget, legislation requiring payment of benefits or entitlements to any person or government meeting requirements established by such law, as social security benefits and veterans' pensions.

Section 401 of the Congressional Budget and Impoundment Control Act of 1974 placed restrictions on the enactment of new entitlement authorities since they are not subject to budgetary control.

See *backdoor authority*. VI.B.1.

entropy.   1. the portion of a system's energy, per degree of absolute temperature, that cannot be converted to work. 2. in medicine, diminished capacity for useful change, as occurs with depression or aging. 3. absence of form, order, pattern, or differentiation; the ultimate state reached in the degradation of the matter of the universe; compare *erosion*.

Most spontaneous changes, those occurring in nature, are accompanied by an increase in the entropy of the *system;* the growth of life and work of the living reduce natural disorder. I.C.

environment.   1. the sum of all external conditions and influences affecting the life, development, and, ultimately, the survival of an organism. 2. the whole world in which humans live.

An environment is properly defined with reference to a particular *system, population,* or *organism.* It then includes short- and long-term physical, social, and other factors and conditions directly or indirectly interacting with the object system, but not the part of the whole world which does not interact with the object. I.C.

environmental health.   a *healthful* environment; physical, biologic, and social conditions in an environment conducive to health. II.D.

environmental health services.   measures, techniques, and programs for the establishment, maintenance, and improvement of the healthfulness of the environment. VII.B.2.a.

environmental impact statement.   report prepared by a federal agency on the probable environmental impact of proposed governmental action likely to significantly affect the quality of the human environment.

Environmental impact statements are required by the National Environmental Policy Act and were intended as tools for decision making. Since courts first enjoined actions for which adequate statements were not prepared, they have also become a major tool in the struggle to preserve environmental quality. VII.B.2.a.

Environmental Protection Agency (EPA).   the agency of the U.S. government which administers environmental protection programs for control of air pollution, noise, solid waste disposal, and water pollution. III.D.1.

enzootic.   of disease afflicting animals in a limited area; contrast *epizootic*. VIII.C.

epidemic.   rapid spreading of a *contagious* disease in an area or *population;* occurring in extensive outbreaks or with episodic unusually high *incidence* at certain times and places: by extension, rapid increase in the occurrence of other phenomena, as accidents or suicides. Compare *ecdemic, endemic,* and *epizootic*.

Small outbreaks of rare diseases, as three cases of typhoid fever in one city, are epidemics since a few cases is still an unusually high incidence. See *air pollution epidemic.* VIII.C.

Epidemiologic Intelligence Service (EIS). the part of the *Centers for Disease Control,* Department of Health and Human Services, responsible for investigating epidemics and for a variety of related *public health* functions.

EIS officers for years have been assigned to state health departments where they bridge federal and state *vital statistics* and disease control programs. Many are in the *Commissioned Corps.* III.D.1.

epidemiology. 1. the study of diseases as they affect populations. 2. the sum of all physiologic, social, and environmental factors controlling the presence or absence of a particular disease, as the epidemiology of cancer which includes dietary, genetic, occupational, and other factors.

This science and its practice began with the study of the *incidence* and *prevalence,* distribution, causes, and control of infections, and epidemic disease, see *W.H. Frost, J. Snow,* and *R. Virchow.* *Epidemiologists describe health status and disease, see *vital statistics,* and assess the effects of control measures and health services.

See *association, at risk, morbidity, mortality, prevalence,* and *risk factor.* VIII.C.

episode. an acute exacerbation of a chronic disease; an event, of whatever length, having a distinct effect on a person's life or the course of an illness; synonym, *epidemic.* VIII.C.

episodic care center. a program providing ambulatory and emergency services to anybody who seeks and can provide payment for them; many synonyms, doc-in-a-box, urgent care center, urgicenter, and walk-in clinic.

Episodic care centers function like *emergency rooms,* but are separate from hospitals, with which they may have backup *affiliation* arrangements. They are ordinarily open outside regular business hours, do not make appointments, and may refer patients back to their *personal physician* for follow-up care. Unknown before the 1980s, their appearance was prompted by the doctor surplus and corporate takeover of medical care. The eventual place of *convenience medicine, as it is known, in the health system remains to be determined, probably surviving only when combined with *comprehensive continuous* care. III.B.1., VII.C.4.

epizootic. 1. of diseases afflicting animals in many areas, widely dispersed and rapidly spreading; contrast *enzootic.* 2. an outbreak of such a disease; compare *epidemic.* VIII.C.

equipment. a person's or program's fixed assets, or one of them, other than land and building; contrast *supplies.*

The distinction between equipment and *facilities,* both of which are *capital goods,* is somewhat arbitrary; equipment is usually purchased already made, facilities require construction. III.B.2.

equity. fairness, justice, equality; see *accessibility.*

What constitutes equity in health care, and which people have any right to it, both remain undefined. VIII.B.3.

equivalency testing. examination intended to compare an individual's knowledge, experience, and skill, however acquired, with the knowledge, experience, and skill acquired by formal education or training.

Successful completion of equivalency tests may give course credits toward an academic degree without taking the courses, or a license which requires academic training without the training.
See *proficiency testing.* III.A.

ergonomics. human factors engineering, biotechnology; the application of biology and engineering to adjustment of machine to man; the design of operations and equipment to take into account human physical and mental needs.

Ergonomics is important in occupational health where it may reduce effort, injuries, and exposure to noise and other hazards. I.A.2.c.

Erhard Seminar Training (est). a program of seminars in which one may acquire self-awareness and growth.

The seminars are brief, expensive, intense, large group experiences which help one take responsibility for one's own being. Means to this end include physical privation, guided meditation (group hypnosis?), and confrontations and indoctrination by the group trainer. V.

erosion. 1. a lesser god of *entropy.* 2. wearing away, usually through superficial destruction of a surface area, whether by inflammation and trauma in medicine or by weather and man in the *environment.* I.C.5.

error. mistake, false result, failure, defect; deviation from correct or approved procedure or practice; deficiency or imperfection in structure or function; difference between the observed or calculated value of a quantity and the true value.

Error is common in health care, not necessarily *negligent,* and never entirely preventable. It takes many forms, as *bias, sampling error,* and *systematic error,* and names, as *false negative* and *false positive.* V., VIII.D.

essential. 1. in medicine, without known cause, compare *idiopathic.* 2. in nutrition, necessary to an organism's life but not producible by it, as an essential amino or fatty acid which must be obtained from the diet.

Essential hypertension is unexplained rather than necessary (most essential hypertension is simply the upper part of the normal distribution of blood pressures). 1. III.B.1.a. 2. I.A.2.a.

Essentials for Residencies in Family Medicine. the requirements which family medicine residencies must meet for accreditation. Often referred to as "*the essentials."

They are adopted by the *Accreditation Council for Graduate Medical Education* of the American Medical Association after preparation by the Residency Review Committee. The essentials consist of the requirements for all accredited residencies, the general requirements, and the special requirements for family practice published in the annual Directory of Residency Training Programs Accredited by the ACGME (Chicago: American Medical Association, annual). III.C.

established name. the name given a drug or pharmaceutical product by the United States Adopted Names Council; synonyms, *generic name* and nonproprietary name; compare *brand name.*

This name is usually shorter and simpler than the chemical name, and the one most commonly used in scientific literature and medical education. An example would be penicillin, a well-known antibiotic. An established name for drugs is required by section 502(e) of the Federal Food, Drug and Cosmetic Act. III.B.3.

eternal care. euphemism, *death.* *eternal care unit (ECU). slang, heaven. As in, "What became of Mr. Smith?" "Oh, he transferred to the ECU." VIII.B.2.a.

ethical drug. a drug that is advertised only to physicians and other prescribing health professionals, rather than to the public; synonym, *prescription drug.* Drug manufacturers which make only or primarily such drugs constitute the *ethical drug industry. III.B.3.

ethics committee. an interdisciplinary group formed by a health program to consider issues of *medical ethics* arising from the program's operation; synonyms, hospital ethics committee (HEC) and infant bioethics committee; compare *institutional review board.*
　These consulting groups assist in resolving unusual or complex ethical problems, as poor *quality of life* or use of scarce resources, affecting the care of patients within the program. They are voluntary, educational, and advisory. They should not interfere with the primary responsibility of the patient, family, and physician for whatever specific problem may be at issue.
　See *Baby Doe.* III.B.1., III.C.

ethology. the study of *behavior,* particularly the study of animal behavior and the empirical study of human character and ethics. V.C.

ethylene dibromide (EDB). a pesticide used as a fumigant against insects in citrus fruit, grain, and soil.
　Residues of EDB at levels ranging from 2 to 177 parts per billion were found in foods bought in New York City markets in 1983–1984. EDB has been shown to be *carcinogenic* and *mutagenic* in animals and to inferfere with reproduction. In 1984 the Environmental Protection Agency recommended maximum EDB contents of 900 parts per billion (ppb) in raw grains for human consumption, 150 ppb in processed grain products like flour, and 30 ppb in ready-to-eat products like cereal. EDB is also used as an antiknock agent in leaded gasoline and in the production of some dyes and pharmaceuticals. I.A.2.a., I.C.

etiology. synonym, *cause;* the study of the origin of disease. II.B.1.a.

The European Pharmacopoeia. a *pharmacopeia* jointly produced by a convention of collaborating European countries which have undertaken to make their individual pharmacopoeias, as *The British Pharmacopoeia,* consistent with the group effort. III.B.3.

euthanasia. the act or practice of killing hopelessly or painfully sick individuals, *active euthanasia, or of allowing them to die without all possible treatment, *passive euthanasia, for reasons of mercy.
　Turning off the respirator supporting a body which has suffered brain death is not euthanasia. The distinction between active and passive is difficult because active efforts may be needed to maintain a passive posture.
　See *hospice.* V.B.

evacuation. 1. elimination, *emission,* removal. 2. the withdrawal of the sick or wounded, materials, or both as from a battle area.
　In military medicine, an evacuation hospital is a mobile unit designed to provide a facility as near the front as possible for major procedures and preparation and sorting of casualties for further evacuation to the rear.
　See *MASH* and *triage.* VII.C.3.

evaluate. express numerically, appraise, rate; examine and judge concerning worth, *quality, efficiency,* or condition.

Whether the process of evaluation must include feedback to the evaluated and responsibility for correcting identified deficiencies to qualify as true evaluation is comparable to the old argument about whether planning by definition includes plan implementation. Certainly good evaluation systems are formally organized, close the loop, and have the flexibility to focus on identified weaknesses. VI.D., VIII.D.

evidence of insurability. any statement or proof of a person's physical condition or occupation establishing his acceptability for insurance. IV.B.

exam, examination. determination, inspection, search, or test, whether for diagnosis, licensure, or other purpose.
See *National Board Examination* and *physical exam.* V.A.

excess coverage. see *limit on liability.*

excise tax. a single-stage commodity tax levied on a commodity only once as it passes through the production process to the final consumer.
An excise tax is narrowly based with enabling legislation that specifies precisely which products are taxed, as well as the tax rate. Sales taxes, by contrast, are more broadly based. Their tax base comprises many commodities and legislation designates commodities not subject to tax. Excise taxes are common on cigarettes, liquor, and automobiles and gasoline, and are sometimes levied in hopes of discouraging the use of the product taxed. Revenues may be set aside from general revenues and used for purposes related to the taxed product. Thus an excise tax on cigarettes might discourage smoking and revenues could be used for cancer screening. IV.C.

exclusion. a specific hazard, peril, or condition listed in an insurance policy for which the policy will not provide benefit payments.
Preexisting conditions, as heart disease, diabetes, hypertension, or a pregnancy which began before the policy was in effect, are common exclusions. Exclusions are often permanent in individual health insurance, temporary (commonly one year) for small groups in group insurance, and uncommon for large groups capable of absorbing the extra risk involved. IV.A.

excursion factor. maximum extent to which a *threshold limit value* may be exceeded.

exercise. repeated exertion or use of a function, power, or organ, ordinarily to develop or maintain capacity, skill, or *fitness;* one or more activities regularly undertaken to achieve prowess or as practice of an ability.
*Aerobic exercise, or *aerobics, as running and swimming, uses oxygen provided by the lungs, heart, and blood vessels at the rate they supply it once a steady state is reached. By thus stressing them, it develops their capacity. *Anaerobic exercise, as weight lifting and some calesthenics, does not rely on simultaneous oxygen supply and primarily strengthens muscles. A great variety of therapeutic exercises are available for stretching, limbering, and strengthening many parts of the body.
See *Bates method.* I.A.1.

expense. 1. in insurance, the cost, other than paying losses to an insured, of doing business, including acquisition and administrative costs. Expenses are included in the *loading.* 2. in accounting, the cost of goods, services, and facilities used in the production of current revenues.
Cash paid for *supplies* is an expenditure for an *asset.* It is recorded in accounting records as a cost. As the supplies are used, the asset is converted into an expense. 1. IV.B. 2. VI.C.2.

experience book (E-book). a book in which a practitioner or program records practice experience; synonym, *problem index.*

Such books in standard format with cross-referencing typically code patients, their diagnoses, see *ICD-9-CM,* and the *services* provided, see *CPT,* for each *encounter.* They document experience for such purposes as *certification* or *accreditation,* application for hospital privileges, and research. They are well replaced by computer systems which often combine automated accounting. VIII.C.

experience rating. a method of establishing health insurance premiums in which the premium is based on the average cost of actual or anticipated health care used by various groups and subgroups of subscribers and thus varies with their experience or with such variables as age, sex, or health status. The most common way of establishing premiums for health insurance in private programs, compare *community rating.* IV.A.

experiment. synonym, *trial.*

experimental design. the logical framework of a *trial* or *study.*

Experimental design seeks to assure obtaining or detecting real effects and to avoid artificial or ambiguous observed differences. VIII.D.

experimental group. see *control group.*

experimental health service delivery system (EHSDS). a program, developed with support from the Health Services and Mental Health Administration, DHHS, using general health services research authority, to develop, test, and evaluate the organization and operation of coordinated, community-wide health service management systems in various kinds and sizes of communities.

EHSDS sought to improve access to services, moderate their costs, and improve their quality. This small program in the early 1970s was one of several generally unsuccessful efforts to organize the disparate health programs of a community into a coherent system; compare *community health network* and *comprehensive health planning.* III.B.1.

experimental medical care review organization (EMCRO). an organization assisted by a program initiated in 1970 by the National Center for Health Services Research and Development, Department of Health and Human Services (now the National Center for Health Services Research).

The program, a forerunner of the *PSRO* program, helped medical societies create formal organizations and procedures for reviewing the quality and use of medical care in hospitals, nursing homes, and offices in defined communities. The use of explicit criteria and standard definitions was required of all EMCROs, but the particular approach to review was up to the individual organization. Ten such organizations were supported, only some of which actually reviewed services, and the program ended with enactment of the PSRO program, now the *PRO (peer review organization)* program. IV.D.2.

experimental psychology. use of experimental methods to obtain psychological data, solve problems in *psychology,* or study psychologic phenomena; compare *clinical psychology.* III.C.

experimenter bias. investigator behavior or expectations that are inadvertently communicated to subjects or affect the objectivity of observers such that they influence experimental findings. VIII.D.

expert. 1. someone from out of town with a bunch of slides. 2. "x," an unknown quantity, and "spurt," a drip under pressure.

According to *Ryan's law, anyone making three correct guesses consecutively will be established as an expert.

See *expert witness*. VIII.B.2.

expert witness. a witness qualified to speak authoritatively by reason of special training, skill, or familiarity on a scientific, technical, or professional matter; slang, synonym, hired gun.

Physicians conventionally qualify as expert witnesses on medical matters. Expert witnesses differ from others in several respects: they were not usually originally party to the events at issue, their expertise as well as their honesty may be questioned, and their interpretation or opinion of facts may be sought in addition to the facts (and be opposed by other experts). VIII.B.3.

explanation of benefits (eob). the clause in an insurance policy stating the coverage or benefits, exclusions, and so forth. IV.B.

explanatory model. the understanding that a physician, patient, or family has of an illness's causes, natural history, and proper care.

It is not obvious to physician or patient that their explanatory models of the same illness are never the same and often not even similar; the physician's is usually a *medical model* and the patient's an intuitive *biopsychosocial* approach. III.C.

exploitation. unjust or improper use of another person for one's own advantage; in *adult protective services* law, improper use by a *caretaker* of government funds paid to the adult or caretaker for care of the adult, as when the drunken child drinks the aged *incompetent* parent's Social Security check. I.B.2., VII.B.3.a., VIII.B.3.

exposure. 1. subject to something that may have detrimental effects, as weather, radiation, allergens, infectious agents, or occupational hazards; the amount of such thing received, compare *dose*. 2. in law, public display of sexual organs before the opposite sex for gratification or erotic purposes; synonym, indecent exposure; 3. in insurance, *risk*, vulnerability to *loss*.

Exposure may be quantified, as in radiology the exposure is the x-ray dose delivered in rads, and be limited, as by occupational safety and health standards. The distinctions between total exposure, exposure per unit time, and exposure per unit receiver are important because the effects of equivalent total exposures may vary with the time course over which exposure is given and with who receives it. Exposures are not necessarily deleterious, but their effects may be long delayed.

See *threshold exposure*. I.C., IV.B., VII.B.3.

extended care facility (ECF). previously used in Medicare to mean a *skilled nursing facility* which qualified for participation in Medicare. In 1972 the Social Security Act was amended to use the more generic term skilled nursing facility in both Medicare and Medicaid.

Medicare coverage is limited to 100 days of posthospital extended care services during any *spell of illness*. These 100 days are sometimes still referred to as the *extended care facility benefit. Thus Medicare coverage in a skilled nursing facility is limited in duration, must follow a hospital stay, and must be for services related to the cause of the hospital stay. These conditions do not apply to skilled nursing facility benefits in Medicaid. III.B.1.

extended care services. in Medicare, *skilled nursing facility* services provided for up to 100 days for a *spell of illness* after a hospital stay and for the condition for which the patient was hospitalized.

Coverage is for skilled nursing facility inpatient nursing care provided or supervised by a registered professional nurse, bed and board associated with the nursing care, needed physical, occupational, or speech therapy, medical social services, ordinary drugs, biologics, supplies, appliances, and equipment, services of an intern or resident of a hospital with which the facility has a transfer arrangement, and other services necessary to patient health.

See *intermediate care*. VII.C.5.b.

extended duration review. see *continued stay review*.

extern. a medical student who helps with care of hospitalized patients.

Externs often do an *intern's* job, with or without pay or additional supervision, rather than the clerk's job on a *rotation* usually done by a student. IV.A.1.

external benefit, externality. synonym, *social benefit*.

external cost. a cost not borne by the producer, as a *social cost* or one borne by the consumer; antonyms, external or social *benefit* and *internal cost*.

Some external benefits and costs, unlike externalities, may be controllable by the producers, although they lack incentive to do so, as pollution. VII.D.1.

external validity. the applicability of experimental findings beyond their original experimental occasion or setting without its specific subjects, conditions, or measurements; compare *validity*. VIII.D.

externality. something affecting the cost or benefit of an economic activity, but outside the direct control or responsibility of the economic units involved and independent of market mechanisms, as the weather; the effects of such things. *External economy is a factor or effect favorable to the economic units, a *positive externality; *external diseconomy is detrimental or negative. Used generally in its plural form, externalities; synonym, *spillover*. Compare *internal cost* and *social cost*.

An external economy affects the participating economic units, an external benefit or cost does not, but the distinction is illusive and irregular. VIII.B.1.

externship. the state or position of being an extern; the period of an extern's service.

See *COSTEP*. IV.A.1.

extra cash policy. an insurance policy which pays cash benefits to hospitalized individuals in fixed amounts unrelated to their medical expenses or income.

Such policies are typically sold separately from whatever other health insurance people have and have high *loadings*. IV.B.2.

eye bank. see *blood bank*.

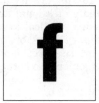

facility. any building or physical plant and, usually, its *equipment.*
Health facilities are a major *health resource.* They include hospitals, nursing homes, ambulatory care centers, and a variety of other kinds of buildings. As used in *certificate of need* and comparable regulatory programs, they do not usually include the offices of individual practitioners. III.B.1.

factitial, factitious. induced by deliberate human action, with or without intention, to produce a lesion or disease; not *natural* or spontaneous; compare *functional.* II.B.1.a.

factitious disorder. see *Munchausen syndrome.*

factoring. the practice of one individual or organization selling accounts receivable or unpaid bills to a second party at a discount. The latter organization, the *factor, ordinarily assumes full risk of loss if the accounts prove uncollectible, compare *collection agent.*
Factoring is common where delays experienced in collecting from a payment program are long or the patients are hard to collect from. In such cases the improved cash flow is worth the *discount* in the amount received by the provider. Because factoring is subject to *fraud* and *abuse,* its uses have been regulated. IV.A.

fair rental system. a method for reimbursing nursing homes for *capital* using a simulated rent based on the current value of assets in lieu of separate payments for *depreciation,* return on equity, and even interest payments.
Such systems, in use in 1986 in West Virginia and Maryland, replace traditional cost-based and flat rate systems, and have the advantage of recognizing increasing value of assets without requiring sale or lease transactions.

Read Cohen, Joel, and John Holahan, "An Evaluation of Current Approaches to Nursing Home Capital Reimbursment" (*Inquiry*, 23(1): 23–39, Spring/1986). III.B.1.

faith healing. a system or practice of treating disease by religious faith or prayer, as *Christian Science.*

One does not usually heal oneself, but goes to one who has the power, a *shaman.* V.

Falk, Isidore S. U.S. bacteriologist and health services researcher, 1899–1984. His contributions to the study of the costs of medical care in the 1930s and his conceptualization of a health system built around capitated group practices were methodologic and theoretical miracles which include among their progeny *health maintenance organizations.* VIII.A.1.

fallout. see *radioactive fallout.*

false negative (FN). an erroneous or deceptive negative reaction to a *test;* contrast *true negative* and *false positive.*

In assessing a screening or diagnostic procedure, it is important to know how many false and true negatives and positives it gives in normal use.

See *efficiency* and *predictive value, sensitivity,* and *specificity.* VIII.D.

false positive (FP). an erroneous or deceptive positive reaction to a *test;* contrast *true positive* and *false negative.* VIII.D.

falsifiable hypothesis. a *hypothesis* stated in sufficiently precise fashion that it can be tested by acceptable rules of logic and empirical and statistical evidence, and thereby found to be either right or wrong. An *unfalsifiable hypothesis is one that is so general and/or ambiguous that all conceivable evidence can be "explained" by it. VIII.D.

familial. occurring among or pertaining to the members of a family, as a familial disease.

Many familial conditions are not *genetic* or *hereditary,* distinctions often lost. I.A.1., I.B.2.

family. 1. generically, a group with things in common or similarities, whether past and future, genes, residence, sex, or interests. 2. in family medicine, a basic social unit whose members have a commitment to nurture each other, "characterized by two generations of persons bound together by marriage, blood, or adoption, who are emotionally dependent upon one another and responsible for their development, stability, and protection" (*Pinney and Slipp, 1982*). 3. in law, variable, as for census purposes, a group of two or more persons related by blood, marriage, or adoption who are living together. 4. in insurance, a *covered* individual and his *dependents.*

Families nurture their members physically and emotionally, and share resources, including shelter, time, and money. A healthy family is one whose members see it as cohesive and offering the nurturing necessary for personal growth and sustenance in the face of life's tasks; compare *functional family.* An individual's family is the people he identifies as such.

For demographic purposes a family is usually a group of people sharing a common household. A relationship (not necessarily by blood or marriage ties) is implied. This may include people temporarily residing away from home.

Families have many definitions, structural and functional, and forms, whether consisting of single individuals, having a single parent, skipping generations, or being blended or reconstituted and based on a marriage of people previously married. One's *family of origin or orientation is the one of one's birth; the *family of procreation has one's children. I.B.1.

Family Adaptability and Cohesion Evaluation Scales (FACES). a set of self-report scales designed to measure individual family members' perceptions of the two major parameters of functioning in a family: adaptability and cohesion.

Scores are obtained for various facets of adaptability, including the handling of assertiveness, control, discipline, negotiation, roles, rules, and system feedback, and similar aspects of cohesion, including the nature of independence, family boundaries, coalitions, time, space, friends, decision-making, and interests and recreation. I.B.1.

family-centered family. family in which "there is a strong emphasis on the importance of the whole family as a unit, and individuals are submerged to the needs and functions of the family group" (*Pinney and Slipp,* 1982) rather than those of an individual, the adults, or the children. I.B.1.

family chart. a record, especially a medical record, of a family's history, present structure and functioning, problems, and progress.

Family charts may consist of individual member charts, but are more than the sum of the parts since they contain organized cross-referencing among members and family data, like genograms, not usually found in traditional histories and physicals. Whether or not all individual charts are filed or presented together at each encounter with a family member, knowledge of the whole family should be readily available in a single organized file. This is typically an appendage to an index family member's chart, whether the first seen, the father's, or mother's. V.

family constellation. see *sibling position.*

family developmental task. see *developmental task.*

family ganging. the practice of requiring or encouraging a patient to return for care to a health program with his whole family, even if the rest of the family does not need care, so the program can charge the patient's *third party* for care given to each member of the family.

The practice and term originated and is most common in *Medicaid mills,* which may have the mother of a sick child bring in all her other children for care, whether or not they need it. IV.C.2., VIII.B.2.a.

family health center. any place that treats families; specifically, a limited form of *community health center* supported briefly by the Department of Health and Human Services in the 1970s, then the Department of Health, Education, and Welfare. III.B.1.

Family Health Foundation of America (FHFA). a nonprofit foundation founded in 1958 and funded by contributions from family physicians, dividends from the *AAFP*'s membership insurance programs, and grants from other foundations.

It supports research and education in family medicine, and the *Family Practice Working Party.* V.C.

family history. in a traditional individual medical *history,* pertinent facts about the person's family, usually limited to recording the principal diseases suffered by his blood relatives. There is no standard form or scope.

Family medicine uses more historical and current structural and functional information, recorded in *genograms* and *family charts,* for family work and other purposes, still without standardization. II.A.1.

family life cycle. the sequence of developmental events families pass through as they mature.

Achieving these stages enlarges and ensures family life, but the effort may provoke critical incidents, cause family problems, and provoke symptoms in family members. There are many versions of the life cycle, usually differing only in details.

Read Carter, Elizabeth A. and Monica McGoldrick, *The Family Life Cycle: A Framework for Family Therapy* (New York: Gardner Press, Inc., 1980). I.B.1.

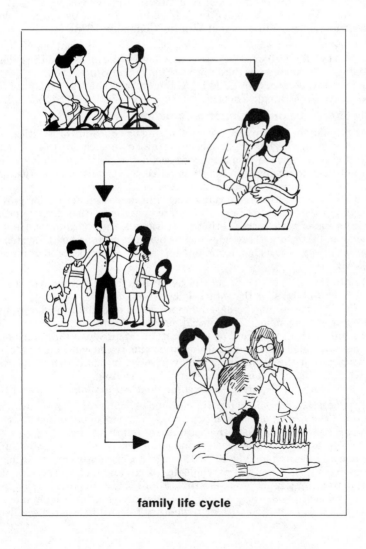

family life cycle

family medicine. the medical *specialty* devoted to the maintenance of the health of families and their members; the body of knowledge, techniques, and skills used in caring for families.

Family medicine shares with medicine, pediatrics, obstetrics, and psychiatry the provision of a large amount of *primary care,* and with preventive medicine, public health, and occupational health its focus on *health maintenance* rather than disease. The family physician uses his special knowledge of how the functioning of communities and families determines the health of families and their members, along with general medical knowledge and the assistance of other specialists and professionals, in treating both individuals and their families. Effective family practice requires both *comprehensive* and *continuous* care; combines knowledge of the behavioral, biologic, and clinical sciences; and uses *biopsychosocial* and *relational models,* as well as the *medical model,* of health and disease.

Read Medalie, J.H., ed., *Family Medicine—Principles and Applications* (Baltimore: The Williams and Wilkins Company, 1978). III.C.

family myth. "beliefs based on kernels of historic reality but elaborated and shared by all family members that help determine and shape the rules governing relationships in the family" *(Pinney and Slipp, 1982).*

Read Anderson, S. A., and D. A. Bagarozzi, "The Use of Family Myths as an Aid to Strategic Therapy" *(J Fam Ther,* 5(2): 145–54, 5/83). I.B.2.

family of orientation, origin, or procreation. see *family.*

family physician. 1. a physician specializing by education or practice in family medicine, whether or not specially trained for such practice. Sometimes limited to physicians who are *board certified* in family medicine, whether or not they are engaged in family practice. 2. casually, and particularly in lay use, a *personal physician* or *general practitioner.*

The family physician assumes continuing responsibility for providing *comprehensive* care to the families in his practice, either directly or by coordination of the efforts of other professionals and *consultants.* He is physician of first contact, provides means of entry into the health system, and serves his patient as medical manager, educator, advocate, and counselor. III.A.1.

family planning. deliberate control by an individual or couple of the number of child births, or the intervals between them.

The planning may be based on individual or social considerations and use various physiological, physical, or chemical means, as contraception, rhythm method, *abortion,* or sterilization. Family planning may seek to avoid unwanted births, control the interval between children, or the age at which parents have children. It may involve, in addition to *birth control,* sex education, and genetic and marital counseling.

See *National Reporting System for Family Planning Services.* I.B.1.

family practice. 1. medical practice devoted primarily or exclusively to maintaining the health of the families and their members enrolled in or using the practice. 2. practice of the specialty of family medicine.

Such practice includes acute and chronic care of the illnesses suffered by the families and individuals in the practice, preventive medicine for those who are not sick, and the psychologic, social, and dietary services needed for maintaining functioning families. Family practice provides *comprehensive* and *continuous* care, although special problems may be managed using either consultation with or temporary referral to other specialists. V.

family therapy. therapy concerned with improving family structure and functioning, often by working with as many family members as possible simultaneously.

The problem with which therapy is concerned may present through an individual, and therapy will affect all family members individually, but the focus is the family. Family therapy differs in major ways from analytic and most other individual therapy; little use is made of insight, intervention is flexible and directive, practitioners are not usually physicians, and training is ordinarily done under direct observation. There are many schools of family therapy defined, including behavioral, Bowen, conflict resolution, conjoint, extended, interactional, psychoanalytic, social network, strategic, and structural; and various types of therapists. V.

Farr, William. English physician, 1807–1883. He was the creator of modern *vital statistics*. His reports from the Registrar-General's office provided ammunition for *sanitary* reform during the middle and later nineteenth century. II.C., VIII.A.1.

fascinoma. slang, an interesting *case*. VIII.B.2.a.

fatality rate. see *mortality rate*.

fat doctor. slang, a physician specializing in care of people with obesity, see *bariatrics*.

Fat doctors are rarely *endocrinologists* or otherwise especially trained. Some use fairly poisonous, expensive, and irrational hormone regimens. III.A.1., VIII.B.2.a.

favorable selection. see *skimming*.

fecundity. see *birth rate*.

Federal Employees Health Benefits Program (FEHBP). the group health insurance program for U.S. government employees.

The largest employer-sponsored *contributory* health insurance program in the world, FEHBP is voluntary for the employees. About 80 percent of those eligible choose coverage. It was established under the Federal Employees Health Benefits Act of 1959 (P.L. 86-382, codified at 89 U.S. Code), began operation in 1960, and is administered by the U.S. Civil Service Commission. Every employee may choose upon employment or during *open seasons* among: two government-wide plans, a *service benefit* plan administered by Blue Cross and Blue Shield, and an *indemnity benefit* plan; 15 employee organization indemnity plans for organization members; and a variety of *health maintenance organizations*. Each plan is a *FEHBP plan. IV.C.

Federal Food, Drug, and Cosmetic Act (FD&C Act). the principal law regulating the *safety, efficacy, labeling*, and *packaging* of *foods, drugs, biologics*, and *cosmetics* in interstate commerce in the United States.

The FD&C Act was originally enacted in 1907 and is codified in Title 21 of the U.S. Code. It is administered by the *Food and Drug Administration*. VII.B.2.e.

Federal Insecticide, Fungicide, and Rodenticide Act (FIFRA). the federal law authorizing the regulation of *labeling*, use, and *exposure* to *pesticides*.

The law has been administered primarily by the Environmental Protection Agency in consultation with the Department of Agriculture and OSHA. Its provisions have been used, in preference to those of the *OSHAct*, for protecting farm workers by such measures as field reentry standards and pesticide labels. I.C.

Federal Register.   an official daily publication of the U.S. government providing a uniform system for making available to the public proposed and final *rules*, legal notices, and similar proclamations, orders, and documents having general applicability and legal effect. The Register publishes material from all federal agencies.
See *notice of proposed rule making*. III.D.1.

Federal Security Administration (FSA).   original name for the *Department of Health and Human Services*.

Federal Trade Commission (FTC).   the agency of the U.S. government responsible for the regulation of trade and commerce.
It enforces the Sherman antitrust laws and regulates business practices, including advertising. The FTC has given recent important attention to professional services, because professional societies and ethics limit advertising, restrict *competition*, and fix prices through *relative value schedules*. III.D.1.

Federation Licensing Examination (FLEX).   a standardized licensure test for physicians, developed by the Federation of State Medical Boards for nationwide use.
Nearly all states now use the FLEX as their exam at least for *FMGs*. It is based on test material developed by the *National Board of Medical Examiners* and is a 3-day exam with the days corresponding roughly to the parts of the National Board Examination: *basic science, clinical science,* and clinical competence. A score of 75 is typically required for passing, although there is some variation among states in the score required for licensure. III.A.1.

Federation of State Medical Boards (FSMB).   the national association of state medical licensing boards.
It provides common services to the various states, as development and administration of the *Federation Licensing Examination*. III.A.1.

fee.   a *charge* or *price*, particularly for public or professional services. VII.D.1.

Fee and Cost Index Program.   a proposed American Medical Association program designed to help physicians determine fees; a successor to *relative value scales*. IV.A.

feedback.   see *biofeedback* and *evaluate*.

fee for service.   a method of *charging*, in which a physician or other practitioner bills for each *encounter* or *service*.
With fee for service, expenditures increase if fees increase, if more units of service are charged for, or if more expensive services are substituted for less expensive ones. This contrasts with salary, *capitation*, and *prepayment* systems, where expenditures do not change with the number of services actually used. The fee for service system is used by physicians, dentists, podiatrists, chiropractors, optometrists, and most *solo practitioners*.
See *fractionation* and *unbundling*. IV.A.

fee schedule.   a listing of *charges* or established *benefits* for specified medical or dental procedures, as a physician's or third party's usual or maximum charges for the listed *procedures*.
See *relative value scale*. IV.A.

fee screen.   a schedule of maximum amounts which a payment program will pay for listed services and procedures without special justification.
Screens are sometimes based on *usual* or *prevailing charges*. IV.B.

fee splitting.   sharing of the fees for professional services without informing the patient, as when a specialist shares his fee with a referring physician.

Fee splitting is an unethical, and in some jurisdictions an illegal, way of soliciting business, because the patient pays the referring physician twice and cannot rely on him to choose the specialist with only the best interests of the patient in mind. IV.A.

feldsher.   in the Soviet Union and other countries, a medical worker with training and responsibilities intermediate between those of nurse and physician; compare *nurse practitioner* and *physician assistant.*

Most feldshers practice *primary care,* often independently in rural areas. III.A.4.

fellow (F).   1. a member of an incorporated scientific or professional society, as a Fellow of the American College of Physicians (FACP) or Fellow of the Royal College of Surgeons (FRCS). Fellowship is often limited to those with special qualifications, as election, seniority, or *board certification.* 2. a physician who has completed residency and been granted a stipend and position for further study and research in a subspecialty, as a cardiology fellow. III.A.1.

fellow-servant doctrine, rule.   the common law principle that an employer or master is not liable for injuries to an employee or servant caused or contributed to by the *negligence* of a fellow servant, as long as the employer has exercised due care in selection of employees.

Availability of this defense, along with that of *contributory negligence,* to employers helped make compensation through tort law for occupational *impairments* ineffective, and led at the turn of the century to the creation of *workmen's compensation* programs. VII.B.2.d., VIII.B.3.

fertility rate.   see *age-specific fertility rate* and *birth rate.*

fetal death.   a *stillbirth* in which death occurred before labor and delivery; an intrauterine death. I.A.1.

fiduciary.   relating to or founded upon a trust or confidence.

A *fiduciary relation, an important concept in law, exists where an individual or organization, a *fiduciary, has an explicit or implicit obligation to act in behalf of another person's or organization's interests in matters which affect the other person or organization. A physician has such a relation with his patient and a hospital trustee with a hospital. Because a fiduciary relationship with a *provider* obligates one to act in the interests of the provider, people with such relationships are defined as providers, rather than as *consumers,* by federal *health planning* law. VIII.B.3.

fifth pathway.   one of the four ways U.S. *foreign medical students* and *graduates* enter *graduate medical education* or practice in the United States.

The fifth pathway provides a year of clinical training, often comparable to an *externship,* sponsored by a U.S. medical school to students who obtain their premedical education in the United States, complete undergraduate medical education abroad, and pass a screening exam approved by the *Coordinating Council on Medical Education.* Successful completion of the year makes the student eligible for a U.S. *internship* or residency, i.e., for the *match.* These students generally complete formal course work in a foreign school, but may not receive a degree if they do not perform required social service in the host country; the sponsoring U.S. school generally does award the candidate a degree. III.A.1.

file. in insurance, claim *benefits.* IV.B.

Finagle factor. changing the universe to fit the equation. VIII.B.3.

Finagle's laws. 1. the likelihood of something happening is inversely proportional to its desirability. 2. once a job is fouled up, anything you do to improve it only makes it worse. VIII.B.3.

final epidemic. nuclear war.

Man may yet kill himself and seems more likely to do it this way than by spoiling and exhausting his environment. This epidemic is only preventable.

Read Adams, Ruth, and Susan Cullen, eds., *The Final Epidemic: Physicians and Scientists on Nuclear War* (Chicago: The University of Chicago Press, 1982. 254 pp. $4.95, softbound). II.C., VIII.C.

first aid. immediate and temporary care given the victim of an accident or illness until *medical care* can be obtained.

See *cardiopulmonary resuscitation.* VII.B.3.a.

first-dollar coverage. *coverage* by an insurance policy which begins with the first dollar of expense incurred by the insured for the covered *benefits;* coverage without *deductibles,* although it may have *copayments* or *coinsurance;* compare *last-dollar coverage.* IV.B.

fiscal agent, intermediary. a contractor that processes and pays provider claims on behalf of a state Medicaid agency.

Fiscal agents are rarely *at risk,* but rather serve as an administrative unit for the state, handling the payment of bills. They may be insurance companies, management firms, or other private contractors. Medicaid fiscal agents are sometimes also Medicare *carriers* or *intermediaries.* IV.C.2.

fiscal year (FY). any 12-month period for which annual accounts are kept. The U.S. fiscal year is October 1 through September 30; the calendar year and July 1 through June 30 are also common. VI.C.2.

fit. 1. a seizure or other brief episode of illness or activity. 2. trained, suited, or qualified for an object or design. 3. *healthy.* 4. in biometry, the agreement of probable and actual data or of curves from explanatory equations and actual experience.

Physical fitness includes endurance, suppleness, balance, strength, speed, and skill or coordination, and requires *exercise* and other effort to create and maintain. 3. I.A.2.b., 4. VIII.D.

fixed benefit. an *indemnity benefit,* payable by reason of occurrence of a covered event, the amount of which is independent of the expense incurred; compare *scheduled* and *unscheduled benefit.*

Such policies also may specify an *aggregate indemnity, a maximum payable benefit per unit time or event. IV.B.2.

fixed cost. in accounting, a *cost,* as real estate, that does not vary in total as the level of production or activity changes over a limited range, the *relevant range.

In the long run and with large enough changes in production, all fixed costs become *variable costs.* VI.C.1.

flat maternity. in insurance, a single inclusive *maternity benefit* for all charges resulting from a pregnancy, childbirth, and any complications. A limit, as $2000, may apply per pregnancy or year.

See *swap* and *switch maternity.* IV.A.

flexible residency. a first-year *residency* cosponsored by residency programs in more than one specialty, usually allowing the resident the choice of pursuing further training in either specialty.

The first year of *graduate medical education* used to be the *internship* but now comes in several, evolving forms, compare *transitional year.* III.A.

Flexner Report. (Abraham Flexner, U.S. educator, 1866–1959) a 1910 study of the 155 medical schools then existing, made for the Carnegie Foundation for the Advancement of Teaching, and published under the title *Medical Education in the United States and Canada.*

It helped cause, and guided, major reforms and standardization of both medical education and statutory requirements for physicians in these two countries.

Read King, Lester S., "The Flexner Report of 1910" (*JAMA,* 251(8): 1079–86, 2/24/84). III.A.1., VIII.A.2.

Flick, Lawrence F. Philadelphia physician, 1856–1934. He organized the first tuberculosis society in the United States. He thus created the pattern for the *voluntary health agency,* a valuable *institution* for mobilizing the forces of the community for control of disease. III.B.4., VIII.A.1.

Fliedner, Theodor (1800–1864) and Friederike. German pastor and wife. They began formal training of women as nurses, founding a school in 1833 visited and copied in England by *Florence Nightingale.* III.A.2., VIII.A.1.

fluoridation. addition of controlled, small amounts of fluorine salts to public water supplies to reduce the *incidence* of dental caries in people using the water.

Appropriate fluoride levels in water reduce cavities; excess amounts, whether from *natural* sources or *pollution,* cause mottling of tooth enamel. VII.B.2.a.

fluoride. any gaseous, solid, or dissolved compound containing fluorine.

Fluorides are *emitted* into air or water from a number of industrial processes, including steel, aluminum, glass, and brick manufacturing. Fluorides in the air damage vegetation and, indirectly, livestock. I.C.1., I.C.5.

fog. see *particle.*

folk medicine. lay or nonprofessional medical understanding and practice, learned through personal experience and tradition rather than from scientific teaching.

Colds from cold feet and treatment with chicken soup are folk medicine. Practitioners range from everybody's parents to *curanderos* and *shamans.* III.C.

follow-up. 1. pursue closely and continuously; strengthen an effect by further action; repeat or reexamine. 2. in medicine, maintain contact with a case; a case so followed.

Follow-up follows a diagnosis or service and may be for further therapy or for study of the results.

See *workup.* V.B.

fomite. an inanimate object, as cloth or a dish, that is *contaminated* with *infectious* organisms and serves in their transmission; compare *vector.* I.C., VIII.C.

food. any substance containing or consisting of *nutrients,* which can be ingested or otherwise assimilated by a living organism and contributes to the maintenance of life; synonym, nutriment.
This includes water and minerals. Some definitions are limited to organic substances which can be used for energy or tissue building. The Federal Food, Drug, and Cosmetic Act defines food as, "(1) articles used as food or drink for man or other animals, (2) chewing gum, and (3) articles used for components of any such article." The three main types of food are protein, carbohydrate, and fat.
See *diet, health, natural,* and *organic food.* I.A.2.a.

food additive. anything added to food in processing; an *additive* found in food.
Food additives are defined in the Federal Food, Drug, and Cosmetic Act in an odd, elaborate way which includes *food irradiation* and are regulated by the Food and Drug Administration. They serve a variety of purposes, as antioxidants, antispoilants, coloring agents, emulsifiers, minerals like iodide to prevent goiter, preservatives, and vitamins. They present several problems, as *carcinogens* or *mutagens.*
See *Delaney amendment* and *generally recognized as safe.* I.A.2.a.

Food and Agricultural Organization (FAO). the agency of the United Nations responsible for international programs to improve and assist agriculture and to receive and distribute food. I.A.2.a, III.D.2.

Food and Drug Administration (FDA). the agency within the Department of Health and Human Services responsible for regulating the *safety, efficacy, labeling,* and packaging of *food, drugs, biologics,* and *cosmetics* offered for sale in the United States. I.A.2.a., III.D.1.

food chain. successive feedings of one organism on another in a constant and recurring series, each feeding being referred to as *trophic level.
At each feeding, matter or energy is transferred from a producer to a consumer animal or vegetable species within an *ecosystem.* Food chains are not strict linear series but constitute an interdependent *system,* a *food web. I.A.2.a.

Food, Drug, and Cosmetic Act of 1907 (FD&C Act). the principal federal authority for regulation of the *labeling* and *advertising* of *food, biologics, drugs,* and *cosmetics* offered for sale in interstate commerce.
The act has been amended on many occasions, and like most basic federal legislative authorities, is usually referred to without the "of 1907." The act's often arcane language is now so surrounded by court interpretation in case law that it rarely means what it says and cannot be changed without ruining the careers of the few lawyers who understand it. I.A.2.a., III.B.3., VIII.B.3.

food irradiation. *exposure* of spices, fruit, meat, or other food to gamma rays or high energy electrons to kill insects, bacteria, viruses, or other *contaminants,* or to prevent sprouting.
Irradiation does not make food *radioactive* and is *safe, effective,* and inexpensive. The Federal Food, Drug, and Cosmetic Act was amended in 1958 to define it as a food additive rather than a food handling process, as freezing or canning. This imposed requirements for safety testing more appropriate to chemical additives and for *labeling* of irradiated foods that have

limited development and use of the technology in the United States. I.A.2.a., I.C.3

food waste. animal and vegetable *waste* resulting from the handling, storage, sale, preparation, cooking, and serving of foods; synonym, garbage. I.C.4.

foot zone therapy. synonym, *Ingham Reflex Method of Compression Massage.*

foreign medical graduate (FMG). a physician who graduated from a medical school outside the United States and, usually, Canada (whose schools have the same *accreditation* as U.S. schools).

U.S. citizens graduating from schools abroad are known as *US-FMGs. Foreign graduates of foreign schools are distinguished as *F-FMGs. The term is occasionally defined as, and nearly synonymous with, any graduate of a school not accredited by the Liaison Committee on Medical Education. FMGs constitute about 20 percent of all U.S. physicians.

See *Coordinated Transfer Application System, Educational Commission for Foreign Medical Graduates, fifth pathway, J visa, labor certification, schedule A,* and *visa qualifying examination.* III.A.1.

foreign medical student (FMS). a student at a medical school outside the United States and Canada, whether a U.S. citizen (*US-FMS) or not. III.A.1.

forensic. legal, as in *forensic medicine, the medical specialty concerned with the relation and application of medical facts to legal problems; synonyms, legal medicine and medical jurisprudence. III.C.

formula grant. a grant of federal funds, usually to states but sometimes to other governmental units or private organizations, in which the grant amount is based on a formula which divides total funds available among eligible recipients using such variables as the number and average income of the populations served. IV.C.

formulary. a list of drugs, usually intended to include a sufficient range of medicines to enable users to prescribe medically appropriate treatment for all reasonably common illnesses; occasional synonym, *pharmacopeia.*

A hospital formulary lists, typically by generic name, all the drugs routinely stocked in the hospital pharmacy. *Substitution* of a *chemically equivalent* drug in filling a prescription by *brand name* for a drug in the formulary is often permitted. A formulary may also be used to list drugs for which a *third party* will or will not pay, or drugs which are considered appropriate for treating specified illnesses.

See *American Hospital Formulary Service* and *compendium.* III.B.3.

forward funding. see *advance appropriation.*

foster care. supervised *care* for orphaned, neglected, or delinquent children, or for persons with *mental disorders,* usually in a substitute home, a *foster home, or occasionally in an institution on a full-time or *day-care* basis; compare *boarding home.*

Foster homes are ordinarily approved by a government or social service agency which arranges and supervises their care. VII.C.1.

foundation. a philanthropic organization established, by endowment or with some other provision for future maintenance, for some purpose like making grants to support research.

Foundation, *charity,* and *institute* are somewhat irregularly used and occasionally synonymous. III.B.4.

foundation for medical care. synonym, *medical foundation.*

Fox's laws. *house staff* slang, three aphorisms describing hospital patients: 10 percent of the population has 90 percent of the disease, nice guys get cancer, and trash survives. Fox's identity is lost, his chart having been signed out to an illegible signature years ago. III.B.3.

Fracastoro, Girolamo. Veronese physician, 1478(?)–1553. As early as 1546 in *De Contagione* he enunciated a rational theory of infection as due to the passage of minute bodies from the infector to the infected. These hypothetical seeds had the power of self-multiplication. Fracastoro also wrote a poem on syphilis, which described the disease precisely, and gave one of the first good descriptions of typhus fever. I.A.1., VIII.A.1.

fractionation. *charging* separately for several services or components of a service previously subject to a single charge or not charged for at all; synonym, *unbundling.*

The usual effect is to increase the total charge. Thus, it is a response to regulating increases in the charge which is fractionated. VII.D.1.

Framingham Heart Study. a *prospective study* of *risk factors* for cardiovascular disease, based on a *cohort* of 5209 people in Framingham, Massachusetts, who have been followed with routine complete examinations every 2 years since 1948.

Read Dawber, T.R., *The Framingham Study: The Epidemiology of Atherosclerotic Heart Disease* (Cambridge, MA: Harvard University Press, 1980. 257 pp.). VIII.D.

fraud. intentional deceit, deception, or misrepresentation by either providers or consumers to obtain services, payment for services, or program eligibility; compare *abuse.*

Fraud includes the receipt of services obtained by deliberate misrepresentation of need or *eligibility,* providing false information concerning costs or conditions to obtain reimbursement or certification, or claiming payment for services which were never delivered or received. Fraud is illegal and carries a penalty when proved. VI.D., VIII.B.3.

free care. care provided without *charge* or, for some purposes, without *collections;* compare *bad debt.*

The *Hill-Burton* program requires assisted hospitals and other facilities to make available "a reasonable volume of services to persons unable to pay therefor," sections 603(e) and 1604 (b)(1)(J)(ii) of the *Public Health Service Act.* These and supporting requirements are known as the *free care provisions. They have been the subject of much litigation since enactment because for years they were neither honored nor enforced. III.B.1., VII.D.1.

free clinic. a neighborhood *clinic* or health program providing free or inexpensive medical services in a relatively informal setting and style, generally to students, transient youths, or minority groups.

The first free clinic was the Haight-Ashbury Free Clinic, organized in San Francisco in the summer of 1967 by David Smith (U.S. physician). III.B.1.

freedom of choice. in U.S. medicine, the principle that patients should be free to choose their own physicians, other sources of services, and treatment and, by extension, physicians their own therapeutic advice, consultants, and charges.

Historically, this principle reflects the belief that the physician-patient relationship is most effective when voluntary and free of outside constraint. It has been used to oppose government or other organization or regulation of services, not to encourage *competition.* Thus Medicaid law requires that state Medicaid plans do nothing to inhibit freedom of choice. Authority for the Department of Health and Human Services to waive the requirement was enacted in 1981 because the provision had frustrated effective use of *formularies,* program experimentation, and cost control. IV.C.2., V.

free good. see *good.*

Freeman rule. a standard of legal sanity holding that "a person is not responsible for criminal conduct if at the time of such conduct as a result of mental disease or defect he lacked substantial capacity either to appreciate the wrongfulness of his conduct or to conform his conduct to the requirements of the law"; compare *Durham decision* and *M'Naghten rule.*

The rule arises from *U.S. vs. Charles Freeman,* 1966, and is the basis in the Model Penal Code of the *American Law Institute Formulation.* VIII.B.3.

freestanding facility. one not connected to another, ordinarily housing a health program under its own management dedicated to one primary purpose, as a locally owned hospital which is only a hospital. III.B.1.

fresh water. of or belonging to water that is free of sodium chloride, specifically, or salts, minerals, *contamination,* and taste or odor, generally; compare *drinking water* and *water quality.* I.C.5.

Freud, Anna. Austrian psychoanalyst, 1895–1982. Daughter of Sigmund Freud, noted for her contributions to the developmental theory of *psychoanalysis* and its application to preventive work with children. III.C.

Freud, Sigmund. Austrian physician, 1856–1939. Founder of *psychoanalysis.* He modeled and explored the development of the self and showed that some of its dysfunctions had no physical or religious basis, arising instead from badly organized feelings, instincts, defenses, and thoughts. These dysfunctions he treated by exploring and recreating the self with the patient. III.C.

Frontier Nursing Service (FNS). a program of *rural health services* in Kentucky, noteworthy for its age, size, training and use of *nurse clinicians,* and extensive *home health care.* III.A.2., III.B.1.

Frost, Wade H. Epidemiologist, 1880–1938. He developed *epidemiology,* dealt with epidemiological problems in a rigorous scientific manner, and established epidemiology as a science applicable to community health problems. VIII.A.1., VIII.C.

Frye Report. popular name for *Protecting the Health of Eighty Million Americans: A National Goal for Occupational Health* (Special Report to the Surgeon General of the U.S. Public Health Service, HEW, November 19, 1965).

The only significant policy document in *occupational health* in the 1960s, it called for increased research on the occupational environment and estimated the economic costs of occupational disease. VII.B.2.d.

fugitive literature. see *medical literature.*

full-service benefits. see *service benefits.*

fume. see *particle.*

fumigant. a volatile or volatilizable chemical compound used as a disinfectant or *pesticide,* as *ethylene dibromide.* *fumigate. use a fumigant; occasional synonym, *smoke.* I.C.1.

function, functional classification. in the federal *budget* and accounting, organization of *budget authority, outlay* and *tax expenditure* data, and accounts in terms of the principal purposes the funds are intended to serve.

Each specific account is placed in the single function, like national defense or health, that best represents its major purpose, regardless of the agency administering the program. The Congressional Budget and Impoundment Control Act of 1974 requires estimation of budget authority, outlays, and tax expenditures for each function. Functions are subdivided into narrower categories called subfunctions. VI.B.1.

functional. in medicine, changes in normal activity or bodily operation that are not attributable to known physical or structural alterations; compare *organic.*

Functional disorders, usually *psychosomatic,* are real, albeit unexplained. II.B.1.a.

functional family. one "in which there is complementarity between its members, with mutual accommodation to each other's needs, clear and flexible boundaries between individuals, and the ability to resolve conflict and create change in accord with the family's life cycle" (*Pinney and Slipp, 1982*). I.B.1.

funded. in insurance, having sufficient funds to meet future *liabilities;* also used of *trust funds* for *social insurance* programs with sufficient funds to pay covered benefits. *Capital depreciation* is funded if amounts included in an *institution's* reimbursements for capital depreciation are set aside in a fund used for capital purposes rather than being spent on current operating costs. IV.B., VI.A.

fungicide. see *pesticide.*

funny looking kid (FLK). slang, a *child* with a visible *deformity,* usually *congenital.* Typically used in the acronym form for children with subtle or undiagnosed departures from normal. I.A.1.

furfuraceous. branny; having thin light scales. VIII.B.3.

fusion. combination or lack of *differentiation of self* from others or of intellect from emotion.

In the former, *enmeshment* and failure to develop autonomy result. In the latter, intellect remains an infantile appendage of emotion. I.A.2., I.B.1.

Galenus, Plaudius (known as Galen). Greek physician, 130–200. Born in Pergamum in Asia Minor, he later practiced in Rome, where he became physician to the emperor, Marcus Aurelius. Although he did not dissect the human cadaver, he made many valuable anatomic and physiologic observations on animals. His influence on medicine was profound for many centuries. His teleology, "nature does nothing in vain," was particularly attractive to the medieval mind, although stultifying to medical thought and practice. VIII.A.1.

gang visit. slang, an *encounter* with several people simultaneously for which each is charged and would be better served individually, as a visit with all the patients in a nursing home dining room.
　　See *family ganging.* VII., VIII.B.2.a.

garbage. synonym, *food waste.*

gastroenterologist. a physician trained in or practicing gastroenterology. III.A.1.

gastroenterology. the *subspecialty* of *internal medicine* concerned with the instestines and liver. III.C.

gatekeeper. a designated health professional, typically a physician, who provides a patient's *primary care* and whose *referral* of the patient for specialist services is a condition of *third party* payment for such services; compare *lock in.*
　　General practitioners in the British National Health Service and other European countries have long functioned as gatekeepers. Their introduction in *health maintenance organizations* and other U.S. programs is intended to control costs and to improve *continuity* of care by case management.

Read Somers, Anne R., "And Who Shall Be the Gatekeeper? The Role of the Primary Physician in the Health Care Delivery System." (*Inquiry*, XX(4): 301–13, Winter/1983). III.A.1.

gene pool. all reproductively available genes in a breeding *population*, characterized by the alleles that are present and their relative frequency. II.C.

general and administrative cost (G and A). a *cost* that cannot be attributed to an identifiable *cost center, function*, or responsibility; compare *overhead*. VII.D.1.

general duty clause. the provision of the *Occupational Safety and Health Act*, section (5)(a)(1), requiring an employer to "furnish each of his employees employment and a place of employment which are free from *recognized hazards* that are causing or are likely to cause death or serious physical harm to his employees."

Employers must also comply with standards promulgated under the Act's authority. Since standards cannot reach all hazards, the general duty clause, which codifies a common law principle, can be used when standards are not available, and makes clear the employer's general responsibility for the *healthfulness* of the workplace. VII.B.2.d.

generally recognized as effective (GRAE). one of the qualities a *drug* must have if it is not to be considered a *new drug* and thus not subject to the premarket approval requirements of the Federal Food, Drug, and Cosmetic Act.

To be generally recognized as *effective* a drug must be considered so by "experts qualified by scientific training and experience to evaluate the *safety* and effectiveness of drugs" and must have been "used to a material extent or for a material time." The Food and Drug Administration determines that a drug is GRAE, subject to judicial reversal if its determination is arbitrary or capricious. The FDA may require for its determination from drug sponsors the same kind of evidence, consisting of *adequate and well-controlled investigations* by qualified experts, required for approval of a *new drug application*. III.B.3.

generally recognized as safe (GRAS). one of the qualities a *drug* must have if it is not to be considered a *new drug*, or a food must have if it is not to be considered a *food additive*.

A drug which is GRAS or GRAE need not go through the premarket approval procedures prescribed in the Federal Food, Drug, and Cosmetic Act for new drugs. General recognition of the *safety* of a drug must be "among experts qualified by scientific training and experience to evaluate the safety and *effectiveness* of drugs" and may come only after the drug is "used to a material extent or for a material time." III.B.3.

general practice. "the provision of *primary, comprehensive, continuing* whole-patient care to individuals, families, and their community" (The Royal Australian College of General Practitioners, *The Scope of General/Family Practice: The Discipline of Family Medicine* (Jolimont, Victoria 3002, Australia: The Royal Australian College of General Practitioners, 1/81)). V.

general practitioner (GP). a practicing physician who does not specialize in any particular field of medicine, i.e., is not a *specialist;* contrast *family phy-*

sician, a specialist in family medicine, and *primary care* physician, who may be a specialist in any of several specialties.

Generalists, horizontal people in our vertical world, are important people, but the old general practitioners were not trained for it. III.A.1.

general revenue. government revenue raised without regard to the specific purpose for which it may be used.

Federal general revenues come principally from personal and corporate *income* taxes and some *excise* taxes. State general revenues come primarily from personal income and sales taxes. Expenditure of general revenues is determined by legislative *authorizations* and *appropriations.* IV.C.

general surgeon. a physician specializing by *practice* or education in general surgery; a surgeon not engaged in one of the surgical specialties.

In an era of oversupply, without enough surgery to keep them busy, some general surgeons practice general medicine, for which they are not trained. III.A.1.

general surgery. surgery as a whole, not confined to a particular surgical specialty.

General surgery has become limited to surgery not belonging to one of surgery's specialties (colon and rectal surgery, microsurgery, obstetrics and gynecology, ophthalmology, orthopedic surgery, otolaryngology, pediatric surgery, plastic surgery, thoracic surgery, and urology), principally abdominal and *minor surgery.* Most surgeons have at least one year of training in general surgery. General surgeons have three years of residency in general surgery, while the other surgical specialists have their additional years of training in their specific specialties. III.C.

generic drug. a drug known or prescribed by its *established name,* rather than a *brand name.*

A *labeled or *branded generic drug is one prescribed or sold under its generic name with specification of which manufacturer's formulation of the drug is to be used, as propoxyphene (Lilly), rather than simply propoxyphene or Darvon. Manufacturers may sell their branded generics for less than their own brand name versions. III.B.3.

generic equivalents. drug products from different sources *labeled* with the same *generic name.*

Generic equivalents have the same active chemical ingredients, but may have different *inactive ingredients* and compounding, and often have different *brand names.* Generic equivalents are often assumed to be, but are not necessarily, *therapeutic equivalents.* III.B.3.

generic name. the *established,* official, or nonproprietary, name by which a *drug* is known as an isolated substance, irrespective of its manufacturer; synonym, nonproprietary name.

A drug will be approved for marketing under only one generic name, but may be given a different *brand name* by each of its manufacturers. The generic name is assigned by the *United States Adopted Names Council. Prescribing* drugs by generic name instead of by brand name is said to allow considerable cost savings, but controversy continues over whether drugs sold by generic name are *therapeutically equivalent* to their brand name counterparts. Two versions of the same drug, manufactured by the same or different manufacturers, may not, usually for reasons of *bioavailability,* be therapeutically equivalent. Advocates of generic prescribing question whether such differences are common or significant.

See *antisubstitution law, International Nonproprietary Names,* and *Maximum Allowable Cost Program.* III.B.3.

genetic. produced by, or related to, genes, biologically *inherited,* thus *congenital.* I.A.1.

genetic engineering. the science by which the genetics of organisms are made useful to man, typically by changing or *recombining the DNA in which an organism's genetic information is encoded.

See *biotechnology.* I.A.1., III.B.3.

Geneva Cross. synonym, *Red Cross.*

genius. see *intelligence quotient.*

genogram. a formal mapping, included in *family charts,* of family, medical, and other history, built on a family tree, and recording current structure and function, critical incidents, and major medical and life events.

See *proband.* I.B.1., V.

genotype. 1. the hereditary constitution of an organism resulting from its particular combination of genes and their *penetrance.* 2. a class of individuals with the same *genetic* constitution. I.A.1.

geratology, gerontology. the study of *aging.* III.C.

geriatric. of or pertaining to *aging.* I.A.1.

geriatrics. the branch of medicine concerned with *aging,* diseases of the aging, and the care of old people and their illnesses. III.C.

geriatrician, geriatrist. a physician specializing by training or practice in geriatrics. III.A.1.

gerontology. synonym, *geratology.*

Gerson Therapy. (Max Gerson, German physician, 1881–1859) obsolete dietary therapy for cancer, arthritis, and a variety of other chronic ailments. V.

gestalt psychology, therapy. a system of *psychology* and therapy emphasizing the wholeness of experience and that psychologic processes and *behavior* cannot be described adequately by the elements of experience alone, but only by integration into a whole perceptual configuration.

Gestalt psychology was developed by Otto Rank, Wilhelm Reich, Fritz Perls, and others in reaction to behaviorism, atomistic approaches to psychology, and *psychoanalysis.* Therapy relies on sudden learning by insight, rather than by trial and error or association; compare *holistic medicine.* It has survived by flexible growth of its practices, particularly the relatively recent introduction of the use of groups.

Read Perls, Frederick, *Gestalt Therapy Verbatim* (Bantam, 1971). V.

Ginsberg's theorems. 1. you can't win. 2. you can't break even. 3. you can't even quit the game. VIII.B.3.

goal. in health *planning,* a quantified statement of a desired future state or condition, as an infant mortality rate of less than 20 per thousand live births, a physician to population ratio greater than 4 per thousand, or an average access time for emergency medical services less than 20 minutes.

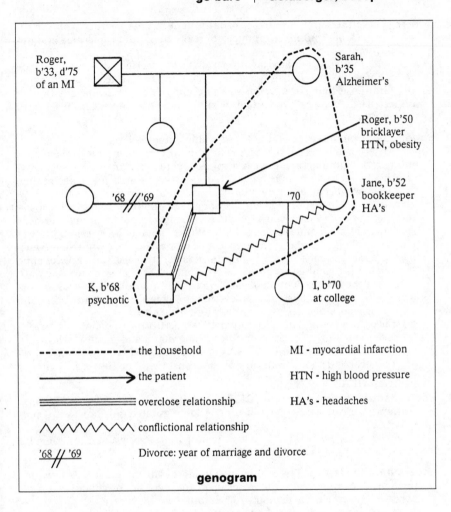

Roger, b'33, d'75 of an MI

Sarah, b'35 Alzheimer's

Roger, b'50 bricklayer HTN, obesity

Jane, b'52 bookkeeper HA's

'68 // '69   '70

K, b'68 psychotic

I, b'70 at college

------------- the household   MI - myocardial infarction

———→ the patient   HTN - high blood pressure

≡≡≡≡ overclose relationship   HA's - headaches

ΛΛΛΛΛΛ conflictional relationship

'68 // '69   Divorce: year of marriage and divorce

genogram

Health planning formulates goals and seeks to achieve them. A goal differs from an *objective* by lacking a deadline, and usually by being long range (5 to 10 years) rather than short (1 to 2 years). VI.A.

go bare. practice without *malpractice* insurance.
Going bare was unheard of until the malpractice crisis of the late 1970s and is still rare, particularly for institutions. It may be done with or without formal *self-insurance.* V.D.

Goldberger, Joseph. U.S. *Public Health Service* physician, 1874–1929. He solved the riddle of pellagra by showing it was a *deficiency disease* due to lack of tryptophan or niacin. Tryptophan is an amino acid lacking in the corn-based diet of the poor in the U.S. south. As with many such contributions, the impact of pellagra and importance of its prevention are forgotten. VII.B.2.e., VIII.A.1.

gomer. hospital slang, a patient, usually male, whose senility, chronic illness, or lack of *compliance* promises to make his care troublesome and unrewarding.

It may have originated as an acronym for "get out of my emergency room," or as a corruption of "gumma" (the characteristic lesion of late syphilis, a disease that once produced many old gomers), but ancient British dialect used "gomeral" for a fool or simpleton. It is ordinarily used with friendly tone. VIII.B.2.

good. anything having a value to individuals and society.

An *economic good, or *commodity, is any product from agriculture, mining, or manufacturing with a market value in a monetary economy, which value derives from being wanted, relatively scarce, and transferable. *Services* are goods, albeit nonmaterial ones and therefore sometimes separated, as in the expression "goods and services." Here usage is inconsistent; goods sometimes being defined as tangible products and services separated as intangible ones. A *free good, or *nonmonetary commodity, is one available in abundance at no economic cost at the point wanted. If transportable, it becomes an economic good after transportation. Economic growth tends to make free goods, as fresh air, clean water, or scenery, into economic goods by reduction of their quality or quantity. A *social good is one which has a higher value to society in general than to any economic unit, and whose market price is therefore difficult to estimate. A *capital good is an economic good, as equipment, structure, or raw material inventory, used for the production of other goods. Land and money technically are not included as capital goods. A *consumer good is a durable or nondurable economic good used directly by consumers for the satisfaction of their own wants. VIII.B.1.

good manufacturing practice (GMP). a federal Food and Drug Administration requirement for how food or other regulated substances are prepared.

Food made with GMP is not considered *adulterated* and may legally move in interstate commerce. I.A.2.a.

good samaritan law. a law or provision in most state malpractice laws which provides that a physician who comes upon an *emergency* by chance and gives needed medical care is exempt from liability for such care.

These laws are intended to keep the threat of a malpractice suit from discouraging a physician (and in some cases other health professionals) from giving care in an emergency where facilities are inadequate or where the needed care lies outside the physician's expertise. Good samaritan laws do not exempt from liability care given in a facility or by a physician who normally treats emergencies. V.D.

gorc. variant, *gork,* from "God only really cares."

Gorgas, William Crawford. U.S. physician, 1854–1920. Known for the eradication of yellow fever and control of malaria in Havana and the Panama Canal Zone, making construction of the Panama Canal possible. He was president of the American Medical Association in 1908, and Surgeon General of the Army during World War I. VIII.A.1.

gork. *house staff* slang, originally an acronym for "God only really knows," and then used of patients with problems which defied diagnosis; variant, *gorc.* It has lost all connection with the original meaning and is used offensively of patients who are, and are likely to remain, comatose. VIII.B.2.a.

governmental immunity. in *malpractice* law, the ancient doctrine that the government cannot be sued for the *negligent* acts of its officers, agents, or employees unless it consents to such suit.

Governmental immunity originated in common law, and the principle has been firmly established that a state cannot be sued without its consent. Like *charitable immunity,* governmental immunity has been limited as states and the federal government have enacted statutes, as the Federal Tort Claims Act, specifying how they may be sued. V.D.

grace period. in insurance, a specified period, typically 30 days, after a premium payment is due on an insurance policy, during which time the policyholder may make the payment and the policy protection continues. IV.B.

graduate medical education. medical education after receiving the medical doctorate or equivalent degree, including education received as an *intern, resident,* or *fellow,* and *continuing medical education.*

This contrasts to graduate school education after college leading to a masters or doctoral degree, what is known as *undergraduate medical education* in medicine. Graduate medical education may include supervised practice, research, and even teaching, as well as didactic learning. III.C.

Graduate Medical Education National Advisory Committee to the Secretary (GMENAC). a committee appointed in 1976 by the Secretary of the Department of Health and Human Services to make recommendations on the supply of and requirements for physicians, their specialty and geographic distribution, and methods for financing graduate medical education.

The GMENAC reports were most important for reversing federal policy from supporting an increasing supply of physicians to attempts to limit supply. III.D.2.

graduate nurse (GN). a *registered nurse* educated in a *baccalaureate degree program.*

Such nurses have more didactic (and often less *clinical*) training than graduates of *associate degree* and *diploma* programs. Supervisory nursing jobs are sometimes open only to graduate nurses. Sometimes "graduate nurse" refers to a nurse who has finished any kind of training program but has not passed the state board exam. They put GN after their names in charting and are paid less than RNs. III.A.2.

grandfather clause, provision. one which exempts people or things from the requirements of a law or regulation if they are already established when the requirements become effective.

Grandfather clauses may permit continued eligibility or coverage for individuals or organizations receiving benefits under a law despite a change in the law which would otherwise make them ineligible. For example, they may permit licensure of existing practitioners who cannot meet educational requirements of a new licensing law. III.B.3.

Graunt, John. see *Petty, William.*

green screen. administrative slang, limit consideration of which services a health program will provide to those which will make money.

Other considerations, as availability of resources and community need, apply only to services which make it through the green screen. VI.A., VIII.B.2.a.

Greyhound therapy.   the psychiatric practice of buying particularly difficult, refractory, or dangerous patients one-way bus tickets to faraway places. Sometimes also practiced by police and other social service agencies. II.B.2., III.C.

group.   in *group insurance,* a set of *subscribers* eligible for group insurance by virtue of a common identifying attribute, as common employment or membership in a union, association, or other organization. Groups considered for insurance are usually larger than nine people. IV.B.

group insurance.   any *insurance* plan by which a number of employees of an employer and their *dependents,* or members of a similar homogenous group, are insured under a single policy, issued to their employer or the group, with individual *certificates of insurance* given to each insured individual or family.

Individual employees may be insured automatically by virtue of employment, only on meeting certain conditions (employment for over a month), or only when they elect to be insured (and usually to make a contribution to the cost of the insurance, see *contributory insurance).* Group health insurance is typically *experience rated* and less expensive for the insured than comparable individual insurance, because an employed population is generally healthier than the general population, and because of lower administrative costs, especially in marketing and billing. Note that the policyholder or insured is the employer not the employee. IV.B.

group practice.   a formal association for joint provision of services of three or more physicians or other health professionals, with income from the practice pooled and redistributed to the members of the group according to some prearranged plan (often, but not necessarily, through partnership); compare *solo practice.*

Groups may be single specialty or multispecialty and vary in size, composition, and financial arrangements. They include *health maintenance organizations, preferred provider organizations,* and other *prepaid group practices.* III.B.1., V.

guardian.   a person lawfully charged by a court, will, or statute with care of a *minor* or other *incompetent* person, the *ward, and usually also charged with managing the property and rights of that person. VII.B.3.

guideline.   synonym, *criterion* or *policy.*

gum farmer.   slang, *periodontist.* III.A.3., VIII.B.2.a.

gundeck physical.   a fast or fake *physical examination,* written as though done more completely than was actually the case.

In the Navy gundecking something hides it from inspection. Gundeck physicals are done when a hundred recruits must be completely examined in an hour. V.A., VIII.B.2.a.

gynecologist.   a physician specializing by practice or education in gynecology; a specialist in obstetrics and gynecology who limits his practice to gynecology. III.A.1.

(gyn).   the part of *obstetrics and gynecology* devoted to the study and care of women's diseases, particularly of their sexual organs. III.C.

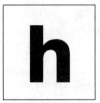

habilitate. to make capable. *habilitation. bringing to a state of *fitness,* as by treatment or training, overcoming *congenital handicaps* and *developmental disabilities;* compare *rehabilitation.* V.B.

habitat. in ecology, the particular *environment* in which a specific organism or *community* of organisms naturally lives; an artificial environment in which people and other organisms can live under surrounding inhospitable conditions; a space used for human domestic activities.

Local environmental conditions, current technology, and the lifestyle or culture of the community largely determine the design and construction of local habitats or settlements.

See *biomass.* I.C.

habituation. 1. gradual adaptation to *environment,* accompanied by learning what stimuli and responses to expect from the environment. 2. development of a *habit, a *behavior* pattern fixed by repetition. 3. development of tolerance to the effects of a drug, poison, or other *exposure,* acquired by repeated use or contact and sometimes accompanied by *addiction.*

See *drug dependence.* I.A.2.

half-life ($t_{1/2}$). the time required for half of something which *decays,* loses activity, or disappears from a defined space to do so, as for a dose of a drug to be half cleared from the body or for a *radioactive* isotope to lose half its activity. The half-life of the remaining half is not necessarily the same as it was for the first half. I.A.1

halfway house. a residential facility for the formerly institutionalized, as mental patients, addicts, or prisoners, which facilitates their readjustment to private life and independent living; compare *deinstitutionalization, partial hospitalization,* and *shelter.* III.B.1.

halo effect. the effect (usually beneficial) which the manner, attention, and caring of a provider have on a patient during a medical encounter regard-

243

244 **Hamilton, Alice | Harvey, William**

less of what medical procedures or services the encounter actually involves; compare *Hawthorne effect* and *placebo*. VIII.D.

Hamilton, Alice. U.S. industrial hygienist, 1868–1970. She devoted her attention to toxicology, studied lead poisoning, and helped make *occupational health* a concern of the community.

Read Sicherman, Barbara, *Alice Hamilton: A Life in Letters* (Cambridge: Harvard University Press, 1984. 460 pp.). VII.B.2., VIII.A.1.

handicap (HC). "a disadvantage for a given individual, resulting from an *impairment* or *disability*, that limits or prevents the fulfillment of a role that is normal (depending on age, sex, and social and cultural factors) for that individual" (*International Classification of Impairments, Disabilities, and Handicaps*. Geneva: World Health Organization, 1980); irregularly synonymous with *deformity*, disability, and impairment.

Federal education legislation has required assisted schools to provide proper education for handicapped children. The Architectural Barriers Act requires buildings built with federal assistance to be constructed in such a way that the handicapped can use them, as with ramps and doors wide enough for wheelchairs. I.A.1., II.

handicapped individual. "any person who (i) has a physical or mental *impairment* which substantially limits one or more of such person's major life activities, (ii) has a record of such an impairment, or (iii) is regarded as having such an impairment" (section (7),(B), the Rehabilitation Act of 1973, 29 U.S.C. 706 as amended).

The act is a good example of the nuances of legal definition. Within the act itself the definition is at times limited to people who "can reasonably be expected to benefit in terms of employability from *vocational rehabilitation* services," or to exclude "any individual who is an *alcoholic* or *drug abuser* whose current use of alcohol or drugs prevents such individual from performing the duties of the job in question or whose employment, by reason of such current alcohol or drug abuse, would constitute a direct threat to property or the safety or others." An alcoholic in *remission*, discriminated against because he was an alcoholic, is a handicapped individual because of (iii): he is perceived as impaired. One who is currently drunk is not a handicapped individual, unless the job is mattress testing. One need not be handicapped to be a handicapped individual, as long as one has a record of having been handicapped or is perceived as such. I.A.1., II.

hanging crepe. portraying a patient's *prognosis* as worse, and more certainly so, than it actually is, typically as almost certainly fatal. Often also used, inaccurately, to describe accurate portrayal of a certainly fatal prognosis.

This approach to communicating prognosis protects the physician's image, shields him from liability, and defends against anxiety. It prepares the family for the worst and allows them to gather and begin mourning. It is also dishonest and will eventually tell the patient he is dying at a time when, with his, his physician's, and his family's best effort, he might well survive.

Read Siegler, Mark, "Pascal's Wager and the Hanging of Crepe" (*N Engl J Med*, 293: 853–7, 10/23/75). II.B.3.

Harvey, William. British physician, 1578–1657. His brilliant inductive reasoning and experiments, described in his 1628 *De motu cordis*, established him as the true discoverer of the circulation of the blood. He was also one of the first to doubt the doctrine of preformation of the fetus. II.C.

Hawthorne effect. the fact that changing the conditions of production, as altering the workplace, whether for better or worse, will increase productivity. Occasionally, in medicine, the beneficial effect an encounter has on a patient which is independent of the encounter's medical content; compare *demand characteristic, halo effect,* and *placebo.*

The name comes from classic industrial management experiments at the Hawthorne Plant of the Western Electric Company; increasing lighting increased productivity more than decreasing the lighting did, but both increased it. The effect confounds *health services research* since it suggests anything works. VIII.D.

hazard. an adverse chance; a danger or *peril* of injury, loss, or acquiring disease; a thing or condition which is the source of, or increases, such chance or danger, as slippery floors, *exposure* to *asbestos,* or *noise.*

Wage differentials for workers engaged in particularly *hazardous work are known as *hazard pay. There is no regular distinction between ordinarily and particularly hazardous work. Workers have a fairly well established common law right to refuse such work.

See *health hazard, moral hazard, recognized hazard, safety hazard, target health hazard,* and *synergism.* I.C.

hazardous air pollutant. a *pollutant* for which no ambient *air quality standard* is applicable because any of its presence in the air may cause or contribute to an increase in death or serious illness, as *asbestos,* beryllium, and mercury. I.C.1.

hazardous waste. see *waste.*

heal. to make sound, well, or whole; to restore to health; compare *care* and *cure.*

Sometimes the hardest things get the simplest definitions. V.B.

healer. anyone who cures, or professes healing powers. Usually applied to *Christian Science* practitioners and others outside conventional medicine. III.A.

health. 1. "a state of complete physical, mental, and social well-being and not merely the absence of *disease* or *infirmity*" (World Health Organization). 2. the condition of being sound in body, mind, or spirit, free of disease and disability, and in an optimum state of equilibrium with the environment. 3. general condition or degree of well-being, as in poor health; compare *welfare.* *healthful. beneficial to health. *healthy. well, having health, as healthful air, healthy people.

The concept of health as an equilibrium which maintains the structural and functional integrity of the organism is probably more useful than the political ideal of the WHO. Health has many dimensions, compare *mental health,* and much cultural variability. Measurement is usually negative in terms of *morbidity* and *mortality,* since they are easier to assess than *health status.* I., II.

health and accident insurance (H&A). see *accident and health insurance.*

Health and Nutrition Examination Survey. see *National Health and Nutrition Examination Survey.*

health authority. a government-owned corporation organized to carry on governmental health programs, managed according to business principles by an appointed or elected board, and usually to some extent independent of the government.

Relatively uncommon in the United States, although some public hospital systems, as in Miami and New York City, are run by health authorities and public authorities are common for other services, as transportation. In Great Britain, the *National Health Service* is run by regional health authorities (RHA), which in turn rely upon area health authorities (AHA). In 1982–1983 the latter were replaced by smaller district health authorities (DHA). VI.C.

health card.   an identification card, similar to a credit card, included in some *national health insurance* proposals, which would be issued to each covered individual or family.

The card would be used at the time of service in lieu of cash payment. The individual would subsequently receive a bill for any *cost sharing*. Health cards, it is said, would simplify eligibility determination, billing and accounting, and the study of use of services. The idea presents interesting *confidentiality* problems, particularly with respect to the Federal Credit Disclosure Act. IV.D.

health care.   any conscious effort to influence events to improve individual health, as *medical care;* the collective health of families or communities, as *public* and *occupational health;* or the healthfulness of people's various environments, as *environmental health.* Often a synonym for medical care, as "the provision of advice, therapy, education, etc., by qualified professionals to improve or maintain the health of one or more patients" (*NAPCRG, 1978*).

health care delivery system.   a *system* for providing health care; usually the whole of the medical resources and programs serving an area, person, or group, whether or not coordinated or working together in any real degree. *Alternative health care delivery systems are then any other, new, unusual, or uncommon ways of organizing the resources and programs needed to provide health care to such an area, person, or group, as a health maintenance organization.

Alternative health care delivery system is an ill-defined, well-avoided, buzz phrase in medical politics, standing for any coherent effort to do better than the free market system. VII.C.2.

Health Care Financing Administration (HCFA).   the agency within the Department of Health and Human Services which administers federal health financing and related regulatory programs, principally the *Medicare, Medicaid,* and *Peer Review Organization* programs. III.D.1., IV.C.

health care provider.   "any individual who *renders* health services within the field of his/her qualification" (*NAPCRG, 1978*). III.A.

health care system, health services system.   "the organizational structure through which health care is provided" (*NAPCRG, 1978*); compare *health care delivery system.* VII.C.2.

health care technology.   the *technology* of *health care;* the means, methods, and language of promoting health and preventing, diagnosing, and treating disease.

The emphasis is usually on the things used, particularly the new and expensive ones, as *CT scanners.* Society's response to these and such ethically important technologies as safe, simple *abortions* has been *technology assessment* and occasional efforts at legal control. Most technology is still controlled only by market forces.

See *medical technologist.* III.C.

health department. an office or division of a city, county, or state responsible for enforcement of health and *sanitation* laws and for operating *public health* programs. III.D.2.

health education. 1. the act or process of developing knowledge of health and disease, or healthful skills, behavior, or character, especially by formal instruction. 2. the field of study and profession concerned with such education.

Health education is given in schools and other group settings and to patients and other individuals, using a variety of instructional media and methods. It may provide *health information,* promote healthful behavior, see *health promotion,* or concern itself with the creation of healthful environments.

See *activated patient.* VII.B.2.a.

Health Education Assistance Loan Program (HEAL). a federal program of loan guarantees for private loans to medical students with interest rates tied to those of 91-day U.S. Treasury bills, about 20 percent in 1981. III.D.1.

Health Education Information Retrieval System (HEIRS). a collection of literature related to health education, indexed and accessible by the *HEIRS Thesaurus of Health Education Terminology* (prepared by the editorial staff of *Health Education Monographs,* the official publication of the Society of Public Health Educators, published by the Bureau of Health Education of the Centers for Disease Control, and available from the National Technical Information Service, HRP-0014366, 1975). V.C., VII.B.2.b.

health educator. an individual with training or experience in, or who practices, health education.

In the United States most health educators are trained at the master's degree level. III.A.4.

health facility. any *facility* used in the provision of health care. Usually limited to facilities built primarily for providing health care, thus does not include a school with a nurse's office, factory with an *infirmary,* or office building with a physician's office.

See *bed, boarding home, capital, certificate of need, clinic, Hill-Burton, institutional health services, JCAH, Life Safety Code, modernization,* and *proprietary hospital.* III.B.1.

health fair. a voluntary program, lasting a few days at most, which offers health education and medical *screening* to self-referred participants at little or no cost.

In 1984 as many as 2 million people attended health fairs in malls, community centers, and parking lots, undergoing about 20 million blood chemistry tests. The value of these programs remains to be demonstrated.

Read Berwick, Donald M., "Screening in Health Fairs: A Critical Review of Benefits, Risks, and Costs" (*JAMA,* 254(11): 1492–9, 9/20/85). VII.B.2.b.

health food. food with, or said to have, healthful or therapeutic properties; any food sold in a health food store.

Many, but not all, are *natural* or *organic.* Most offer several unproven benefits. These are usually not mentioned in the *labeling;* doing so would subject them to Food and Drug Administration scrutiny. However, books, magazines, and testimonials available in the same stores amply instruct the shopper. Health foods are not just nutritious; they make you healthy, increase longevity, or improve your sex life. I.A.2.a.

healthful. see *health.*

health hazard. a *hazard* or danger to health, particularly one which may cause disease rather than injury; compare *safety hazard.*

The disease resulting from a health hazard may be acute or chronic, have a long latency or *incubation* period before developing, particularly if the original *exposure* is brief, and may be difficult to diagnose early. *Occupational health* is concerned with workers' health, both in the course of work and after leaving it, either for the day or after retirement. In *safety,* the concern is primarily the time the worker is working. Since occupational health hazards may act more slowly on the body than safety hazards, may compound the effects of nonoccupational health hazards, as smoking, may be of many different kinds which act simultaneously, and may manifest themselves when the worker is no longer at his job, the task of preserving workers' health must necessarily be more complicated than that of assuring workers' safety. Health hazards can be grouped in four types: physical— *noise,* heat, vibration, and *radiation;* chemical—*dusts,* poisonous fumes and gases, toxic metals and chemicals, and *carcinogens;* biologic—bacteria, fungi, and insects; and *stressful*—physical, psychologic, and *ergonomic.* I.C., VII.B.2.d.

health hazard appraisal. *prognosis* for the well; prediction, based upon study of an individual's present physiology, *behavior,* and situation, of his *longevity* and probability of developing diseases for which he is *at risk;* compare *multiphasic screening.* VII.B.2.b.

health index. a measure of *health status.*

Health indices summarize data describing two or more aspects of an individual or group to give an approximation of health, as *longevity* and *maternal mortality.*

See *indexed* and read National Center for Health Statistics, *Clearinghouse on Health Indexes: Cumulated Annotations, 1976.* (U.S. DHEW Publ. No. (PHS) 78-1225. Washington: U.S. Government Printing Office, 9/78). II.C.

health information. 1. facts and intelligence concerning health. 2. that part of *health education* concerned wth developing knowledge of health and disease.

See *health promotion.* V., VII.B.2.b.

health insurance. insurance against loss by illness or accidental injury to the insured.

Such insurance usually covers medical costs of treating the disease or injury and may cover other losses, as of earnings. It may be either *individual* or *group insurance.* IV.B.

Health Insurance Benefits Advisory Council (HIBAC). an advisory council to the Department of Health and Human Services which makes recommendations on *policy* in the administration of Medicare and Medicaid.

The council consists of 19 nongovernmental *experts* in health-related fields who are selected by the Secretary of DHHS and hold office for terms of 4 years. It is authorized by section 1867 of the Social Security Act. IV.C.1.

Health Insurance for the Aged and Disabled. the *social insurance* program authorized in 1965 by Title XVIII of the Social Security Act and known as *Medicare*. IV.C.1.

health maintenance. care and services devoted to creating and maintaining optimum health in individuals and families.

Such care includes *self-care, screening,* and *prevention.* Health maintenance is difficult because it is hard to obtain *compliance* when there is no problem, and hard to deal with aspects of life which affect health but are not ordinarily medicine's concern, like social connectedness, education, and vocation.

See *checkup* and *Lifetime Health Monitoring Program.* V.C., VII.B.3.b.

health maintenance organization (HMO). a health program with four essential attributes: (1) an organized *system* for providing health care in a geographic area, which accepts responsibility to provide or otherwise assure the delivery of; (2) an agreed upon set of *basic* and *supplemental health services* to; (3) a voluntarily *enrolled* group of persons; and (4) for which services the program is reimbursed through a predetermined, fixed, periodic prepayment made by or on behalf of each person or family unit enrolled without regard to the amounts of actual services provided (from section 1301 of the *Public Health Service Act*).

An HMO is responsible for providing health services required by enrolled individuals or families and specified in the contract between the program and the enrollees. Prototype HMOs were the Kaiser-Permamente system of *prepaid group practices* and the early *medical foundations.* They demonstrated the ability to provide high-quality medical services for less money than the rest of the medical system because of low hospitalization and surgical rates, and preventive care.

See *group practice, health care delivery system, individual practice association, qualified, skimping,* and *skimming.* III.B.1.

health manpower. people providing *health care,* whether as individual practitioners or employees of health programs, and whether or not professionally trained or subject to public regulation.

Facilities and manpower are the principal *resources* used in producing health services. U.S. health manpower law divides the health professions in four major groups: medicine, osteopathy, and dentistry (*MODs); veterinary medicine, optometry, podiatry, and public health (*VOPPs); nursing; and *allied health personnel.*

See *academic health science center, capitation, certification, Coordinating Council on Medical Education, credentialing, foreign medical graduate, graduate and undergraduate medical education, internship and residency, practice, professional,* and *proficiency and equivalency testing.* III.A.

Health Manpower Education Initiative Award (HMEIA). a Department of Health and Human Services grant or contract to a health or educational entity for a health manpower program which will improve the distribution, *supply, quality, use,* and/or *efficiency* of health personnel and the *health care delivery system.*

These awards were authorized in 1971 through section 774 of the Public Health Service Act. Support has been provided for such activities as development of *area health education centers,* training of *physician assistants,* and identification and encouragement of disadvantaged students with a potential for training in the health professions. III.A.

health officer. an agent, usually of a city, county, or state, responsible for enforcement of health and *sanitation* laws and for operating *public health* programs. III.A.5.

Health/PAC Bulletin. see *Health Policy Advisory Center.*

health planning. *planning* concerned with improving health and health care, whether undertaken comprehensively for a whole community, see *comprehensive health planning*, or for a particular population, type of health service, or health program.

Some definitions include all activities undertaken for improving health, as education, traffic and environmental control, and nutrition, as responsibilities of the planning process. Other uses limit planning's responsibility to conventional health services and programs, *public health*, or *personal health services.* U.S. health planning policy, funding, and operations were largely defined by the National Health Planning and Resources Development Act of 1974, P.L. 93-641. Although the federal statute was repealed in 1986, many states continue their own programs.

See *budget, goal, health systems agency, management, objective,* and *state health planning and development agency.* VI.A.

Health Policy Advisory Center (Health/PAC). a consumer and labor-oriented, radical center of thought about the organization and operation of the U.S. health care system. III.B.1.

health professional. see *professional.*

Health Professions Student Loan Program (HPSL). a program of federal funding for loans from medical schools to students for tuition and other expenses.

Created in 1963, the program was attractive because of low interest rates, delay of interest and payback until 9 months after completing residency, and partial forgiveness of obligations by service in health manpower shortage areas. III.A.1.

health promotion. encouraging consumer *behaviors* most likely to optimize health potential through *health information*, preventive programs, and access to medical care (from *Medical Subject Headings*); *health education* and other organizational, political, and economic efforts intended to change behavior and *environments* in ways which will improve or protect health. VII.B.2.a.

health provider. see *provider.*

Health Research Group. an organization founded by Ralph Nader (U.S. lawyer and consumer advocate) which studies and represents public health interests. It is particularly known for its publications, participation in the legislative process, and monitoring of regulatory agencies. III.B.4.

health resource. any *resource* available for or used in the provision of health care.

This includes *capital, health manpower, health facilities, equipment,* and *supplies.* Resources, available or used, can be measured and described for an area, see *medically underserved area,* population, see *medically underserved population,* or individual program or service. III.

health service area (HSA). a geographic *region* appropriate for the effective *planning* and development of health services.

Section 1511 of the *Public Health Service Act* requires that health service areas be delineated throughout the United States. The governors of the various states designate the areas using requirements specified in the law respecting geography, political boundaries, population, health resources, and coordination with areas defined for other purposes. In each area, planning is then done by a designated *health systems agency*.

See *catchment area, locality,* and *medical trade area.* VI.A.1.

Health Service, Inc. (HSI). a stock insurance company organized in Illinois by *Blue Cross plans* to serve as a national enrollment agency, assist individual plans in negotiating contracts, and serve large national accounts in which two or more plans are involved. While HSI and *Medical Indemnity of America* are separate companies with separate boards of directors, they have an integrated administration and a common president. II.B.1.

health services research. *research* concerned with the organization, operation, financing, effects, or other aspects of health services; contrast *biomedical research.*

In a sense, health services research concerns itself with the form, and biomedical research with the content, of medicine. VIII.D.

health spa. any place which provides, as one of its primary purposes, services or facilities intended to help customers improve their health, physical condition, or appearance through weight change, exercise, or other means, as a reducing salon, exercise gym, health studio, or health club. Originally, a mineral spring resorted to for cures.

Spas are enormously variable in cost and program content. They are subject to FTC regulation of their advertising and sales practices. Their charges are ordinarily not *medical deductions* for tax purposes. V.

health status. the state of *health* of a specified individual, group, or population, as Ohioans, a health maintenance organization membership, or an employer's employees.

Health status may be measured with people's subjective assessment of their health, or with one or more *health indices,* as the *incidence* or *prevalence* of major diseases. These are, of course, measures of disease status, used as proxies in the absence of measures of health, and are being replaced by measures of physical ability and functioning, as days lost from work. Health status conceptually is the proper *outcome measure* for the *effectiveness* of a population's medical care, although attempts to correlate health status and *available* medical care have proved difficult and generally unsuccessful. Measures of available health resources or services, as a physician to population ratio, cannot measure health status.

See *National Health Survey, performance status,* and *vital statistics.* II.C.

health survey. a program for studying a *group* or *population* to assess its health status, conditions influencing or influenced by its health, and the health services available to and used by it.

See *National Health Survey.* II.C.

health system. the health resources and programs providing health services to a given area or population; compare *alternative health care delivery system* and *system.*

A health system is a regularly interacting and interdependent whole but not usually consciously organized or under unified control. III.B., VII.

health system plan (HSP). a long-range health *plan* prepared by a health systems agency for its health service area specifying the health *goals* considered *appropriate* by the agency for the area and its health system.

The HSPs are prepared after consideration of national guidelines issued by the Department of Health and Human Services, as well as study of the characteristics, resources, and special needs of the health service area, see section 1513 of the *Public Health Service Act.*

See *annual implementation plan.* VI.A.1.

health systems agency (HSA). a health *planning* and resources development agency designated under the terms of the National Health Planning and Resources Development Act of 1974.

The act requires the designation of an HSA in each of the health service areas in the United States. HSAs are nonprofit private corporations, public regional planning bodies, or single units of local government, and are charged with performing the health planning and resources development functions listed in section 1513 of the Public Health Service Act. The legal structure, size, composition, and operation of HSAs are also specified in the act. HSA functions include preparing a *health system plan* and an *annual implementation plan,* making grants and contracts, reviewing and approving or disapproving proposed uses in the agency's area of a wide range of federal funds, and making recommendations respecting proposed new and existing *institutional health services* to *state health planning and development agencies.* HSAs replaced existing areawide *comprehensive health planning* agencies and *regional medical programs.* VI.A.1.

healthy. see *health.*

heart disease. any disease or condition affecting the heart or blood vessels; a lay, collective term for a variety of quite different clinical entities, of which the most important is atherosclerosis, "hardening" of the coronary or heart's arteries.

Heart disease, the nation's leading cause of death, along with *cancer* and strokes, was the reason for creation of the *Regional Medical Program.* II.B.2.

heavy metal. a metallic element with high atomic weight, including arsenic, cadmium, chromium, *lead,* and *mercury.*

Generally toxic in low concentrations to plant and animal life, such metals are often persistent in the environment and exhibit biologic accumulation. I.C.

hematologist. a physician trained in or practicing hematology. III.A.1.

hematology. the *subspecialty* of either *internal medicine* or *pathology* concerned with the blood. III.C.

hemodialysis. see *dialysis.*

herbicide. see *pesticide.*

Henle, Jacob. German anatomist, 1809–1885. Best known for his contributions to our understanding of the microscopic structure of the body. Equally important was his work on *contagions,* which recognized that communicable diseases are caused by minute living organisms. He actually first set out the conditions later known as *Koch's postulates. R. Koch* studied under Henle at the University of Gottingen.

See *G. Fracastoro.* I.A.1., VIII.A.1.

herd effect, immunity. the protection a whole *population* of animals or humans receives when enough individuals are immune to an *infectious* disease that the disease will not spread in the population and infect *susceptible* people, even if introduced.

Herd immunity may not exist for highly *virulent* diseases like influenza but will protect the population for less virulent diseases like whooping cough if 60 percent to 80 percent are immunized.

heredity. *genetic,* and sometimes *familial* or cultural, transmission of characteristics from ancestor to descendant; an individual's genes or genetic complement, and sometimes also his familial and cultural inheritance. I.A.1.

hibakusha. Japanese, "explosion-affected person"; a survivor of the nuclear bombing of Hiroshima and Nagasaki in 1945. The *hibakusha* experienced an immersion in a sea of death that left a sense of permanent death taint and endless anxiety associated with invisible contamination.

See *final epidemic* and *nuclear winter,* and read Lifton, Robert Jay, *Death in Life: Survivors of Hiroshima* (New York: Random House Inc., 1986). II.B.2.

high level. see *radioactive waste.*

high option. in a *Federal Employees Health Benefits Plan* and some other insurance policies, the more complete of two or more levels of insurance which may be chosen by the *subscriber.*

In such options, benefits covered often are the same with the high option requiring less *cost sharing* and offering more generous time or quantity limits. The premium for the high option is higher than for the *low option* to pay for the more generous package. IV.C.

Hill-Burton. legislation, named after its original sponsors, and the programs operated under it for federal support of construction and *modernization* of hospitals and other *health facilities.*

The original law, the Hospital Survey and Construction Act of 1946, P.L. 79-725, which has been frequently amended, provided for surveying state facility *needs,* developing plans for construction of hospitals and public health centers, and assisting in constructing and equipping them. State Hill-Burton programs are now administered by *state health planning and development agencies,* and provide grants, loans, or loan guarantees for the following purposes: modernization of facilities, construction of outpatient facilities, construction of inpatient facilities in areas with recent rapid population growth, and conversion of existing medical facilities for provision of new health services.

See *free care.* III.B.1.

hip-pocket hysterectomy. slang, unnecessary removal of the uterus. VIII.B.2.a.

Hippocrates of Cos. Greek physician, ca. 459–355 B.C. The ideal physician and therefore called the father of medicine. His name is associated with the *Hippocratic Collection,* although no single work can be with certainty ascribed to him. The Hippocratic book, *Airs, Waters, and Places,* was the basic *epidemiologic* text for more than two millennia. VIII.A.1.

Hippocratic Oath. an oath attributed to Hippocrates of Cos and his school which has since been the ethical guide of the medical profession:

I swear by Apollo the physician, by *Aesculapius,* Hygeia and Panacea, and I take to witness all the gods, and all the goddesses, to keep according to my ability and my judgment the following oath:

To consider dear to me as my parents him who taught me this art; to live in common with him and if necessary to share my goods with him; to look upon his children as my own brothers, to teach them this art if they so desire without fee or written promise; to impart to my sons and the sons of the master who taught me and the disciples who have enrolled themselves and have agreed to the rules of the profession, but to these alone, the precepts and the instruction. I will prescribe regimen for the good of my patients according to my ability and my judgment and never do harm to anyone. To please no one will I prescribe a deadly drug, nor give advice which may cause his death. Nor will I give a woman a pessary to procure abortion. But I will preserve the purity of my life and my art. I will not cut for stone, even for patients in whom the disease is manifest; I will leave this operation to be performed by practitioners (specialists in this art). In every house where I come I will enter only for the good of my patients, keeping myself far from all intentional ill-doing and all seduction, and especially from the pleasures of love with women or with men, be they free or slaves. All that may come to my knowledge in the exercise of my profession or outside of my profession or in daily commerce with men, which ought not to be spread abroad, I will keep secret and will not ever reveal. If I keep this oath faithfully, may I enjoy my life and practice my art, respected by all men and in all times; but if I swerve from it or violate it, may the reverse be my lot. V.D.

hired gun.   slang synonym, *expert witness.*

history, history and physical (H&P).   an account or record of a patient's present and past health, medical status and events, and characteristics which are likely to affect his health.

The traditional medical history records a *chief complaint,* description of the present illness, *past medical history, family history, social history, review of systems,* and *physical examination.* History taking and physical diagnosis are among the great *clinical* skills of medicine. V.A.

history of work.   see *occupation.*

hold harmless provision.   1. a clause in a law or regulation preventing a government, institution, or individual from suffering additional expenses or loss of benefits as a result of a change made by the law or regulation. 2. in insurance, a provision offering the insured protection in disputes between the insurer and the provider of a covered service.

Without such a provision an institution would be responsible for expenses not previously anticipated due to an expanded caseload or less generous coverage provisions, or an individual might lose previously covered benefits. On the other hand, the use of hold harmless provisions creates confusion, heterogeneity, and inequity in eligibility, coverage, and responsibilities under a statute. 1. VIII.B.3. 2. IV.B.

holiday relief care.   see *respite care.*

holistic.   an approach to the study of the individual in totality, rather than as an aggregate of separate physiologic, psychologic, and social characteristics.

holistic medicine.   medical theory and practice based on *holism, a theory holding that a whole cannot be analyzed without residue into the sum of its parts or reduced to discrete elements, i.e., that the whole is greater than the sum of the parts; compare *gestalt psychology*.

Whether or not holistic medicine treats the person in some special way, it also has come to mean medical practice which selects, from the whole array of *alternative medicines,* whatever will help in a particular situation. V.

Holmes, Oliver Wendell. U.S. physician and author, 1809–1894. As early as 1843 he saw that the mysterious *puerperal* fever was *contagious* and carried by the hands of the obstetricians, which they for years denied, see *I.P. Semmelweis.* He suggested precautions intended to keep the hands clean, see *antiseptic.* He also fathered a fine justice of the U.S. Supreme Court. V.C., VIII.A.1.

homebound. confined to the home, as by *disability.*

Eligibility for Medicare and other *home health care* is in some degree dependent on being homebound and has led those paying the bills to consider defining it as "totally bedridden." II.

home health agency. an organization which provides home health services.

To participate in Medicare an agency must provide skilled nursing services and at least one additional therapeutic service (*physical, speech,* or *occupational therapy,* medical social services, or home health aide services) in the home as well as meet applicable *conditions of participation.* Such agencies may be part of hospitals or health departments or free-standing organizations. III.B.1.

home health aide. anyone employed to provide homemaker services, usually minimally trained and not subject to licensure or certification. III.A.4.

home health care (HC, HHC). health services provided an individual in the home.

Home health services are provided to aged, disabled or sick, or convalescent individuals who do not need institutional care. The services may be provided by a *visiting nurse association,* home health agency, hospital, or other organized community group. They may be quite specialized or comprehensive including nursing services, speech, physical, occupation, and rehabilitation therapy, homemaker services, and social services. Medicare covers such services only if provided by a home health agency. In Medicaid states do not have to restrict coverage of home health care to services provided by home health agencies. VII.C.1.

homemaker. synonym, *home health aide.*

homemaker service. a nonmedical support service like cooking and assistance with the *activities of daily living* given a *homebound* individual who is unable to perform such tasks unassisted.

Such services are not covered by Medicare and only rarely by Medicaid, or most other health insurance programs, but are included in some social service programs. Homemaker services are intended to preserve independent living and normal family life for the aged, disabled, sick, or convalescent.

See *alternatives to long-term institutional care* and *meals on wheels.* VII.C.1.

Homeopathic Pharmacopeia of the U.S. one of the three official *compendia* in the United States recognized in the Federal Food, Drug, and Cosmetic Act. III.B.3.

homeopathy (homeo). a system of medicine expounded by Samuel Christian Hahnemann (German physician, 1755–1843), based on the simile phenomenon (*similia similibus curantur,* "likes treat likes").

Cure of disease is effected by minute doses of drugs that produce the same signs and symptoms in a healthy person as are present in the disease for which they are administered. This is said to stimulate bodily defenses against these signs and symptoms. Homeopathy is now rarely practiced in the United States but still found in Europe and Asia. The Hahnemann Medical College now trains *allopathic physicians.*

See *concordant, inimic,* and *tissue remedies.* V.

hometown medical and dental care. in the Veterans Administration (VA) health program, outpatient medical or dental treatment paid for by the program and provided eligible veterans in their own communities by VA-approved doctors or dentists of their own choice.

Hometown care is covered when it cannot be given by VA facilities, or when the health of the patient or distance to be traveled gives sufficient justification. III.D.1.

home visit. an *encounter* by a physician or other provider with a patient in his home; synonym, house call.

Home visits are no longer much used for emergencies and acute illnesses, and have become more costly. They remain useful in effective management of incurable and chronic illness, and are still commonly made by nurses and other therapists employed by visiting nurse associations, home health agencies, and hospices. VII.C.1.

horizontal categorization. see *categorization.*

hospice. a program providing palliative, supportive, and *respite care* for terminally ill patients and their families, either directly or on a consulting basis with the patient's physician and other community agencies, as *visiting nurse associations.*

Originally a medieval way station for pilgrims and travelers where they could be replenished, refreshed, and cared for; now an organized program of care for people going through life's last station. The whole family is considered the unit of care. Emphasis is placed on symptom control, and preparation for and support before and after death—including the mourning process. Comprehensive services are provided by an organized interdisciplinary team available around the clock. Hospices originated in England and are now common in the United States. III.B.1.

hospital. a *health facility* whose primary function is to provide *inpatient* diagnostic and therapeutic medical services and related nursing, dietary, and *ancillary services* for a variety of medical conditions, both surgical and nonsurgical.

Most hospitals also provide some outpatient services, particularly *emergency care.* Hospitals are classified by *length of stay* (short-term or long-term); as *teaching* or nonteaching; by major type of service (general, psychiatric, tuberculosis, maternity, children's, or ear, nose, and throat); and by control (government, *proprietary,* and *voluntary*). Most U.S. hospitals are short-term, general, nonprofit community hospitals.

See *affiliated hospital.* III.B.1.

hospital-based physician. a physician who spends the predominant part of his practice time in one or more hospitals, instead of in an office setting, or in providing services to hospital patients.

Hospital-based physicians conventionally include anesthesiologists, pathologists, and radiologists, and sometimes directors of medical education, emergency physicians, and those staffing outpatient departments, but not surgeons or *house staff*. Such physicians often have special financial arrangements with the hospitals where they practice, whether a salary or percentage of hospital charges collected in addition to their own charges. See *professional and technical component*. III.A.1.

hospital component. see *professional component*.

hospital day. a *day* spent in a hospital.

hospital insurance program (Part A, HI). the *compulsory* portion of *Medicare* which automatically enrolls all persons aged 65 and over entitled to Social Security benefits or railroad retirement, persons under 65 who have been eligible for *disability* for over 2 years, and insured workers and their *dependents* requiring renal *dialysis* or kidney transplantation.

The program pays, after various *cost-sharing* requirements are met, for inpatient hospital care and care by *skilled nursing facilities* and *home health agencies*. The program is financed from a separate *trust fund* funded with a contributory or *payroll tax* levied on employers, employees, and the self-employed. IV.C.1.

Hospital International Classification of Disease Adapted for Use in the United States (H-ICDA). see *International Classification of Diseases, Adapted for Use in the United States*.

hospital privilege. synonym, *staff privilege*.

hospital staff. synonym, *medical staff*.

host. 1. an organism on or in which another, a *parasite*, lives and from which the other obtains nourishment during all or part of its existence; compare *infestation*. 2. the recipient of a transplanted organ or tissue. 3. the tissue *invaded* by a tumor. 4. in *teratology*, a relatively normal fetus to which a less complete fetus or fetal part is attached. I.A.1.

hot line. telephone assistance for people in need of crisis intervention.

Usually staffed by trained lay people with mental health professional assistance or backup. These well publicized, anonymous, telephone services are answered 24 hours a day to help people facing suicide or similar personal crises. III.B.1.

house call (HC). synonym, *home visit*.

house officer (HO). a member of a *house staff*. III.A.1.

house physician. a house officer or other physician employed by and constantly available at a hotel, hospital, or other institution. III.A.1.

house staff. the physicians employed by or in training at a hospital; a hospital's *interns, residents,* and *fellows*. Members of the house staff are called house officers. Occasionally applies to physicians salaried by a hospital who are not receiving any *graduate medical education*. III.B.1.

Howard, John. British humanist, 1726–1790. He was responsible for reform of conditions in prisons and *lazarettos,* which were *reservoirs* of *epidemic* fevers frequently afflicting armies and the merchant marine. VIII.A.1.

Howard Hughes Medical Institute (HHMI). a private, nonprofit *charity* endowed by Howard Hughes (U.S. industrialist) and one of the few still underwriting substantial support of medical research, principally by funding a few selected investigators and research centers. III.B.4.

human capital. see *capital.*

humanistic medicine. medical practice and culture which respects and uses the understanding that the patient is more than his disease, the professional more than a scientifically trained mind using technical skills, and both are whole human beings interacting in the healing effort.

A person is more than his body; he is a unique interdependent relationship of body, mind, emotions, culture, and spirit. Health and disease are not matters of the moment but have an intricate past, present, and future; physical disease, pain, suffering, aging, and even death may frequently be valuable, meaningful events in an individual's life. V.

Hyde Amendment. an amendment to *appropriations* legislation for federal health programs restricting federal funding for *abortions,* particularly in the Medicaid program, authored by U.S. Representative Henry Hyde (R-IL).

First passed in 1976, the enacted amendment differed from both Mr. Hyde's and the Senate's original versions. It allowed use of federal funds only when continued pregnancy would endanger the life of the mother or when pregnancy followed immediately reported rape or incest. The authors of the amendment and this dictionary are unrelated. IV.C.2.

Hygeia. see *Asclepius.*

hygiene (hyg). 1. the science of the principles, methods, and practices concerned with the preservation and improvement of *health.* 2. conditions or practices, as of cleanliness, conducive to health.

Hygiene is often British and nearly obsolete. Its many aspects include the study of personal hygiene, domestic hygiene, community hygiene, industrial hygiene, and mental hygiene. III.C.

hygienist. one trained in hygiene; usually a *technician,* see *dental hygienist.* III.A.4.

hyperactivity. excessive, abnormal, and usually uncontrollable activity; now renamed *attention-deficit disorder;* compare *specific learning disability* and *minimal brain dysfunction.*

Hyperactivity is a rare severe behavioral disturbance of children and a common label for children with inadequate parents or teachers, see *blaming the victim.* II.B.2.

hyperkinetic syndrome. synonym, *attention-deficit disorder.*

hypersusceptibility. great *susceptibility.* In occupational health, often a synonym for *accident proneness.*

hypnosis. an altered state of consciousness, characterized by increased memory and suggestibility; compare *meditation.* *hypnotherapy. therapy using hypnosis. *hypnotic. relating to hypnosis or, usually, sleep, which hypnosis superficially resembles (a hypnotic drug induces sleep not hypnosis). *hypnotism. the study and practice of hypnosis.

Hypnosis was first practiced by Mesmer (Austrian physician, 1734–1815) and later named by James Braid (British physician, mid-1800s). The nature and mechanisms of hypnosis are poorly understood. People are variable in the degree to which they may be hypnotized and usually cannot be without wanting to. Hypnosis may be self-induced, though this ordinarily requires training; generally it is induced by and dependent upon a hypnotist, to whom the increased suggestibility is directed. Hypnosis may be used for anesthesia, changing habits and symptoms, reviewing "forgotten" experiences and feelings, and producing amnesia; as such it is a powerful therapeutic tool. However, it is unreliable and occasionally dangerous, and its teaching and practice irregular and unregulated. V.

hypochondria. 1. the regions of the body beneath the rib margins, the classic Greek seat of melancholy and complaint. 2. a chronic condition characterized by preoccupation with one's body, its symptoms, and the illnesses it must have; synonym, *hypochondriasis.*

Hypochondriacal moments and behavior are common; true hypochondria is a depressing chronic disorder of unknown cause. The sufferer knows he is sick but cannot perceive that the illness is hypochondria. II.B.2.

hypothesis. a conjecture or supposition put forth to account for known facts; a tentative assumption made for the sake of argument or experiment; an interpretation or explanation of a situation taken as a ground for action. See *falsifiable hypothesis* and *null hypothesis.* VIII.D.

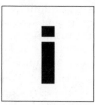

identified patient. a family member presented as and kept sicker than is actually the case in service to abnormal family structural or functional needs, as an asthmatic child whose attacks detour parental conflict into concern for the child; compare *scapegoat*.

The identified patient may or may not have any real disease or any consciousness of his role. *Family therapy* may start by separating the patient from the underlying problem, which usually cures him but can bring the problem to the surface elsewhere. VII.A.1.

idiocy. an old legal term for *congenital* profound to severe *mental retardation;* compare *imbecility*. A man is not an idiot if he can tell his parent's name, his age, or such common matters. I.A.1.

idiopathic. of unknown or obscure cause. II.B.1.

illegitimacy ratio. the number of *births* occurring out of wedlock per thousand total births in a given population and period, usually a year. VIII.C.

illness. usually synonymous, *disease;* can be differentiated by saying illness is present when an individual perceives himself as *sick* and disease is present when identifiable by objective, external criteria. II.

imagery. *meditation* in which the mantra or focus is an image of the subject's own design, invented around his disease.

Patient imaging of their bodies combating illnesses such as cancer has been found to increase their response to conventional medical therapy. V.

imbecility. an old legal term for *acquired mental retardation,* typically *senile dementia* and usually to the point of *incompetence*.

Mental functioning in one who has lost mental powers through age and/or chronic illness is somewhat different in quality from one in whom they never developed. Thus the legal distinction between imbecility and *idiocy* is useful although their measures are the same. I.A.1

immune. safe from attack; protected against a disease by an innate or acquired resistance.

An *immune response is an *allergic* response to a germ or other agent
of disease or an antigen involved in disease, which protects the responding
organism against the disease, i.e., develops *immunity in the organism.
See *herd immunity.* I.A.1.

immunization. the creation of immunity, usually by vaccination against a
particular disease; synonym, *vaccination.* VII.B.3.b.

impaired physician. a practicing physician with an impairment, as alcoholism, drug addiction, or senility, which may compromise the quality of his
practice; usually not used for physicians who are not practicing because of
some disability or who have an uncompromising impairment, as a missing
leg.

Many state medical associations have organized programs for identifying and assisting such physicians who often do not recognize or admit their
impairment. III.A.1.

impairment. 1. deterioration, or lessening; "any loss or abnormality of psychologic, physiologic, or anatomical structure or function" (*International
Classification of Impairments, Disabilities, and Handicaps.* Geneva: World
Health Organization, 1980); synonym, incapacity; casually synonymous, *disability, disorder, handicap,* or *injury.* 2. in environmental health, *contamination* or *pollution* of any portion of a natural resource, sometimes limited
to resources which cannot subsequently be used for their original purpose,
as contamination of an *aquifer* that permanently impairs it as drinking
water. 3. in *workmen's compensation,* a pathologic *condition* caused by work-
related injury or disease whether or not associated with a wage loss.

Workmen's compensation often pays impairment benefits for damage
which does not produce a wage loss, as a lost finger. In this context a disability becomes an impairment with a wage loss. Impairment benefits are
often *scheduled.* Impairment without loss of income, and thus without disability in the eyes of workmen's compensation, is a major consequence of
chronic occupational diseases like *brown lung.* II. VII.B.2.d.

impoundment. in the federal budget, any executive branch action or inaction that precludes the *obligation* or expenditure of *budget authority* provided by Congress.

An *impoundment resolution is a resolution of the House of Representatives or the Senate which expresses disapproval of a deferral of budget
authority proposed by the president. Passage of an impoundment resolution by either house of Congress disapproves the proposed deferral and requires that the budget authority be made available for obligation.
See *rescission.* VI.B.1.

impurity. foreign matter *naturally* present in small amounts in a substance
which reduces its quality; compare *adulterate,* which is preferred when foreign matter is added to a substance. I.C.

inactive ingredient. a constituent of a drug product with no therapeutic effect; a part of a product which does not actively or directly serve the product's purpose.

Most drugs contain multiple therapeutically inactive chemicals for color,
flavor, preservation, fill, and a variety of other purposes. These inactive
ingredients may actively produce *allergic* reactions or other *side effects* in

particular patients. The hundreds of chemicals approved by the Food and Drug Administration as inactive ingredients in prescription drugs need not be listed in the *labeling*. They include acetone, activated altapulgite, beeswax, many common foods and flavors, glycerin and lactose, 12 inks, shellac, and tall oil.

Read Brown, J.L., "Incomplete Labeling of Pharmaceuticals: A List of Inactive Ingredients" (*N Engl J Med*, 309(7): 439–41, 8/18/83.) III.B.3.

in-and-out surgery. see *surgicenter*.

incapacity. synonym, *impairment*.

incaparina. a new protein food made of a mixture of corn and cottonseed meal and enriched with vitamins A and B.

Developed by the Institute of Nutrition for Central America and Panama for use by the poor of Central America, incaparina was an early attempt to add balanced protein to an area's diet from otherwise unusable sources. I.A.2.a.

incidence. 1. in epidemiology, the number of cases of a disease or other event beginning during a specified period of time, ordinarily expressed as an incidence rate which gives new cases per 1000 or 100,000 population *at risk* in a particular area and specified time, typically a year; compare *prevalence*.

$$\text{Incidence rate (episodes per 1000 population)} = 1000 \times \frac{\text{new episodes reported during the year}}{\text{survey population at the middle of the year}}$$

2. in economics, the distribution of a tax among groups, usually income groups, in the population. *Nominal incidence is the distribution mandated by law, as a specified division of a payroll tax between employers and employees. *Ultimate incidence is the distribution after allowing for the income effects of the tax. 1. VIII.C. 2. VIII.B.1.

incident report. a report of an accident, error, or unusual event occurring in a hospital or other inpatient health facility that is made a part of the *record* of any patient and personnel involved. V.D.

incombustible waste. see *waste*.

income. the gain or return, usually measured in money, from one's business, labor, or capital invested.

As an example of the complexity of operational definition of income, the IRS 1040 form should be considered as a specific definition of income. Welfare and other programs distinguish *earned income (wages or net earnings from employment) and *unearned income (support or maintenance furnished in kind or cash; annuities, pensions, retirements, or disability benefits; prizes, gifts, and awards; proceeds from insurance policies, support, and alimony payments; inheritances; and rents, dividends, interest, and royalties). Note that fringe benefits of employment, as an employer's contribution to the cost of health insurance, are often not considered as income for tax purposes, thus enhancing their real value.

See *resources*. I.A.2.c.

income elasticity. see *elasticity*.

incompetence. lacking *competence*.

incubation. 1. the act or process of hatching or developing, as eggs or bacteria. 2. the phase of an *infectious* disease from the time of inoculation to the appearance of symptoms, the *incubation period, an example of a *latency period*. 3. the growth or maintenance for laboratory purposes of bacteria, cells, or other biologic material. 4. in ancient Greek medicine, sleep within the temples of healing gods for the purpose of curing disease. I.A.1.

incur. in insurance, to become liable for a *loss,* claim, or expense.
Cases or losses incurred are those occurring within a fixed period for which an insurance plan becomes liable whether or not yet reported, adjusted, and paid. Losses incurred but not reported (IBNR) are covered by primary *reserves.* IV.B.

indecent exposure. see *exposure.*

indemnity, indemnity benefit. in health insurance, a *benefit* in the form of cash payments rather than services; compare *fixed* and *scheduled benefit,* contrast *service benefit.*
The indemnity insurance contract often defines maximum amounts payable for covered services, and may also have *cost-sharing* provisions. After the provider of service has billed the patient, the insured person submits to the insurance company proof that he has paid the bills and is reimbursed by the company as much of the costs as are covered, making up the difference himself. In some instances, the provider of service may complete the necessary forms and submit them to the insurance company directly for reimbursement, billing the patient for costs which are not covered.
See *aggregate indemnity* and *superbill.* IV.B.2.

independent laboratory. see *laboratory.*

independent practice. practice in which the practitioner serves without supervision, taking personal responsibility for patient care; compare *private* and *solo practice.* V.

independent professional review (IPR). synonym, *medical review,* required by Medicaid for inpatients in long-term care facilities. V.C.2.

independent variable. see *variable.*

index case. a case of a disease whose identification leads to investigation of other cases in the same *epidemic,* family, or area.
See *proband.* II.

indexed. describes an amount which is regularly adjusted in proportion to changes in an *index (a measure of something), as Social Security payments are now indexed to (adjusted to reflect changes in) the *Consumer Price Index.*
See *health index.* IV.

***Index Medicus* (IM).** a bibliographic citation index of recurring publications pertaining to medicine and related fields by *Medical Subject Headings* and author.
The index has been published continuously since 1869, currently by the U.S. National Library of Medicine. It is now computer generated.
See *Medlars.* III.C.

indication. something that points out or to, as in medicine a symptom, sign, or occurrence in a *problem* which reveals its cause, diagnosis, appropriate treatment, or prognosis; compare *contraindication.* V.B.

indigent. poor, needy; irregularly used, see *medically indigent.*

indirect association.   see *association.*

indirect cost.   a cost which cannot be identified directly with a particular activity, service, or product of the program experiencing the cost.

Indirect costs, or *overhead,* are allocated among the program's services or *cost centers,* usually in proportion to each one's share of *direct costs.* VII.D.1.

indirect encounter.   "an encounter in which there is no physical or face-to-face meeting between the patient and the professional, as telephone encounter or written encounter" (*NAPCRG, 1978*).

indirect provider.   see *provider.*

individual insurance.   insurance covering an individual, and usually his dependents, rather than a group.

Individual health insurance usually offers *indemnity benefits* and has higher *loadings* than group insurance. IV.B.2.

individual practice.   see *practice.*

individual practice association (IPA).   a legal entity which has entered into an arrangement with providers, a majority of whom are licensed to practice medicine or osteopathy, for provision of their services.

The IPA may be a partnership, corporation, or any other legal entity. The arrangement between it and the providers must require that they provide their professional services in accordance with a compensation plan established by the entity. The IPA arrangement must also encourage team practice, sharing of medical records and equipment, and continuing medical education. The term originated and is defined in the Health Maintenance Organization Act of 1973, section 1302(5) of the Public Health Service Act. IPAs are one source of professional services for *health maintenance organizations* and are modeled after *medical foundations.* III.B.1.

individual practice plan.   synonym, *individual practice association* or *medical foundation.*

individual retirement account (IRA).   see *Keogh plan.*

industrial.   of or pertaining to industry; caused by work or processes used in industry; generally synonymous with occupational.

industrial accident rate.   nonspecific name for any of several *rates* measuring the *incidence* or *prevalence* of occupational disease and injury.

The Bureau of Labor Statistics of the Department of Labor publishes two good examples, *recordable* occupational injuries and illnesses per 100 man-years worked and disabling work-related injuries per million man-hours worked. VIII.B.2.d

industrial development bond.   see *bond.*

industrial health service.   largely obsolete synonym, *occupational health service.*

industrial hygiene.   the branch of *preventive medicine* concerned with *occupational safety and health;* the recognition and control of environmental *hazards* with adverse effects on the health and efficiency of workers. III.C., VII.B.2.d.

industrial hygienist.   a practitioner of industrial hygiene; compare *inspector.*

The training and qualifications of industrial hygienists are not well standardized, but most have a master's degree in science or public health with particular emphasis on industrial hygiene. III.A.5.

industrial injury rate. see *industrial accident rate.*

industrial medicine. synonym, *occupational medicine.*

industrial physician. one who practices solely or primarily *occupational medicine;* synonym, occupational physician.

About 3 percent of physicians practice occupational medicine, with or without residency training and whether part- or full-time. Industrial physicians, particularly among occupational health workers, have struggled with the inherent conflict between the interests of their employers and their patients. III.A.1.

infant. 1. a *child* in the first stage of life. 2. in medicine, a child in the first year of life or, occasionally, the first two years. 3. in law, synonym, *minor;* compare *age* and *neonate.* I.A.1.

infant mortality rate. the number of infant deaths reported per 1000 *live births* in a given area or program per year.

A common measure of *health status,* the infant mortality rate varies among countries partly because the definition is somewhat variable.

See *birth, neonatal,* and *perinatal mortality rate.* II.C.

infection. 1. invasion of a living body by other organisms, usually *pathogens,* as bacteria, fungi, viruses, protozoa, insects, or helminths (worms). 2. a disease produced by infection. An *infection committee in a health program, as a hospital, works to control *nosocomial, puerpural,* and other infections.

See *communicable disease, contagion, G. Fracastoro, J. Henle, infestation,* and *R. Koch.* I.A.1.

infectious disease. the subspecialty of internal medicine concerned with infections. III.C.

infernal medicine. slang, *internal medicine.*

infestation. properly, the presence of *pests* or *parasites* on the surface of a *host* or in its *environment;* commonly, synonym, *infection,* usually by parasites. I.A.1.

infirmary. 1. specifically, a health facility serving a nonmedical residential institution, as a school or prison, usually on a short-term, nonintensive basis. 2. loosely, a clinic or hospital. III.B.1.

inflation. an increase in the volume of available money and credit relative to goods, resulting in a substantial and continuing rise in the general price level. *inflationary spiral. a continuous rise in prices sustained by the fact that wage and price increases stimulate each other. VIII.B.1.

informed consent. voluntary *consent* given after adequately understanding the nature, risks, benefits, and alternatives to a proposed course of medical action. Patient refusal of possibly beneficial treatment is known as *informed refusal when voluntarily undertaken with similarly adaquate understanding of the situation.

Physicians have a duty in law, arising out of the *fiduciary* nature of the physician-patient relationship and the patient's right to self-determination, to obtain informed consent prior to treatment. It is preferably obtained in writing after disclosure, intelligible to the patient, of the diagnosis, or *differential,* the *risks,* the *prognosis* with and without treatment, and the available alternatives, if any. There are exceptions in emergencies, when relying on the *therapeutic privilege,* for rare, minor, unknown, or commonly known risks, and for trivial, common, or safe treatment.

Read Miller, Leslie J., "Informed Consent" (*JAMA,* 244(18,20,22,23): 11–12/80). V.B., VIII.B.3.

Ingham Reflex Method of Compression Massage. a system of therapy using finger pressure accompanied by massaging motions applied to specific zones of the foot for diagnosis and treatment of a variety of ailments; synonyms, *foot zone therapy, reflexology, zone therapy.*

It is said to work by eliciting beneficial reflex action through nerve endings connecting the feet to various organs of the body. The method was derived by William H. Fitzgerald (U.S. otolaryngologist) from eastern practices related to *yoga,* and elaborated in the 1930s by Eunice D. Ingham. V.

Inglefinger Rule. (Franz Inglefinger, U.S. physician and medical editor) a policy of the *New England Journal of Medicine,* and some other *reviewed* journals, which provides that the journal undertakes review for publication only with the understanding that neither the substance, data, pictures, nor tables submitted have been published or will be submitted for publication elsewhere prior to publication or rejection by the journal. The restriction does not apply to brief publication necessary for public health purposes, abstracts published in connection with scientific meetings, or news reports based solely on formal and public oral presentations at such meetings.

The rule seeks to keep original work out of the news until after the successful scientific review required for publication, and to protect the work's newsworthiness for the benefit of the journal. III.C.

inhalation therapist, therapy. see *respiratory therapist, therapy.*

inherit. to derive or acquire from an ancestor, whether by *genetic, familial,* or cultural means. I.A.1.

inimic remedies. in *homeopathy,* remedies whose actions are antagonistic; compare *concordant* and *tissue remedies.* V.

injury. 1. traumatic (in insurance) or *iatrogenic* (in *malpractice*) damage to the body, typically of external origin, usually unexpected and undesigned by the injured. 2. in law, any wrong or damage done to another, whether to his person, rights, reputation, or property. II.B.1.a.

inpatient. a patient who has been *admitted* at least overnight to a hospital or other health facility which assumes responsibility for his room and board for the purpose of receiving diagnostic, therapeutic, or other health services; contrast *outpatient.* VII.C.S.

inpatient care. the health care given inpatients. VII.C.5.

inpatient surgery. see *ambulatory surgery.*

in-plant noise. indoor occupational noise; compare *occupational air.* I.C.2., VII.B.2.d.

input measure. a measure of the *quality* of services based on the number, type, or quality of *resources* or inputs used in production of the services; compare *output measure.*

Medical services are often evaluated by measuring the education of the provider, the *accreditation* of the facility, the number of personnel involved, or the dollars spent as proxy measures for the actual quality of the service.

Input measures are inferior to *process* and outcome measures because they are indirect and do not consider actual results, or outcomes, of services. They are used because people are accustomed to them and they are easily obtained. VII.D.2.

inquest. in law, a judicial hearing, as a *coroner's* inquest, for the purpose of determining how a death by violence or unknown cause occurred, i.e., whether death was natural, accidental, suicidal, or homicidal. VII.B.3.

insanity. 1. in law, a *mental disorder* of such severity that the individual is not *competent* to manage his affairs and fulfill social duties, cannot distinguish right from wrong, is *committable,* or cannot reasonably be held responsible for his acts. 2. in medicine, obsolete synonym, *mental illness.*

Insanity as used in law is different from in medicine (where mental illness is the more common term). In law it concerns only the relation of the person to the act which is the subject of judicial investigation. It is also subject to variable and elaborate definition.

See *American Law Institute Formulation, Durham Rule,* and *M'Naghten Rule.* 1. VIII.B.3. 2. II.B.2.

insecticide. see *pesticide* and *chlorinated hydrocarbon.*

inspector. one who views or examines, usually closely and officially to ascertain *quality* or compliance with *standards.*

In occupational health, *safety inspectors are used by federal and state governments to enforce Occupational Safety and Health Act safety standards. They are often *safety professionals.* *Health inspectors, concerned with *health standards,* may be *industrial hygienists.* Inspectors are increasingly concerned with both *safety* and health, another aspect of the gradual merging of the traditional, arbitrary separation of the two. III.A.6., VII.B.2.d

instantaneous sample. see *sample.*

institute. an organization for the promotion of a cause; an association, center, or program for *research,* education, and related services concerned with a particular subject; compare *charity* and *foundation.*

Irregularly used; institutes are commonly public organizations, as the National Institutes of Health, sometimes private nonprofit organizations, and ordinarily primarily concerned with funding and doing research. III.D.3.

Institute of Medicine of the National Academy of Sciences (IOM). the part of the National Academy of Sciences concerned with health and health care.

The academy is a private nonprofit organization chartered by the federal government. The institute functions fairly independently of it, choosing its own members who in turn set institute policy and guide its activities. III.D.2.

institution. a valiant attempt to keep an inspiration alive. VIII.B.2.b.

institutional health service. a health service delivered on an *inpatient* basis by a health maintenance organization, hospital, nursing home, or other inpatient health facility; usually includes services delivered on an *outpatient* basis by inpatient facilities.

The National Health Planning and Resources Development Act of 1974 defined them as services and facilities subject under *Department of Health and Human Services* rules to *section 1122* review, and required that all institutional, but not noninstitutional, health services be subject to *certificate-of-need* review and periodic review for *appropriateness.* VII.C.5., VI.A.2.

institutional licensure. a proposed *licensure* system, not presently in use in the United States, in which health programs would be generally licensed and then be free to hire and use personnel as each saw fit, whether or not they met usual, individual licensure or *certification* requirements. III.B.1., VII.D.2.

institutional provider. in Medicare, a hospital, skilled nursing facility, home health agency, or other *provider* which receives cost-related reimbursement from *intermediaries;* contrast *supplier.* III.B.1., IV.C.1.

institutional review board (IRB). a committee organized by a medical school, hospital, or other program engaged in research using human subjects to review and approve research proposals to assure that they are ethical, and adequately inform and protect their subjects.

Approval by an IRB, which must conform to National Institutes of Health regulations, is required by the Public Health Service Act before federal funding may be awarded for research using human subjects. The IRBs are multidisciplinary with representation from the lay community outside the program. They often concern themselves with the scientific quality, as well as the ethics, of proposals.

Read Levine, Robert J., *Ethics and Regulation of Clinical Research* (Baltimore: Urban & Schwarzenburg, 1981). VIII.D.

institution for mental disease (IMD). an inpatient facility that treats primarily patients needing psychopharmacological drugs, i.e., patients with psychiatric illnesses; compare *ICF/MR*.

This may include hospitals or nursing homes with many young patients, locked wards, or patient populations more than half of which have *psychiatric diagnoses.* Medicaid does not cover patients aged 22–65 cared for in IMDs. II.B.2., IV.C.2.

insulin certification. see *antibiotic certification.*

insurable risk. a *risk* which has the following attributes: it is one of a large homogeneous group of similar risks; the *loss* produced by the risk is definable and quantifiable; the occurrence of loss in individual cases is accidental or fortuitous; the potential loss is large enough to cause hardship; the cost of insuring is economically feasible; the chance of loss is calculable; and it is sufficiently unlikely that loss will occur in many individual cases at the same time. IV.B.

insurance. a contractual relationship in which one party, for a consideration, agrees to reimburse another for *loss* to a person or thing caused by designated contingencies; synonym, assurance. The first party is the *insurer;* the second, the *insured;* the contract, the *insurance policy;* the consideration, the *premium;* the person or thing, the *risk;* the reimbursement, the *benefit;* and the contingency, the *hazard* or *peril.*

Insurance is a formal social device for reducing the risk of losses for individuals by spreading the risk over groups. Insurance characteristically, but not necessarily, involves equitable contributions by the insured, pooling of risks, and the transfer of risks by contract. Insurance may be offered on either a *profit* or nonprofit basis, to *groups* or individuals.

See *antidiscrimination law, prepayment,* and *social insurance.* IV.B.

insurance clause. the part of an insurance policy which sets forth the parties to the contract, the losses *covered,* and the benefits payable. IV.B.

insurance commissioner. the state official charged with the enforcement of laws pertaining to insurance in a state; sometimes called a superintendent or director.

The commissioner's title, status in government, and responsibilities differ from state to state, but all states have an official with such responsibilities regardless of title. The commissioner may also be responsible for regulating *prepayment* programs like *Blue Cross/Blue Shield* and *health maintenance organizations.* IV.B.

insurance policy. a written contract of insurance between an insurer and the insured. IV.B.

insurance pool. an organization of insurers or *reinsurers* through which particular types of *risks* are shared or pooled.

The risk of great *loss* by any particular insurance company is transferred to the group as a whole, the insurance pool, with premiums, losses, and expenses shared in agreed amounts. The advantage of a pool is that the size of expected losses can be predicted for the pool with much more certainty than for any individual party to it. Pooling arrangements are used for *catastrophic coverage* or high risk populations like the disabled. Pooling may be done within a single company by pooling the risks insured under several policies so that high losses *incurred* by one policy are shared with others.

See *assigned risk.* IV.B.

insured. the individual or organization protected in case of loss under the terms of an insurance policy.

The insured is not necessarily the *risk,* the person whose losses from *accident* or *sickness* are covered. In *group insurance* the employer may be the insured, the employees the risks. IV.B.

insurer. the company, party, or trust fund contracted by an insurance policy to pay losses or provide services. IV.B.

integrated sample. see *sample.*

intelligence quotient (IQ). a standardized numerical measure of intelligence; a ratio of an individual's performance on a standardized mental test to the average performance of individuals similar in age and, to some degree, other factors affecting intelligence, as achievement and language.

The most common IQ is obtained by dividing the mental age by the chronological age up to age 16 and multiplying by 100. Scores are generally adjusted to a *mean* of 100 and *standard deviation* of 15. The most common among many U.S. measures is the Stanford-Binet test. IQ classification is irregular, but generally *mental retardation* occurs below 70, and then dull normal, 70–90; normal, 90–110; superior, 110–125; very superior, 125–140; and genius, over 140. I.A.2.

intensity of service. the quantity of services provided to patients per day, admission, or diagnosis in a given health program or other comparable setting.

Intensity may be expressed by a weighted index of services provided, or statistics indicating the average number of laboratory tests, surgical procedures, or x-rays per patient or patient day. Intensity is a function of the type of program and its *case mix.*

See *diagnosis related group.* VII.D.2.

intensive care. concentrated services for critically ill patients; informal, intensive care unit.

Intensive care is continuous close medical and nursing attention using complex equipment and therapeutic regimens. Nurses, particularly, often have special training and responsibilities, see *critical care*. VII.C.5.a.

intensive care unit (ICU). a specialized nursing unit in a hospital for seriously ill patients needing intensive care.

Some units are limited to certain types of patients, as coronary care, surgical intensive care, and neonatal intensive care units.

See *progressive patient* and *special care*. III.B.1.

interactional approach, interactional family therapy. *family therapy* which seeks "to change transactions and communication patterns in the dysfunctional family which affect the *identified patient*. Attention is paid to verbal and nonverbal behavior, its timing, and also the congruence between these two levels. The focus is on modification and change of behavior and not on cognitive insight or emotional catharsis" (*Pinney and Slipp, 1979*). V.

intercurrent. of something, as an acute illness, occurring in the midst of, and usually *complicating*, another thing, as an existing illness. II.

intermediary. a public or private organization which enters into an agreement with the secretary of the Department of Health and Human Services under the *Hospital Insurance Program* (Part A) of Medicare, to pay *claims* and perform other functions for the program with respect to such providers, usually a *Blue Cross plan* or private insurance company; compare *carrier* and *fiscal agent*. IV.C.1.

intermediary letter (IL). one of a numbered series of letters from the *Health Care Financing Administration*, Department of Health and Human Services, to the intermediaries in the Medicare program which provide *administrative* direction or *policy*.

HHS has used these letters to make much of Medicare's policy since it was enacted. IV.C.1.

intermediate care. chronic, simple medical and nursing inpatient services.

Intermediate care is largely defined by what may and may not be done in an *intermediate care facility*. It includes assisting with *activities of daily living*, giving medications, and other maintenance services, but not *rehabilitation*, intravenous care, or tube feedings, which constitute *skilled care*.

See *level of care*. VII.C.5.b.

intermediate care facility (ICF). a facility recognized by Medicaid and licensed under state law to provide regular health-related care and services to individuals who do not require the degree of care or treatment which a hospital or *skilled nursing facility* is designed to provide, but who, because of their mental or physical condition, require care and services above the level of room and board which can be made available to them only through institutional facilities.

Public institutions for care of the *mentally retarded* or people with related conditions are considered ICFs for the mentally retarded (ICF/MR). The distinction between "health-related care and services" and "room and board" is difficult to make but important because ICFs are much more regulated than institutions not providing health-related care and services. Intermediate care is the lowest level of inpatient care paid for by Medicaid and other health payment programs. III.B.1.

intern. one who serves an *internship*.

internal cost. a *cost* recognized and borne by the producer; contrast *social cost* borne by someone else and therefore not reflected in the price of the good or service produced; compare *direct cost* and *external cost*. *Internalization of a cost occurs when a social cost is made into an internal one, as *workmen's compensation* internalizes the cost of occupational injuries and illness. VII.D.1.

internal medicine (IM). the science and specialty devoted to the study and care of the internal organs and the nonsurgical care of diseases of adults.
   The term is from the German "innere medizin," where it was introduced about 1882 to distinguish medicine based on experimental work in physiology and chemistry from *clinical medicine* based on observation of the *natural history* of disease. General internal medicine is one of the *primary care* specialties. Its subspecialties with *certificates of special competence* are cardiology, endocrinology and metabolism, gastroenterology, hematology, infectious disease, medical oncology, nephrology, pulmonary disease, and rheumatology. III.C.

International Classification of Disease (ICD). a system for classifying and reporting disease developed by the *World Health Organization* and now in its ninth edition (ICD-9).
   Diseases are grouped in major categories which include the infections, neoplastic, traumatic, undiagnosed, and those of the organ systems. Each entity is given a numerical code of up to four digits. The ICD is revised about once a decade. II.B.2.

International Classification of Disease, Adapted for Use in the United States (ICDA). an official U.S. Public Health Service adaptation of the *International Classification of Disease* for use in the United States.
   The ICD is used for international *vital statistics* purposes and easier to use in its various adapted versions. A further revised and expanded version of ICDA, known as Hospital-ICDA, was developed by the *Commission on Professional and Hospital Activities* and is widely used in hospitals and the *Professional Activity Study*. III.B.1.

International Classification of Disease for Oncology (ICD-O). a two-axis topography and morphology coding system for tumors, identical with the relevant parts of the *Systemized Nomenclature of Medicine* and ICD-9. II.B.1.

International Classification of Disease, Ninth Edition, Clinical Modification (ICD-9-CM). an adaptation of the *ICD-9* for use in clinical rather than public health settings.
   This version is widely used in the United States for reporting diagnoses, *Current Procedural Terminology* being used to report services.
   Read *International Classification of Disease, Ninth Revision, Clinical Modification*. (3 vols., Ann Arbor, Michigan: Edwards Brothers, Inc. 1981.) II.B.1.

International Classification of Health Problems in Primary Care (ICHPPC, PriCare). an adaptation of the *International Classification of Disease* for use in ambulatory and primary care settings.
   Now in its second edition (ICHPPC-2), it is almost entirely compatible with the ninth edition of the international classification (ICD-9). ICHPPC-2 was prepared by *WONCA* and published in 1980 by the Oxford University Press. II.B.1.

International Nonproprietary Names (INN).   a registry of generic names for drugs. III.B.3.

International System of Units (SI).   an extension of the metric system based on seven fundamental physical quantities approved by the General Conference on Weights and Measures in 1960 (the acronym comes from the French name, "Le Système International d'Unités").

The SI, expanded for use in medicine, has been adopted in most European countries and Canada. The *General Conference on Weights and Measures consists of the signers, including the United States, of the 1875 Meter Convention and operates the International Bureau of Standards created by the convention. The seven physical quantities, with their base units and symbols, are length (meter, m); mass (kilogram, kg); time (second, s); amount of substance (mole, mol); thermodynamic temperature (Kelvin, K); electric current (ampere, A); and luminous intensity (candela, cd).

Read Lundberg, George D., et al., "Now Read This: The SI Units Are Here" (*JAMA*, 255(17): 2329–39, 5/2/86). II.

internist.   a physician specializing by practice or education in internal medicine or one of its subspecialties. III.A.1.

internship.   any period of on-the-job training which is part of a larger educational program. In medicine, dentistry, podiatry, and some other health professions, usually a one-year program of *graduate medical education.*

Nearly all physicians take internships, although they are not required for licensure in all states. Most hospitals require successful completion of an internship for granting of *staff privileges. Residencies* now often begin the first year after graduation, eliminating internships as separate entities. A *rotating internship provides experience (*rotations*) in several specialties, a *straight program primarily in only one.

See *extern.* III.A.

interval sample.   see *sample.*

intervening variable.   something occurring between an antecedent circumstance or *independent variable* and its consequent or *dependent variable,* and modifying the relation between the two.

Appetite can be an intervening variable determining whether or not a given food will be eaten. The intervening variable may be inferred rather than empirically detected. VIII.D.

in the quotes.   see *quotes.*

in-training examination.   an annual exam and examination program administered by the American Board of Family Practice for residents training in family medicine.

It is designed to assist residents and faculty in assessing their progress and program in comparison to national standards. III.C.

invalid.   1. suffering from disease or disability, sickly; of, relating to, or suited to one who is sick. 2. one who is sick or disabled. 3. to remove from work or active duty because of sickness.

Invalid is primarily applied to people with long-term, ordinarily acquired, disability which limits self-sufficiency. I.A.1.

invasive.   1. tending to spread, especially to healthy tissue, as malignant cancer. 2. of a diagnostic or therapeutic *procedure* which requires entering the body by an unusual route or amount; antonym, *noninvasive.*

Most surgery is invasive. Drawing blood is not; introducing catheters or scopes is. The term could, but does not usually, apply to procedures which disrupt function rather than physical structure. VII.D.2.

investigation. synonym, *study* or *research.*

investigational new drug (IND). a drug available solely for experimental purposes intended to determine its *safety* and *effectiveness* and not yet approved by the Food and Drug Administration for marketing to the general public.

Use of an IND is limited to experts qualified by training and experience to investigate its safety and effectiveness. Use of the drug in humans requires approval by the FDA of an *IND application which provides reports of animal toxicity tests, a description of proposed clinical trials, and a list of the names and qualifications of the investigators. See *new drug* and *new drug application.* III.B.3.

involuntary commitment. see *commitment.*

iridology. the study of the iris of the eye, particularly its color, markings, and changes, as they are associated with and diagnose disease; medical palmistry.

An intelligent look at any part of a person will tell of him, but better to look at all of him. V.

irradiation. see *food irradiation.*

irresistible impulse test. the rule that a person is not responsible for a crime if he acts through an uncontrollable impulse due to a *mental illness.*

Introduced in 1922, the test is now used only in a few states; compare *American Law Institute Formulation.* VIII.B.3.

itinerant surgeon. a surgeon, often a subspecialist, who operates in several separate communities, entrusting pre- and postoperative care to general surgeons or other physicians practicing full-time in each community.

This now uncommon practice was used to make specialized services available in communities otherwise without them but left patients in the care of physicians not fully qualified to care for them; safer to take the patient to the surgeon. III.A.1.

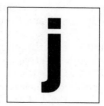

Jekyll-and-Hyde syndrome. a disturbed, excessively dependent pattern of relations between an elderly, disabled person and his primary *caretaker*. The syndrome is characterized by physical disease, deterioration, and personality change after discharge from the hospital, and improvement after readmission. The patient generally has a negative attitude and only one relative doing most of the work. The syndrome is managed by a modicum of separation, as by occasional brief nursing home admissions for *respite care*.

Read Boyd, R.V., and J.A. Woolman, "The Jekyll-and-Hyde Syndrome" (*Lancet* 2(8091): 671–2, 9/23/78). I.B.1., II.B.2.

Jenner, Edward. English country practitioner, 1749–1823. He discovered and introduced *vaccination* against smallpox. This important discovery was published in 1798 under the title, *An Inquiry Into the Causes and Effects of the Variolae Vaccinae.* VII.B.3.b., VIII.A.1.

jin shin jyutsu. see *shiatsu.*

Joint Commission on Accreditation of Hospitals (JCAH). a private nonprofit organization whose purpose is to encourage attainment of uniformly high *standards* of institutional medical care.

Comprised of representatives of the American Hospital Association, American Medical Association, American College of Physicians, and American College of Surgeons, the organization establishes guidelines for the operation of *hospitals* and other health facilities, and conducts survey and *accreditation* programs. A staff of medical inspectors visits hospitals by invitation and examines the operation of the hospital, the organization of its medical staff, and its patient records. Hospitals with 25 or more beds are eligible for review. On the basis of inspection reports, the hospitals may be granted "full accreditation," "provisional accreditation," or none. Accreditation has been used by, or adopted as a requirement of, specific public programs and funding agencies. Thus hospitals participating in the Medicare program are deemed to have met most *conditions of participation* if they are accredited by the JCAH. III.B.1.

Joint Commission on Mental Illness and Health. a multidisciplinary agency incorporated in 1956, representing 36 national agencies in the *mental health* and welfare fields.

It conducted a study of U.S. mental health needs from 1956 to 1961 required by the U.S. Congress in the Mental Health Study Act of 1955. The final report of the Commission, "Action for Mental Health," led to legislation in 1963 authorizing the development of *community mental health centers.* III.B.1.

joint purchasing agreement. a formal arrangement among two or more health programs to combine their purchasing of professional *services, equipment,* or *supplies.*

The agreements simplify purchasing or result in *economies of scale* intended to lower costs to the programs. The purchased services or supplies may be shared or simply distributed among the programs. III.B.1.

joint underwriting association (JUA). an organization consisting of all insurers authorized by a state to write a certain kind of insurance, usually some form of *liability* insurance like *malpractice insurance.*

Such associations are used to write *risky* or undesirable insurance. They may be *exclusive, which means individual carriers cannot write such insurance, or *nonexclusive, allowing them to do so. The JUA approach has been used in several states to assure the availability of malpractice insurance. A JUA may develop rates, issue policies, employ a service company to handle the insurance and do claims adjustment, assume *reinsurance* from its members, and cede reinsurance. IV.B., V.D.

J visa. a special visa category authorized by the U.S. Information and Education Exchange (Smith-Mundt) Act of 1948.

Individuals with J visas may be admitted to the United States to pursue a full-time program of study, as *residency,* but must be absent from the United States for two years after their studies have ended before they can reenter as immigrants. The J visa is a product of the concept of the educational exchange initiated by the Fulbright program. In 1970, the requirement for return to country of origin was legislatively eliminated for *foreign medical graduates* coming to the United States on private funds as long as they were not from a country where their special skills were in short supply. Waivers may be obtained for physicians from countries where their skills are in short supply if the home country has not objected to immigration to the United States. Waivers are rarely, if ever, denied, primarily for lack of objection from home countries.

See *labor certification* and *schedule A.* III.A.1.

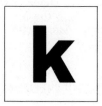

Kaiser-Permanente. see *health maintenance organization.*

kardex. a card file maintained on a *nursing service* with a card for each patient showing current *orders* for the patient's care.

Separate kardexes are often maintained for medications and *procedures.* The kardex is not typically part of the patient's *chart,* which does not usually have any similar summary of what is currently being done for the patient. V.B.

Kelley, Florence. U.S. administrator, 1859–1932. A pioneer in social reform, she made important contributions to the improvement of *maternal and child health* (MCH). She was one of the creators of the Children's Bureau, which administered federal MCH programs and worked to improve conditions of industrial employment. VII.A.1., VIII.A.1.

Keogh plan. a plan, available since 1963, under the Self-Employed Individual's Tax Retirement Act or Keogh Act, which permits a self-employed individual, as a *private physician,* to establish a formal retirement plan for himself and to obtain tax advantages similar to those available for *qualified* corporate pension plans.

Self-employed individuals annually can set aside up to 15 percent of earned *income* or $7500, whichever is less, and take a *tax deduction* for it. They, as well as individual retirement accounts, are also now available to employed people.

See *private corporation.* I.B.5.

Kerr-Mills. popular name for the Social Security Amendments of 1960, which expanded and modified the federal government's existing responsibility for assisting states in paying for medical care for the aged poor.

The amendments increased federal sharing in state *vendor payments* for medical care in the old age cash assistance program and created a new public assistance category, Medical Assistance for the Aged (MAA). The *medically indigent* eligible for assistance under this program were persons age 65 or over whose *incomes* were high enough that they were not eligible for old age assistance but who needed help in meeting the costs of their medical care. These important precedents were extended by the Social Security Amendments of 1965, which established the *Medicaid* program. IV.C.2.

kickback.   a return of part of a payment, usually because of a secret arrangement or coercion; in medicine, often refers to *fee splitting*, in which the kickback is to the referring physician rather than the paying patient. IV.A.

kiting.   in pharmacy, increasing the quantity of a drug ordered by a *prescription*.

    Either the patient or pharmacist may kite the quantity of the original prescription, as by adding zeros to the number prescribed. When done by a pharmacist, he then provides the patient with the quantity originally prescribed and bills a third party for the larger quantity. When done by a patient, it is usually because of *drug dependency*.

    See *fraud* and *shorting*. III.B.3., IV.A.

Koch, Robert.   German bacteriologist and physician, 1843–1910. Together with *Pasteur*, he created medical bacteriology. He demonstrated spore formation by anthrax bacilli, discovered the organisms of tuberculosis, cholera, and sleeping sickness, placed knowledge of wound infection on a scientific basis, and created the major techniques by which bacteriological studies are pursued.

    See *J. Henle*. I.A.1., VIII.A.1.

Koch's law, postulates.   the four conditions that establish a bacteria, virus, or other microorganism as the cause of a disease: the microorganism must be present in all cases of the disease; it must be capable of cultivation in pure culture; it must, when inoculated from pure culture, produce the disease in *susceptible* animals; and it must be recovered and again grown in pure culture from the inoculated animal. The postulates were actually developed by *J. Henle* and his student, R. Koch. I.A.1.

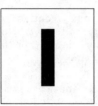

labeling. all labels and other written, printed, or graphic matter upon or accompanying a *food, drug, device,* or *cosmetic* or any of their containers or wrappers, according to section 201(m) of the Federal Food, Drug, and Cosmetic Act.

Labeling for all of these products is regulated by the Food and Drug Administration, while *advertising,* except for prescription drugs, is regulated by the Federal Trade Commission. Labeling must not contain any false or misleading statements and must include adequate directions for use. Courts have found labeling to include all written material associated with a product, as leaflets, books, and reprints of journal articles or other materials that explain or are designed to be used with the product, and point of purchase display material, as place cards and signs. Written material need not be provided the purchaser at the same time as the product to be considered labeling.

See *compendium, package insert,* and *Physicians' Desk Reference.* I.A.2.a., III.B.3.

labeled generic drug. see *generic drug.*

laboratory. 1. a place for scientific experimental work. 2. a place for performing routine tests and examinations of blood, tissue, and other biologic material, and for providing other *pathology* services. 3. by extension, the results of such tests.

The pathologist's laboratory is called a *clinical laboratory to distinguish it from a research laboratory. A laboratory is often a *department* of a hospital. Free-standing laboratories handling specimens from several sources are *independent laboratories. A *laboratory diagnosis is one arrived at by results of laboratory work.

See *medical technologist.* III.B.1.

278

labor certification. a *certification* by the U.S. Department of Labor which certain aliens, as *foreign medical graduates,* must obtain before receiving a visa.

People in occupations which the Department of Labor feels are in short supply throughout the country are given such certification after review of the applicant's qualifications, as *ECFMG certification.* See *J visa* and *schedule A.* III.A.1.

lactovegetarian. see *vegetarianism.*

Laetrile. British trademark for *l*-mandelnitrile-B-glucuronic acid, $C_{17}H_{15}HO_7$, obtained by hydrolysis of amygdalin from peach pits and oxidation of the resulting glycoside.

Laetrile has been widely touted as a cure for cancer, like *orgone* before it, although lack of evidence of its *efficacy* has required the Food and Drug Administration to keep it out of interstate commerce. V.

La Leche League. an organization dedicated to breastfeeding ("la leche" is French for milk), to education of mothers, physicians, and others in the value and ways of nursing, and to support of nursing mothers. I.A.2.a.

Lancisi, Giovanni Maria. Italian clinician, 1654–1720. He came close to the *vector* concept in the epidemiology of malaria and in part anticipated the final solution of this problem. VIII.A.1., VIII.C.

lapsed funds. in the federal *budget,* unobligated *budget authority* that by law has ceased to be available for *obligation* because the period for which it was available expired. VI.B.1.

last-dollar coverage. insurance without upper limits or maximums, no matter how great the benefits payable; compare *catastrophic health insurance* and *first-dollar coverage.* IV.B.

latent. not manifest; dormant, potential. *latency or latent period. any stage of a disease, as the *incubation* period of an infectious illness, when it has no clinical symptoms or signs. II.

lazaretto. obsolete, a hospital for people with contagious diseases; a building or ship used to *quarantine* people. III.B.1.

lead (Pb). a *heavy metal;* a soft, malleable plastic but inelastic element used in paint, gasoline, shields against radioactivity, and many other ways.

Lead, breathed or eaten, is an important health *hazard,* as an air pollutant or when lead-based paint is used indoors, since either may produce lead poisoning. I.C.

learning defect, disability, disorder, disturbance (LD). a specific deficiency in a child's ability to learn a basic academic discipline, as reading (*dyslexia), writing (*dysgraphia), or mathematics (*dyscalculia); compare *attention-deficit disorder* and *minimal brain dysfunction.*

These closely related, poorly understood conditions have been subject to much social and political abuse; see *specific learning disability.* Learning disability and attention-deficit disorder are perhaps separate forms of minimal brain dysfunction. II.B.2.

legal age. synonym, age of majority; contrast *minor.*

legal consent. deliberate, voluntary *consent* by a *competent* person; compare *informed consent.* VIII.B.3.

legal medicine. synonym, *forensic medicine.*

legend. the statement, "Caution: Federal law prohibits dispensing without prescription," required by section 503(b)(4) of the Federal Food, Drug, and Cosmetic Act as a part of the *labeling* of all prescription drugs (and only such drugs). A *legend drug is thus a prescription drug. III.B.3.

Legionnaire's disease. acute infection, principally pneumonia, caused by *Legionella pneumophila,* named after the American Legion members attending the annual convention in Philadelphia in 1976 where the disease was first recognized.

Legionnaire's disease is important in retrospect for the impetus it gave the *swine flu* program, because this early epidemic *episode* resembled the first outbreaks of the 1918 flu at a time when the management of swine flu was being debated. II.B.2.

legislative history. the written record of the writing of an act of Congress.

It may be used in writing *rules* or by courts in interpreting the law, if the act is ambiguous or lacking in detail, to ascertain or detail the intent of the Congress. The legislative history is listed in the *slip law* and consists of the House, Senate, and *conference committee reports* (if any), and the House and Senate floor debates on the law. The history, particularly the committee reports, often contains the only available complete explanation of the meaning and intent of the law. VIII.B.3.

length of stay (LOS). the length of an *inpatient's* stay in a hospital or other health facility.

The *average length of stay (ALOS) is one measure of use of health facilities. It is the average number of *days* spent in a facility by each patient calculated as the total days in the facility for all discharges and deaths occurring during a given period divided by the number of discharges and deaths during the same period. In *concurrent review* a length of stay appropriate for the patient's diagnosis may be assigned each patient upon admission. Lengths of stay vary when measured by age, *diagnosis related group,* and source of payment. VII.D.2.

lesion. a structural or functional injury or alteration due to disease, usually applied to well-defined anatomic changes. II.B.1.b.

level of care. complexity of services needed by a patient or provided by a facility.

The more acutely sick, the higher the level of care required. Level of care is never very specifically or regularly defined. Conventionally, in the United States, it increases from *self-care,* through *ambulatory care* and *home health services, intermediate care,* and *skilled nursing services,* to hospital and *intensive care.*

See *admission certification* and *swing bed.* VII.C., VII.D.3.

liability. something one is bound, by law and justice, to do; an obligation one is bound to fulfill; the probable cost of meeting such an obligation.

Liabilities may be enforced in court. They are usually financial *debts* or can be expressed in financial terms. Benefits which insurance must pay are liabilities. *Current liabilities are those payable within a year; contrast *long-term liability.*

See *defensive medicine.* V.D., VIII.B.3.

liability exam. a *physical examination* done solely for insurance, licensing, employment, or other nonpreventive purpose, as examinations required for children's participation in camp or sports activities.

These exams are done to protect the employer, school, or whoever requires the physical from *liability,* for which they are probably ineffective, rather than for actual patient benefit. V.D.

Liaison Committee on Continuing Medical Education (LCCME). a predecessor of the *Accreditation Council for Continuing Medical Education,* until the latter was formed in 1982. III.A.1.

Liaison Committee on Graduate Medical Education (LCGME). a predecessor of the *Accreditation Council for Graduate Medical Education* until 1982. III.A.1.

Liaison Committee on Medical Education (LCME). a joint committee of the American Medical Association and the Association of American Medical Colleges responsible for *accrediting* 121 U.S. and 16 Canadian medical schools.

Established in 1942, the LCME is recognized for this purpose by the U.S. government and the National Commission on Accrediting. The committee is made up of six representatives from the AMA Council on Medical Education, six representatives from the AAMC Executive Council, two representatives from the public, and one representative from the federal government. While all medical schools are now accredited, there are different types and grades of accreditation which are not constant among schools. In addition to accreditation, the LCME advises medical schools on their programs. Accreditation *criteria* are published in "Functions and Structure of a Medical School" and "Special Criteria for Programs on Medical Sciences." See *CFMA* and *ECFMG.* III.A.1.

license. a permission granted to an individual or organization by competent authority, usually public, to engage in a *practice,* occupation, or activity otherwise unlawful. *Licensure is the process by which a license is granted.

Since a license is needed to begin lawful practice, it is usually granted on the basis of examination, inspection, and/or proof of education or conformity with applicable standards, rather than measures of performance. A license is ordinarily permanent but may be conditioned on annual payment of a fee, proof of *continuing medical education,* or proof of *competence.* Common grounds for revocation of a license include incompetence, commission of a felony whether or not related to the licensed practice, or moral turpitude. Medical licensure in one state may, see *reciprocity,* or may not suffice to obtain a license from another. There is no national licensure system for health professionals, although requirements are often so nearly standardized as to constitute a national system.

See *accreditation, certification, endorsement, Federation Licensing Examination, institutional licensure,* and *national boards.* III.A., III.B.1., VII.D.2.

licensed practical nurse (LPN). a nurse who has graduated from a hospital, technical, or vocational nursing school and been licensed by a state; occasional synonym, licensed vocational nurse (LVN).

LPNs are between *patient care technicians* and *registered nurses* in skill. Licensure is ordinarily by examination and some states still allow *practical nurses* to sit for the exam. Education and licensure are somewhat variable among states. III.A.2.

licensed psychologist. see *psychologist.*

Licentiate of the Medical Council of Canada (LMCC). a physician certified for provincial licensure by the Medical Council, the Canadian equivalent of the U.S. *National Board of Medical Examiners.*

To qualify, candidates must complete medical education and a year of internship and pass the council's exams. They may then be licensed in all Canadian provinces, which have full *reciprocity* with each other and the council. III.A.1.

life. not *death.*

Read Shaw, Margery W., and A. Edward Doudera, eds., *Defining Human Life: Medical, Legal, and Ethical Implications* (Ann Arbor, MI: AUPHA Press, 1983. 379 pp.). I.A.1.

life care community, life care retirement community. a program which combines residential facilities and *long-term care.*

A typical community might have 300 residences and a health center with 50 *intermediate* and *skilled nursing* beds and another 50 personal care beds. A resident would pay a one-time entrance fee of $100,000 to $125,000 and monthly service fees for housing, services, and unlimited access to the health care facility. Up to $90,000 in entrance fees is exempt from federal taxation. III.B.1.

life change event. an occurrence, whether social, psychologic, or environmental, which requires an adjustment or effects a change in an individual's pattern of living.

Essentially synonymous with the more common term, *stressful life event,* this is better for a neutral focus on change rather than a negative one on resulting stress, and worse for omission of the family. I.A.2., I.B.1.

life cost. mortality, morbidity, and suffering associated with a given medical *procedure* or *disease.*

Life costs of *diagnosis* and *therapy* may be contrasted with their financial costs, the money required for their provision. Life costs of treating a disease may be compared with those resulting from the untreated disease, while financial costs are compared with the various monetary costs of not treating the disease. Use of life costs in assessing medical procedures avoids the need for assigning dollar values to mortality and morbidity, as in *cost-benefit analysis.* VIII.B.1.

life expectancy. in epidemiology, the *mean* number of years lived by a group of individuals of a given age, determined by the expected mortality in a specified time and area; the statistically most probable years of survival for a given individual.

Life expectancy is based on *age-specific death rates,* variable for different population categories and groups, and affected by genetic, social, and environmental factors.

Read Brackenridge, R.D.C., *Medical Selection of Life Risks: A Comprehensive Guide to Life Expectancy for Underwriters and Clinicians* (2d ed. New York: Nature Press, 1985. 814 pp.). II.C.

Life Safety Code. a fire safety code prepared by the National Fire Protection Association.

The provisions of this code relating to hospitals and nursing facilities must be met as a *condition of participation* in Medicare and Medicaid. The secretary of the Department of Health and Human Services may accept a state's fire and safety code in lieu of the Life Safety Code if it is imposed by law and will provide adequate protection for patients. The code is based on the Southern Standard Building Code, which contains optimum, not minimum, standards. III.B.1.

life stress event. see *life change event* and *stressful life event.*

life table. a description of the pattern of survival in a population using time-specific survival data and showing the cumulative probabilities of survival of the individuals in the population; in *insurance,* a tabulated statement presenting mortality and morbidity characteristics of a given population, as employed men aged 20–25, and used in *underwriting* to calculate *risks.*

A *current life table is a convenient summary of current mortality rather than a description of the actual mortality experience of any group. Commonly, the death data used for a current life table relate to a period of 1 to 3 years, and the population data relate to the middle of that period. A current life table represents the combined mortality experience by age of a population in a particular short period of time rather than the mortality experience of an actual *cohort,* and assumes a hypothetical cohort subject to the age-specific death rates observed in the particular period. A *cohort or generation life table describes the actual survival experience of a cohort of individuals born at about the same time. Cohort life tables are useful for projections of mortality, studies of mortality trends, and measurement of fertility and reproductivity. Life tables are also named for the length of the age interval in which the data are presented. A *complete life table contains data for every single year of age from birth to the last applicable age. An *abridged life table contains data by convenient intervals of 5 or 10 years of age. II.C., IV.B.

lifetime reserve. in the *Hospital Insurance Program* of Medicare, a reserve of 60 days of inpatient hospital care available over an individual's lifetime for use after one has used the maximum 90 days allowed in a single *benefit period.*

See *spell of illness.* IV.C.1.

limit on liability. in insurance, a limit on dollar coverage contained in an insurance policy or imposed by law.

Malpractice insurance generally contains such limits on the amounts payable for an individual claim or in the policy year, as $300,000 to $500,000, and $1,000,000 to $5,000,000, respectively. *Excess coverage refers to insurance with limits higher than conventional levels. IV.A., V.D.

Lind, James. British physician, 1716–1794. His *Treatise on the Scurvy,* 1773, founded *preventive medicine* by correctly recommending lemon juice be given on long voyages to prevent scurvy, which in that era of global exploration regularly killed many sailors. III.C., VIII.A.1.

list. 1. to enter someone in a *register.* 2. British, the patients cared for by a physician; compare *panel.* V.

Lister, Joseph. English surgeon, 1827–1912. Last and greatest of a Quaker family of physicians, he fathered *antiseptic* surgery by applying Pasteur's germ theories of disease, showing that sterile conditions prevented *nosocomial* infections. I.C., VIII.A.1.

lithotripsy. the crushing of calculi or stones, as kidney stones, to facilitate their removal; synonym, litholapaxy (Gr. *litho,* stone + *lapaxis,* evacuation). *lithotriptor. an instrument for crushing calculi, now by use of ultrasound; synonym, lithotrite. V.B.

litogen.   a drug that does not cause congenital malformations but does cause lawsuits, as the widely used treatment for morning sickness, Bendectin, and vaginal spermicides.

Read Mills, James L., and Duane Alexander, "Teratogens and 'Litogens'" (*N Engl J Med*, 315(19): 1234–6, 11/6/86). III.B.3.

live birth.   complete expulsion or extraction from its mother of a product of conception, at any time during pregnancy, that after separation breathes or shows any other evidence of life, as beating of the heart, pulsation of the umbilical cord, or definite movement of voluntary muscles, whether or not the umbilical cord has been cut or the placenta is attached. Each product of such a birth is considered *live-born; compare *birth* and *stillbirth*.

This definition does not require that the product of conception be viable or capable of independent life and includes very early and patently nonviable fetuses. This means the definition is often not strictly applied and suggests the need for addition of a viability criterion, or use of a different term, as viable birth, which includes such a criterion. I.A.1.

living will.   a statement of an individual's desires respecting medical care made when well and in anticipation of the possibility that disease or injury might leave the individual alive but unconscious or incompetent.

These documents try to avoid *cardiopulmonary resuscitation,* long-term use of respirators to support a body whose brain cannot function or recover, or any modern medical possibility of which an individual disapproves. See *natural death act.* I.A.2.

loading.   in insurance, the amount added to the actuarial value of the *coverage* expected, or to the average amounts payable to the insured, to cover the expense to the insurer of securing and maintaining the business; the amount added to the pure premium needed for anticipated *liabilities* to provide for *expenses,* contingencies, *profits,* or special situations.

Loading costs for *group insurance* range from 5 to 25 percent of premiums and for individual health insurance from 40 to 60 percent. IV.B.

lobby.   attempt, by anyone other than a citizen acting in his own behalf, to influence a government official in the performance of his duty by the provision of information, argument, or other means.

Federal law on lobbying activities, Title III of the Legislative Reorganization Act of 1946, does not define lobbying or lobbyist and has other such loopholes. It does require registration by anyone "who, by himself or through any agent or employee or other persons in any manner whatsoever, directly or indirectly, solicits, collects, or receives money or any other thing of value to be used principally to aid or the principal purpose of which person is to aid...the passage or defeat of any legislation by the Congress." Paid lobbyists are required to register with the House and Senate and file financial reports. VIII.B.3.

local government.   a general purpose political and administrative unit below the federal and state levels, whose authority derives from the state government. This includes counties, municipalities, and their equivalents (parishes, townships, towns, and villages) and excludes regional and district organizations.

Local governments in the United States are as variable as are New York City, Silver Lake, and Scott County. They regularly have environmental and *public health* responsibilities and programs and, to a variable extent, provide direct medical services, usually just to the poor. III.D.2.

locality. in *Medicare,* the geographic region from which a *carrier* derives *prevailing charges* for the purpose of making *reasonable charge* determinations.
A locality is ordinarily a political or economic subdivision of a state. It should include a cross section of the population with respect to economic and other characteristics. Localities have no particular relation to *health service areas* or providers' *medical trade areas.* IV.C.1.

locality rule. in malpractice, a doctrine which bases the standard of care a physician owes a patient on the standard of care generally attained in a specific community or location.
The most restrictive interpretation of this rule is that the measure of a physician's duty of care to a patient is that degree of care, skill, and diligence used by physicians, generally, in the same locality or community in which the physician practices. A less restrictive form holds a physician to the degree of care exercised by physicians, generally, in the same or similar localities or communities. The more expansive rule is now being applied more widely because the early emphasis on locality is inappropriate with modern communication and national standardization of education and practice. V.D.

local medical doctor (LMD). a *referring* physician; practicing physicians are known by the acronym in academic health science centers, ordinarily with condescending tone. III.A.1., VIII.B.2.a.

lock in. an arrangement that requires a patient to seek care from designated providers, typically limiting *freedom of choice* in return for payment for services provided by the providers.
In Medicaid, federal authority and rules for lock in programs were enacted in 1981 to help control excessive use of program benefits, allowing beneficiaries with a demonstrated pattern of *abuse* to be limited to a single primary care physician or pharmacy for a reasonable period of time in nonemergency situations. IV.C.2.

locum tenens. (Latin, one holding a place) one temporarily holding an office or acting as a substitute for another, used especially of physicians.
*Locum tenentes have for generations allowed *solo practitioners* to take vacations.
See *Project USA.* III.A.1.

longevity. long life, length of life; casual synonym, *life expectancy.* I.A.1.

longitudinal study. a *study* in which observations on the same individuals are made at two or more different points in time.
Most *cohort* and *case-control* studies are longitudinal. VIII.D.

long-term care (LTC). health, rehabilitative, or personal services for people who are chronically ill, aged, disabled, or retarded, whether inpatients or at home, provided on a prolonged basis; compare *chronic* and *primary care.*
The term often narrowly refers only to long-term institutional care, as in *nursing homes,* homes for the retarded, and mental hospitals. It is not specifically defined in the United States but might include skilled, intermediate, or home health care continuing for over 60 days. Ambulatory and home health services provided on a long-term basis and *life care communities* are seen as *alternatives to long-term care.* VII.C.5.b.

long-term care insurance. protection against the cost of *intermediate* or *skilled nursing care.*

A little such insurance has become available in recent years but is expensive and limited by actuarial inexperience, the high cost of the care, and the fair chance that, by the time someone realizes he may need such care, he is likely to be right. IV.B.

long-term debt, liability. in accounting, a *debt* that is not expected to be settled within a year; compare *current.* VI.C.1.

loss. in insurance, the basis for a *claim* under the terms of an insurance policy; any diminution of quantity, quality, or value of health or property, resulting from the occurrence of some *hazard* or *peril.*

In health insurance, the loss is the cost of health services required by the *risk.* Reimbursement may be made either to the insured, *indemnity benefits,* or on his behalf to the provider of the services, *services benefits.* IV.B.

Louis, Pierre-Charles-Alexandre. French physician, 1787–1872. He introduced statistical methods in the study of disease, proving the uselessness of *phlebotomy* in pneumonia with numbers and thus largely ending its practice. He was a great teacher whose students included *O.W. Holmes.* VIII. A.1.

Love Canal. a residential area in Niagara Falls, NY, surrounding the Love Canal.

Part of Love Canal was used for years as a *dump* site by the Hooker Chemicals and Plastics Corporation. It was declared a health *hazard* in 1978 because of possible chromosome abnormalities and other toxic effects in residents *exposed* to dumped chemicals seeping into homes, playgrounds, gardens, and water supplies. In 1980, a state of emergency was ordered and 710 families were evacuated, their homes being bought by the federal government; the area was later declared fit for habitation after a cleanup effort. As Hiroshima has become synonymous with wartime use of atomic weapons, Love Canal has become the symbol of *pollution* of residential environments by the dumping of toxic industrial *waste.* I.C.4.

low level. see *radioactive waste.*

low option. the alternative to *high option.* IV.C.

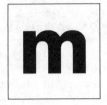

macrobiotics. an attitude toward life and health based on an understanding of the importance of *diet;* the dietary system associated with it.

This extremely specific *vegetarian* diet, largely of whole grains, is derived from the ancient concept of opposing principles Yin (feminine, acid) and Yang (masculine, alkaline). It is said to promote health and well-being, but as practiced is sometimes deficient in *essential* nutrients. V.

magnetic resonance imaging (MRI). synonym, *nuclear magnetic resonance;* introduced in 1984 as the preferred name, presumably to avoid any negative connotation of "nuclear." III.B.2.

mail-order insurance. health, disability, or other individual insurance secured in response to public or personal solicitation by mail and advertising.

It usually requires no physical examination, but rather a statement of health completed by the insured, and is effective upon return of the application by mail and approval by the insurer. The scant health information required, the complexities of medical histories, and the relative difficulty of excluding preexisting conditions have contributed to high premiums and *loading,* and to low rates of claims recovery from mail-order insurance. IV.B.2.

mainstream. educate the *handicapped* in regular classes for those without handicaps.

This educational analogue to *deinstitutionalizing* the mentally ill has produced this equally ugly jargon. II.

mainstream smoke. see *smoke.*

major. antonym, *minor.*

major diagnostic category (MDC). one of 23 groups of related diagnoses, as diseases and disorders of the nervous system (MDC 1) and selected factors influencing health status and contact with health services (MDC 23), used by the Medicare *prospective payment system* to classify and collect the 468 *diagnosis related groups,* each of which is assigned to one of the MDCs, for analytic purposes. IV.C.1.

major medical, major medical expense insurance (mm). insurance against heavy medical expenses resulting from *catastrophic* or prolonged illness or injuries.

Most major medical policies contain a maximum on the total amount that will be paid, as $250,000, and thus do not provide *last-dollar coverage* or complete protection against catastrophic cost. Benefit payments are usually 80 to 100 percent of expenses after the insured has incurred substantial, as $2000, *out-of-pocket* expenses as a *deductible.* IV.B.

major operation, surgery. surgery in which the procedure is hazardous.

Major surgery is irregularly distinguished from *minor surgery* by whether or not it requires a general anesthetic, involves an amputation above the ankle or wrist, includes entering one of the body cavities (abdomen, chest, or head), or requires special surgical skills. V.B.

malathion. an *organophosphate.*

malformation. abnormal development or formation of part of the body; a bad *anomaly* or *deformity.*

Malformations are *congenital;* deformities may be acquired. I.A.1., II.

malignant. see *cancer.*

malinger. to feign or exaggerate illness or incapacity willfully in order to avoid work or other responsibilities.

Malingering may be *fraud* because it is conscious; it is not itself an illness. People with *functional* or *psychosomatic* illness are not malingerers. II.B.1.a.

malnutrition. inadequate *nutrition* due to under- or overnourishment, imbalanced diet, defective digestion or assimilation, or other causes.

It is now stylish to recognize that obesity arising from affluence is malnutrition, but inadequate intake caused by poverty remains the most important problem. I.A.2.a.

malpractice. violation of a *professional* duty to act with reasonable care and in good faith without fraud or collusion; *negligence* or lack of ordinary skill in the performance of a professional act.

Malpractice by a physician is a wrong, or tort, resulting in *injury,* or harm, and arising from a failure either of judgment or to have and use reasonable learning, skill, and experience. Reasonable care is that ordinarily possessed by others of his profession, see *locality rule.* A practitioner is *liable* for damages or injuries caused by malpractice. Such liability may be covered by malpractice insurance. To recover damages for malpractice patients must demonstrate some injury and that the injury was negligently caused.

See *abandonment, charitable immunity, contingency fee, defensive medicine, discovery, good samaritan law, governmental immunity, New Jersey and locality rules, limits on liability, professional liability, res ipsa loquiter, respondeat superior, screening panels,* and *warranty.* V.D.

malpractice insurance. insurance against the risk of suffering financial damage because of malpractice and the cost of defending suits.

See *claims incurred* and *made policies, go bare, joint underwriting association, sponsored malpractice insurance,* and *tail.* IV.A., V.D.

managed care. medical services for which a *third party payer* takes budgetary responsibility.

The manager is ordinarily an insurer, Blue Cross/Blue Shield, or a self-insured employer. Managed care systems include health maintenance and preferred provider organizations, and any other arrangement by which these monopsonists supervise how their money is spent. VI.B.

management. the organization and control of human activity directed toward specific ends; compare *administration*.

Different kinds of management are sometimes described, as *by exception, in which only exceptions from defined *policy* are reported and acted on; and *by *objective*, in which clearly stated objectives are used to guide the management process. VI.

management information system. a data system which produces the information needed for management of a program or other activity.

Such systems are usually automated, produce accounting, productivity, and other data in useful form at appropriate intervals, measure program progress toward *objectives*, and report costs and problems needing attention. VI.C.

management medicine. primary care which combines clinical skills and modern management techniques to maximize patient satisfaction.

Health promotion, quality control, team work, and such may all be used in steering a respectable course between *holistic care* and *health maintenance organizations*.

Read Inglefinger, Franz J., "Management Medicine: The Doctor's Job Today" (an essay in *The Great Ideas Today, 1978*. Chicago: Encyclopedia Britannica, Inc., 1978). V.

maniac. imprecise and misleading term for an emotionally disturbed person; implies violent behavior. Not specifically referable to any psychiatric diagnostic category. II.B.2.

mantra. see *meditation*.

manipulation. the use of the hands in a skillful manner to treat disease, as reducing a dislocation or hernia, or to create health, as improving bodily alignment.

The laying on of hands is basic to health care with remarkable *placebo effect* and many forms; compare *Alexander technique, chiropractic, massage, osteopathy*, and *shiatsu*. V.B.

marginal cost. in economics, the change in the *cost* of producing a service which results from a small or unit change in the quantity of services being produced.

Marginal cost is the appropriate cost concept to consider when contemplating program expansion or contraction. *Economies of scale* result from expansion of a program when marginal cost is negative. VIII.B.1.

marginal tax rate. the tax rate, or percentage, applied on the last increment of *income* for purposes of computing federal or other income taxes.

The marginal tax rate varies with a taxpayer's filing status, as well as his income. The marginal tax rate increases with income for *progressive taxes* and decreases for *regressive taxes*. The marginal tax rate is often referred to as an *individual's tax bracket. IV.C.

Marine Hospital Service. from 1798 until 1902, the agency of the U.S. government responsible for providing medical care to merchant seamen, *quarantine* services at points of entry, and related activities.

In 1902 its functions and name were expanded to Public Health and Marine Hospital Service, and in 1912 it became the *U.S. Public Health Service.* III.D.1.

mark. see *budget.*

markup. in Congress, a congressional committee meeting at which the committee writes law to recommend to the full Congress, makes decisions on appropriations, or otherwise makes *policy.*

Markups take place after public hearings on the subject matter. See *executive session.* VIII.B.3.

marriage. "an institution joining man and woman in special social and legal dependence for the purpose of founding and maintaining a family; a socially sanctioned relationship between two adults (which) determines specific roles, involving reciprocal obligations, duties, (and) rights" (*Pinney and Slipp, 1982*).

Marriage, traditionally defined as permanent, arises out of sexual rather than parental bonds, although many societies combine or confuse the two. The marital dyad is the core of the family, its most important subsystem, and often its weakest link. I.B.1.

Massachusetts General Hospital Utility-Programming System (MUMPS). a pioneering clinical data management system for computers developed in the late 1960s by the National Institutes of Health and Harvard University; compare *COSTAR* and *PROMIS.*

Read Greenes, R.A., "MUMPS: Second-decade Design Considerations" (*Comput Biomed Res,* 14: 104–111, 1981). III.B.2.

massage therapy. 1. in parts of the world (Canada, Scandinavia) a therapeutic approach using massage, hydrotherapy, and *acupressure* for manipulation of the soft tissues of the body to relieve pain and spasm, release tension, and achieve other specific therapeutic results. 2. generally in the United States thought of as a modern version of the oldest profession.

In Canada, massage therapists receive 18 months of formal education after high school, are licensed by some provinces, and reimbursed by some provincial and private health insurance plans. There are several thousand massage therapists in Canada, mostly in private practice. V.

match, the match. common name for the *National Residents Matching Program.*

maternal and child health service (MCH). an organized health or social service for mothers, particularly *family planning* and perinatal services, their children, and, rarely, fathers.

Mothers and children are particularly vulnerable to disease. Their special health needs may be met by educational, nutritional, and preventive activities. Such services are, thus, sometimes separately organized and funded from other health services, as with the U.S. Maternal and Child Health Program, authorized by Title V of the Social Security Act. This program has supported the *Crippled Children's Service* and a variety of *children and youth (C&Y) and *maternal and infant care projects (M&I). MCH became the Maternal and Child Health Block Grant in 1981.

See *S.J. Baker* and *F. Kelley.* VII.A.1.

maternal and infant care project (M&I). see *maternal and child health services.*

maternal mortality rate. the number of deaths reported as caused by complications of pregnancy, abortions, delivery, and of the puerperium. Since 1958 deaths have been assigned to maternal causes only when they occur within one year of the maternal complication. The rate is reported as per 100,000 *live births* in a given area or program per year. II.D.

maternity benefits. any coverage for costs arising from pregnancy, labor, and delivery, and, in some cases, *family planning,* postpartum care, and complications of pregnancy.

Health insurance policies often take special approaches and apply conditions to maternity benefits, see *exclusion,* and *flat, swap,* and *switch maternity.* IV.A.

maximum allowable cost program (MAC). a federal program to limit reimbursement for prescription drugs in Medicaid and other federally assisted programs to the lowest cost at which the drug is generally available.

As originally proposed the program limited payment for drugs to the lowest of the maximum allowable cost (MAC) of the drug, if any, plus a reasonable *dispensing fee,* the acquisition cost of the drug plus a dispensing fee, or the provider's usual and customary charge to the general public for the drug. The MAC was the lowest unit price at which a drug available from several sources or manufacturers could be purchased on a national basis. III.B.3., IV.C.

McCarran-Ferguson Act. the act of March 9, 1945, which declares a general policy that federal laws which regulate or affect business and commerce are not to be interpreted as affecting the *insurance* business unless they do so specifically; synonyms, the McCarran-Wiler Bill (S.1508) and Public Law 15.

Prior to a 1944 Supreme Court decision, insurance was not considered a matter of commerce and thus not subject to federal law. When the Supreme Court found insurance to be a form of commerce it became necessary to clarify the effect on it of existing federal law. The act has the effect of leaving regulation of insurance to the states unless specifically undertaken in federal law and exempting it from much routine federal supervision of commerce. IV.B.

McMaster Model of Family Functioning. a method of evaluating the effectiveness of family functioning which assesses family problem solving, communication, roles, affective responsiveness, affective involvement, and behavior control. It has been used extensively in research and family therapy. V.

meals on wheels. a program which delivers meals to people who are unable to prepare an adequate *diet* for themselves.

Such programs are sponsored by health departments, *VNAs,* churches, and others. They typically use volunteers to deliver a hot, nutritious meal five days a week to poor, housebound, *handicapped* people. I.A.2.a., VII.C.1.

mean. the arithmetic average of a set of observations, the sum of scores divided by the number of scores; synonyms, arithmetic mean, average, and norm; compare *median, mode, normal curve,* and *standard deviation.*

All of these related terms are casually used for any value in the middle of a distribution or range, but each has the indicated proper meaning. VIII.D.

means test. a criterion for eligibility for free or subsidized health care, usually based on a person's *income* and *resources;* an examination of the financial status of a person as a requirement for receiving *social insurance* or other public benefits; contrast *work test.*

Those with incomes above a specified amount become ineligible for the service or may be required to spend a part of their income for services before qualifying, see *spend down.* Means tests are not standardized and are sometimes self-administered by those seeking eligibility. *National health insurance* programs, like other *social security* programs that serve people's needs without regard to income, do not need a means test. IV.C.

measure for coffin (MFC). euphemism, terminal; ordinarily in acronym form, as "After that attack, he's ready to MFC." VIII.B.2.a.

Medex. a *physician assistant* program developed specifically for former military medical corpsmen with independent duty experience; a graduate of such a program; originally an acronym for the French term, *medicin extension.*

Such programs train physician assistants, especially to work with family physicians in rural areas. Most Medex are trained to work with specific physicians. The first such program was begun in 1969 by Richard A. Smith at the University of Washington. The programs generally consist of 3 months of university training and 12 months of preceptorship or apprenticeship. III.A.4.

median. the middle value in a set of values that have been arranged in order from highest to lowest; compare *mean, mode,* and *standard deviation.* VIII.D.

median infective dose (ID$_{50}$). see *dose.*

median lethal concentration (LC$_{50}$). the concentration of a substance in water, air, food, or some other medium that will kill half of insects, animals, or other organisms exposed, see *dose.*

The LC$_{50}$ is a standard measure of the *toxicity* of the substance. I.C.5.

median lethal dose (LD$_{50}$). see *dose.*

Medicaid (Title XIX). a federally aided, state-operated program which provides medical *benefits* for eligible low-income people in need of medical care.

The program, authorized by Title XIX of the Social Security Act and basically for the *poor,* covers only poor people in one of the categories of people covered under welfare cash payment programs—the aged, the blind, the disabled, and members of families with dependent children where one parent is absent, incapacitated, or unemployed. In certain circumstances states may provide Medicaid coverage for children under 21 who are not *categorically related.* Subject to broad federal guidelines, states determine

the benefits covered, program eligibility, rates of payment for *providers,* and methods of administering the program.
See *Kerr-Mills.* IV.C.2.

Medicaid management information system (MMIS). one of the state *management information systems* used in the Medicaid program. IV.C.2.

Medicaid mill. a health program which serves, solely or primarily, Medicaid beneficiaries, typically on an *ambulatory* basis.

The mills originated in the ghettos of New York City and are still found primarily in urban slums with few other medical *services.* They are usually organized to make a *profit,* characterized by their great productivity, and frequently accused of a variety of *abuses,* as *ping-ponging* and *family ganging.* IV.C.2.

Medi-Cal. California's *Medicaid* program.

Medical Activities and Manpower Project (MAMP). a survey of a stratified random sample of U.S. physicians in each of 24 specialties in which respondents completed a questionnaire concerning their training and practice, recorded data on all patients encountered in a 3-day period, and recorded the hours worked and the number of patients encountered in a 7-day period. The study was done at the University of Southern California, hence it is sometimes known as USC-MAMP.

Read Mendenhall, Robert C., et al., "A National Study of Medical and Surgical Specialties. II: Description of the Survey Instrument" (*JAMA,* 240: 1160–8, 9/8/78). III.A.1.

Medical Assistance for the Aged (MAA). see *Kerr-Mills.*

Medical Assistance Program. the health care program for the poor authorized by Title XIX of the Social Security Act, known as *Medicaid.* IV.C.2.

medical assistant. an individual who assists a physician in an office or other medical setting, performing those administrative and/or clinical duties delegated in relation to the individual's degree of training and in accord with respective state laws governing such actions and activities.

Medical assistants have a wide range of duties in many aspects of the physician's practice. Medical assistants have less formal training, independence, and clinical responsibility than *physician assistants.* III.A.4.

medical audit. a professional review of medical practice; usually an organized retrospective evaluation of performance by any of several methods and *criteria,* including chart audit and assessment of *length of stay,* use of consultation, and use of laboratory and x-ray services.

A medical audit is usually concerned with the care of a given illness and is undertaken to identify deficiencies in anticipation of corrective educational measures.

See *concurrent review, medical care evaluation study, quality,* and *risk management.* VI.D.2., VII.D.2.

Medical Audit Program (MAP). an extension of the *Professional Activities Study* (PAS), in which data were displayed in comprehensive quarterly reports by hospital department.

The reports were used by hospital clinical departments in doing medical audit and *utilization review.*

See *Commission on Professional and Hospital Activities.* III.B.1.

medical care. *care* of individuals and their illnesses, usually by physicians or under their direction. Somewhat irregularly used; compare *health care,* and contrast *custodial care* and *first aid.* V.

medical care evaluation study (MCE Study). an early and somewhat less flexible form of *quality review study.* VI.D.2.

medical center. a hospital on the verge of a fund raising campaign. III.B.1., VIII.B.2.b.

Medical College Admission Test (MCAT). a nationally standardized test required or strongly recommended by U.S. medical schools as part of their admission process.

    The MCAT, administered by the Association of American Medical Colleges in Washington, D.C., is designed to provide objective measures of academic ability and achievement through tests of verbal ability, quantitative ability, science knowledge, and general information. It does not try or claim to measure motivation, the nature or sincerity of interest in medicine, or personal characteristics.

    Read Erdmann, J.B., et al., "The Medical College Admission Test and the Selection of Medical Students, the MCAT Malady, and the MCAT Revisited" (*N Engl J Med,* 310(6): 386–9 and 396–401, 2/9/84). III.A.1.

Medical Committee for Human Rights (MCHR). an organization formed in the 1960s to provide medical presence at civil rights and peace in Vietnam demonstrations and forums for radical analysis of medical issues. III.B.4.

medical deduction. the federal income *tax deduction* for expenditures on health care.

    This is the only *national health insurance* program in the United States. No standards are set for health insurance purchased with deducted premiums. Deductible medical expenses are broadly defined, including the services of physicians, dentists, podiatrists, optometrists, chiropractors, and Christian Science practitioners and equipment, *drugs, supplies,* and special diets prescribed by such people. Expenditures on *tax credits* for this version of *Medicredit* amount to billions of dollars annually. IV.D.

medical device. see *device.*

medical ethics. the discipline concerned with, and standards of behavior respecting, what is good and bad and moral duty and obligation in medicine.

    Most *professions* are governed by ethical codes which are surprisingly effective, when considering their lack of enforcement, although not when viewing how they structure, regulate, and restrain the trade.

    See *bioethics* and *ethics committee.* III.C.

medical examiner (ME). a physician duly authorized and charged by a governmental unit, as a city, county, or state, to determine facts concerning causes of death, particularly when unnatural, and to testify about them in court; generally, anyone responsible in a *workmen's compensation, disability,* or other such program for determining medical facts; compare *police surgeon.*

    Medical examiners frequently replace or work with a *coroner,* who may not be a physician. Their principal tool is the *autopsy* and many are pathologists. Your author is a medical examiner; it is unpleasant work. III.A.1., III.D.2., VIII.B.3.

medical foundation. an organization of physicians, generally sponsored by a state or local medical association; synonym, *foundation for medical care.* Foundations are legally independent of their organizing medical associations, set up to conduct peer review programs, serve as *individual practice associations,* or for other purposes. While foundations operating as IPAs are prepaid on a *capitation* basis for services to their patients, they still pay physician members on a *fee-for-service* basis for the services they give. III.B.1.

medical history. see *history.*

Medical Illness Severity Grouping System (MEDISGRPS). a system for rating in four groups the *severity* of patients' illnesses upon admission to the hospital based on physiologic data and defining severity in terms of probability of death.

MEDISGRPS may be used for *case-mix* adjustment but does not use the *Uniform Hospital Discharge Data Set.* II.A.2.

Medical Indemnity of America, Inc. (MIA). a *stock insurance company* organized in Ohio in 1950 by *Blue Shield plans* to serve as a national enrollment agency, to assist individual plans in negotiating contracts, and to serve large national accounts in which two or more plans are involved.

See *Health Service, Inc.* IV.B.1.

medical indigency. the state of having insufficient *income* to pay for adequate medical care without depriving oneself or *dependents* of food, clothing, shelter, and other essentials of living; compare *medically needy.*

Medical indigency may occur when a self-supporting individual, ordinarily able to maintain his *family,* is unable to finance the total cost of medical care in times of illness.

See *spend down.* I.A.2.c.

Medical Information Bureau (MIB). a clearinghouse of information on people who have ever applied for life insurance.

Any adverse medical finding on previous applications to companies subscribing to the service are recorded in code and sent to companies considering new applications. This raises interesting *confidentiality* questions, especially for information produced by medical examinations. IV.B.

medical jurisprudence. synonym, *forensic medicine.*

medical laboratory assistant. an individual who works under the direct supervision of a *medical technologist, pathologist,* physician, or qualified scientist in performing routine laboratory procedures requiring basic technical skills and minimal independent judgment in chemistry, hematology, and microbiology.

Certification is awarded following successful examination. Taking the examination requires a high school diploma or equivalent, either graduation from an American Medical Association–approved school or completion of a basic military laboratory course, and a year of experience. III.A.4.

medical literature. the body of writings on the maintenance of health and treatment of disease.

Medical literature is broadly divided into *the reviewed literature, which is subject to independent critical review prior to publication, costly to the reader, and indexed by *Index Medicus,* and *the throwaway literature, which lacks prior review, is free to the subscriber (completely subsidized by advertising), and poorly indexed. The regular literature, which is found in libraries, is distinguished from *the fugitive literature, which includes many nonrecurring publications, government and private reports, and unpublished works. III.C.

Medical Literature and Analysis Retrieval System (MEDLARS). the National Library of Medicine's computerized system for indexing medicine's literature. *MEDLINE is the on-line part of the system, allowing the user direct computer interaction with the data base for search purposes.

The system is completely computerized and produces *Index Medicus*.

Read Bachrach, C.A., and Thelma Charen, "Selection of MEDLINE Contents, the Development of its Thesaurus, and the Indexing Process" (*Med Inform*, 3(3): 237–54, 1978). III.C.

medically indigent. a person who is too impoverished to meet his medical expenses.

These may be people whose *income* is low enough that they can pay for basic living costs but not routine medical care, or people with generally adequate income who suddenly face *catastrophically* large medical bills. I.A.2.C.

medically needy. in the *Medicaid* program, eligible people who have enough *income* and *resources* to pay for their basic living expenses, and so do not need welfare, but not enough to pay for their medical care.

State Medicaid programs may cover the medically needy with incomes up to 133 percent of the maximum paid a family of similar size by the Aid to Families with Dependent Children (AFDC) program. To be eligible as medically needy, people must be *categorically related* by being in one of the categories of people covered by the welfare cash assistance programs, including the aged, blind, disabled, and members of families with dependent children where one parent is absent, incapacitated, or unemployed. They receive benefits if their income after deducting medical expenses, see *spend down,* is low enough to meet eligibility standards. IV.C.2.

medically underserved area (MUA). an urban or rural geographic location, as a census tract or county, with insufficient *health resources,* particularly manpower and facilities to meet the medical *needs* of the resident population.

*Physician shortage area is defined by measuring the *health status* of the resident population rather than the supply of resources, an area with an unhealthy population being considered underserved. The term is defined and used in the *PHS Act* in order to give priority to such areas for federal assistance. II.C.

medically underserved population. a population with a shortage of personal health services or, occasionally, with poor health.

A medically underserved population need not reside in a particular *medically underserved area;* it is not defined by its place of residence. Thus migrants, Native Americans, or the inmates of a prison or mental hospital may constitute such a population. The term is defined and used in the PHS Act in order to give such populations priority for federal assistance, as in the health maintenance organization and National Health Service Corps programs. II.C.

medical microbiology. see *microbiology*.

medical model. the conceptual system used by most physicians in understanding and caring for disease, a patient, and the combination, an *illness;* compare *explanatory model.*

It is dualistic, separating both patient and disease and mind and body, and reductionist, seeking biophysical explanations for all illness. The model is also remarkably successful. It is informally learned in school and powerfully, but unconsciously, guides and constrains practice. While variably defined, it is concerned with diseases, more than people, for which it seeks causes, preferably single, and gives treatment responsibility to physicians rather than host. This approach to illness is of course used by many psychologists and other nonphysicians. Other models like *self-care,* the *biopsychosocial model,* group approaches, as *Alcoholics Anonymous,* and *family therapy* may be preferred for some illnesses or integrated with the medical model, see *humanistic* and *holistic medicine.* III.C.

medical oncology. the subspecialty of *internal medicine* concerned with cancer. III.C.

medical record. a record kept which properly contains sufficient information to identify the patient clearly, justify his *diagnosis* and *treatment,* and document the results.

The medical record serves as a basis for planning and *continuity* of patient care; means of communication among physicians and others contributing to the patient's care; source of evidence of the patient's course of illness and treatment; basis for review, study, and evaluation; protection of the legal interests of the patient, responsible program, and practitioner; and source of data for use in research and education. Medical records are the responsibility (and usually property) of the provider caring for the patient, to whom the record is not typically available. The content of the record is usually *confidential.* Each different provider in a community caring for a given patient keeps an independent record of that care.

See *incident report, problem-oriented medical record,* and *progress note.* VII.D.

medical records administrator. one who plans and manages systems of administrative and clinical data on patients and their medical records.

The minimum educational requirement for registration is a baccalaureate degree in medical records science or administration from a program *accredited* by the American Medical Association in collaboration with the American Medical Records Association. The administrator is the most highly trained of several types of medical records personnel, including the medical records technician. III.A.6.

medical review. 1. consideration by physicians or others of the need for, quality of, or other aspects of medical care, see *medical audit.* 2. in Medicaid, review by a team of physicians and other health and social service personnel of the condition and need for care, including a medical evaluation, of each inpatient in a long-term care facility.

The Medicaid review team must review care provided in the facility, adequacy of available services, necessity and desirability of the continued placement of patients in the facility, and the feasibility of meeting their needs through alternate services. Medical review differs from *utilization review* by requiring evaluation of each individual patient and an analysis of the *appropriateness* of his specific treatment in a given institution, where utilization review is often done on a sample basis, with special attention to certain procedures, conditions, or *lengths of stay.*

See *admission certification, continued stay review, independent professional review, program review team,* and *quality assurance.* IV.C.2., VII.D.2.

medical school. a school *accredited* by the *LCME* for granting of the Doctor of Medicine degree, ordinarily after 4 years of postbaccalaureate education. There are about 100 medical schools in the United States.
See *academic health science center.* III.B.1.

Medical Sciences Knowledge Profile (MSKP). an examination used by the *Coordinated Transfer Application System* since 1980 to assess U.S. citizens receiving medical education outside the United States. III.A.1.

Medical Signal Code. chapter 3 of the International Signal Code, which allows worldwide communication wherever language or transmission is a difficulty. It is remarkable for the detail which it permits in describing problems and giving medical advice.
See *Deadhead Medico.* Read *International Code of Signals, U.S. Edition, 1969* (U.S. Naval Oceanographic Office, Publ. No. H.O. 102. Washington, D.C., U.S. Government Printing Office, 1969. pp. 97–130). II.

medical staff. collectively, the *physicians* and other *professionals* responsible for medical care in a *health facility,* typically a hospital.
The staff may be full-time or part-time, employed by the hospital or not, and include all professionals who wish to be included, *open staff; or just those who meet various standards of competence, *closed staff. *Staff privileges* may or may not be permanent or conditioned on continued evidence of competence. III.A.1., III.B.1.

Medical Subject Headings (MESH). the thesaurus of indexing terms used by the National Library of Medicine in the *Medical Literature and Analysis Retrieval System* and other indices. III.C.

medical technologist (MT). a *technologist* trained in *clinical laboratory* technology.
Minimum educational requirements for one of several certification programs in medical technology are a baccalaureate degree with appropriate science courses, a one-year structured AMA *accredited* medical technology program, and an examination, or a baccalaureate degree with appropriate science courses and appropriate experience. The medical technologist is the most highly trained of several types of clinical laboratory personnel, including the medical laboratory *technician* and medical laboratory assistant. III.A.4.

medical technology. synonym, *health care technology;* often limited to *clinical laboratory* technology; compare *medical technologist* and contrast *x-ray technologist.*

medical trade area. a *region* from which one or more specified providers draw their patients; similar to *catchment area,* except defined by the patients rather than the providers. III.B.1.

Medicare (Title XVIII). a U.S. social insurance program for people aged 65 and over, for persons who have received social security disability payments for over two years, and for certain workers and their dependents who need kidney transplantation or dialysis.
Medicare is available to *insured* persons without regard to *income.* Mon-

ies from *payroll taxes* and *premiums* from *beneficiaries* are deposited in special *trust funds* for use in meeting expenses incurred by the insured. The program was enacted July 30, 1965, as Title XVIII, Health Insurance for the Aged, of the Social Security Act, and became effective on July 1, 1966. It consists of two separate but coordinated programs: *Hospital Insurance* (Part A), and Supplementary Medical Insurance (Part B). IV.C.1.

Medicare Case Mix Index (CMI). a measure of *complexity* of the mixture of cases cared for by a hospital, calculated by multiplying the proportion of Medicare patients in each of the *diagnosis related groups* by the *diagnosis related group weight.* IV.C.1.

Medicare History File. a longitudinal data set maintained by the Health Care Financing Administration, Department of Health and Human Services, with complete *utilization* and payment records on a 5 percent random sample of Medicare beneficiaries during the period 1974–1977. IV.C.1.

medicine. (1) the art and science of promoting and maintaining health and of *diagnosing* and *treating disease.* III.C.; (2) the branch of medicine concerned with nonsurgical treatment of disease; *internal medicine.* III.C.; (3) a substance used in treating disease, to effect well-being, or for some analogous purpose; a *drug.* III.B.3. (4) in some cultures, an object or potion which gives control over natural or magical forces. I.B.4.

medigap policy. a *supplemental health insurance* policy designed to supplement *Medicare.* IV.C.1.

meditation. 1. in western culture, contemplative thought. 2. in eastern, suspension of thought (and often the consciousness that goes with it) so that other mental activities and forms of consciousness may be used.

Meditation ordinarily requires training and practice. It often produces the *relaxation response,* useful new awareness of self, and enjoyment of sensory perception. It is known in western culture, and as an essential part of many eastern religions and therapies, as *yoga.* The suspension of thought is usually achieved by persistent concentration in a quiet environment and comfortable position on one thing, the *mantra. V.

megamouse experiment. a study done by the *National Center for Toxicological Research* using many mice to determine *carcinogenicity* and other *toxic* effects of chemicals.

Such experiments are important and difficult. Important because a thousand to a million mice may be needed to detect low cancer *thresholds,* as agents that produce only one or two tumors per thousand or million *exposures.* Difficult because of their expense and the lack of comparable animals. VII.B.2.d.

megavitamin therapy. use of large doses of vitamins to treat a variety of mental and other disorders.

A therapeutic approach based on the assumption that for every twisted mind there is a twisted molecule. The most famous example is Linus Pauling's use of enormous doses of vitamin C to prevent and treat colds. Most megavitamin therapy is *quackery. V.

member. a person eligible to receive, or receiving, benefits from a *health maintenance organization* or *insurance policy,* occasionally; compare *insured* and *beneficiary.* Includes both those who have enrolled or *subscribed* and their eligible *dependents.* III.B.1., IV.B.

mens rea.   an intent to do harm
In criminal law, an *insanity defense* may argue that the defendant lacked *mens rea,* the ability to form an intention to do harm. VIII.B.3.

mental age.   see *age.*

mental deficiency.   synonym, *mental retardation.*

mental disease, disorder.   either *mental illness* or *mental retardation;* a general term for abnormal functioning or capacity of the brain, mind, or emotions; the absence of mental health. Operational, any illness or disease included in the American Psychiatric Association's *Diagnostic and Statistical Manual of Mental Disorders.* II.B.2.

mental health.   a state of being, relative rather than absolute, in which a person has effected a reasonably satisfactory integration of his instinctual drives. Operationally, the absence of any identifiable or significant mental disorder; compare, *health.*
   Mental health is a concept influenced by both biologic and cultural factors and highly variable in definition, time, and place. Mental health is demonstrated, and sometimes defined, by an individual's success in interpersonal relations, zest for living, achievements, flexibility, and maturity. It is sometimes perversely used as a synonym for mental illness, as "mental health benefits" in health insurance plans, apparently because it is felt to be more genteel.
   See *community mental health center* and *clinical psychologist.* I.A.2.

mental illness.   any illness in which psychologic, intellectual, emotional, or behavioral disturbances are the dominating feature.
   The term is relative and variable in different cultures, schools of thought, and definitions. It includes a wide range of types (as psychic and physical, neurotic and psychotic) and severities. Mental illnesses do not include *mental retardation,* or the physical diseases of the brain, as strokes.
   See *commitment, competence, Diagnostic Statistical Manual-III, insanity, mental health, mental disorder,* and *B. Rush.* II.B.2.

mental retardation.   significantly below normal intellectual functioning; synonyms, mainly obsolete, include mental deficiency, subnormality, and disability; compare *idiocy* and *imbecility.*
   Retardation may be present at birth or become evident later in life and is always characterized by impaired adaptation in one or all areas of learning, social adjustment, and maturation. Emotional disturbance is often present. Causes include infections in early pregnancy, as German measles; brain infections; injury at or following birth; metabolic or nutritional disorders including malnutrition; chromosomal abnormalities, as Down's syndrome; social and psychologic factors, as emotional deprivation; and inadequate stimulation by the environment in infancy and childhood. The degree of retardation is measured by the *intelligence quotient* (IQ), which is scored so that 100 is average and 15 is a *standard deviation.* The names for levels of retardation are irregular but usually as follows: borderline retardation (70–85), mild (50–70), moderate (35–50), severe (20–35), and profound (under 20). If the IQ is above 50, the person is usually *educable to the fourth to fifth grade level, and adjustment may include independent self-support. The moderately retarded are *trainable, which means they can achieve *self-care,* social adjustment at home, and economic usefulness in a

closely supervised environment, as a *sheltered workshop.* The severely and profoundly retarded usually require institutional care. See *developmental disability.* I.A.1.

mercury. a *heavy metal,* highly toxic to humans if breathed or ingested.

Mercury persists in the environment, showing biologic accumulation in all aquatic organisms, especially fish and shellfish. Chronic exposure to airborne mercury can have serious effects on the nervous system. Industrial mercury pollution comes from pulp mills, chemical companies, and photo processing. I.C.

metacommunication. a message about a message, as when body language, tone, and looks convey a speaker's attitude toward his own message, himself, and the listener. I.B.1.

metapsychology. the branch of theoretical or speculative psychology that deals with the significance of mental processes; the nature of the mind-body relationship; the origin, purpose, and structure of the mind; and similar hypotheses that are beyond the realm of empirical verification. III.C.

metastasis (pl. metastases). the transfer of disease, usually *cancer* or *infection,* from a primary focus to a distant new one by spread of causal agents or cells directly or through blood or lymph vessels; one such distant focus. II.B.2.

methadone. a synthetic narcotic.

It may be substituted for heroin, producing a less socially disabling addiction or aiding in withdrawal from heroin. It may be abused. A *methadone program legally dispenses methadone to narcotic addicts for either maintenance or withdrawal. III.B.3., II.B.2.

"me too" drug. a *drug* that is identical, similar, or closely related to another product for which a *new drug application* (NDA) has been approved.

New drugs introduced by manufacturers without Food and Drug Administration approval on the theory that the NDA holder, or pioneer drug, had become *generally recognized* as *safe* and *effective.* Other "me too" products are marketed with abbreviated new drug applications (ANDAs), which require submission of manufacturing, *bioavailability,* and *labeling* information, but not data relating to safety and effectiveness, which are assumed to be established. III.B.3.

microbiology. the part of biology dealing with bacteria, viruses, and other microorganisms.

*Medical microbiology is the subspecialty of pathology concerned with growing and studying the microbes which cause disease. III.C.

midwife. see *nurse midwife.*

migration bias. see *bias.*

miliary fever. see *J. Caius.*

milieu therapy. socioenvironmental therapy in which the attitudes and behavior of the staff of a treatment program and the activities prescribed for the patient are determined by the patient's emotional and interpersonal needs. This therapy is an essential part of all inpatient treatment but has particular meaning where functional behavior and activities are modeled in psychiatric settings. V.B., VII.C.5.b.

military medicine. health and medical care especially organized for armed forces, the individual soldiers, and the victims of war.

Despite the aphorism that military medicine is to other medicine as military music is to music, it is an ancient field of medical endeavor with special problems, as *quarantine;* institutions, as *MASH;* heroes, as *A. Pare* and *W. Reed;* and language, as *triage.* III.C.

milk bank.   see *blood bank.*

Millis Report.   (John S. Millis, U.S. educator) the report of the Citizens Commission on Graduate Medical Education, chaired by Millis. It was originally published in 1966 by the American Medical Association which had sought formation of the commission (widely reprinted, as *GP,* 34(6), 12/66; 35(1), 1/67; and 36(2), 1/67).

This work, along with the *Willard Report* and the trends in medicine they describe, led to renewed emphasis in the 1960s on *comprehensive* and *primary* care, the development of *family medicine* as a *specialty,* and the gradual *elimination* of internships except as part of *residencies.* III.C.

mineral.   1. an inorganic chemical compound found in nature, especially a solid. 2. irregularly, in medicine and nutrition, an element, particularly an *essential* one.

See *recommended dietary allowance* and *vitamin.* I.A.2.a.

minimal brain dysfunction (MBD).   a disturbance of children, adolescents, and perhaps adults, without signs of major neurologic or psychiatric disturbance, which ordinarily includes *attention-deficit disorder, hyperactivity,* impulsivity, emotional instability, poor motor integration, disturbances in perception, and *learning disability.* The causes are unknown.

Schools and others have found it useful to have a diagnosis for troublesome children with so little wrong that they do not fit any major diagnostic category. The rare child with real MBD may benefit from medication, but the diagnosis must be made with care; compare *specific learning disability.* II.B.2.

minimal care.   1. irregular, room and board, as in a *boarding home;* supervised group living, as in a *halfway house;* or other simple institutional support for barely competent people. VII.C.5.b.

minimum daily requirements (MDR).   see *recommended dietary allowances.*

minister.   1. to care for some need, whether nursing or spiritual. 2. one who cares for spiritual needs; a person of the cloth, whether priest, rabbi, or preacher.

Many modern ministers have substantial training and skill in *pastoral counseling,* which includes much family and marital therapy and help with life's tasks and crises. This valuable resource in many communities is poorly used by *medical model* physicians. 1. V.B., 2. III.A.4.

minor.   a *child* under the age of legal *competence;* one who has not reached the age of majority.

*Majority, the age of legal responsibility, varies by sex and state, often over 18 for women, over 21 for men, and, increasingly, over 18 for both. I.A.1.

minor surgery.   surgery in which the operative procedure is not hazardous to life, as repair of lacerations, treatment of fractures, and biopsies; contrast *major surgery.* V.B.

miracle drug.   synonym, *wonder drug.*

miscarriage.   see *abortion.*

miscellaneous expense.   synonym, *ancillary expense.*

mist. see *particle.*

M'Naghten Rule. the English House of Lords in 1843 ruled that a person was not responsible for a crime if the accused "was laboring under such a defect of reason from disease of the mind as not to know the nature and quality of the act; or, if he did know it, that he did not know that what he was doing was wrong."

This rule still obtains in some states for determining *competence* and responsibility but has been widely succeeded first by the *Durham Rule* and later by the *American Law Institute Formulation.* VII.B.3.

Mobile Army Surgical Hospital (MASH). 1. in *military medicine* a mobile unit designed for early surgical treatment of nontransportable cases; an *evacuation hospital.* 2. a most successful movie and TV show about the mythical *4077 MASH, and thus an important part of how the United States has worked through its Korean and Vietnam war traumas. VII.C.3.

mode. the most frequently occurring observation in a set of observations. Contrast *mean* and *median.* VIII.D.

modeling. "occurs in family therapy when family members identify with and imitate the adaptive behavior demonstrated by the therapist.

"If this behavior is rewarded by positive outcome and repeated often enough, it may become incorporated into the patient's behavioral repertoire and be curative" (*Pinney and Slipp, 1982*). V.A.

modernization. remodeling, renovation or, sometimes, replacement of *health facilities* and *equipment* to bring them up to standards, into compliance with fire and safety codes, or to meet changed *needs* and capabilities; synonyms, *alteration* and *renovation.*

Modernization usually implies no increase in a facility's bed capacity. III.B.1.

Monday morning fever. see *brown lung.*

monitor. observe, measure, record, or evaluate the amount of pollutants in an environment, or the evolution of a phenomenon or condition, in order to ascertain conformity to specified objectives and take corrective action when indicated. Monitoring may be done at random periodically, or continuously by man or machine. II.D., VI.D.2, VII.B.2.

moral hazard. in insurance, the increased risk or danger that something will occur because it is insured; compare *hazard.*

The concept originates in fire insurance; it may be immoral, but insured buildings are more likely to burn than uninsured ones. However, the phenomenon is inherent in insurance; insured health services are more used than uninsured. IV.B.

morbidity. the quality or state of being diseased; the conditions inducing disease. I.A.1.

morbid. pathologic, unwholesome, unhealthy.

morbidity index. synonym, *problem index.*

morbidity rate. ratio of all diseased individuals, or of individuals having contracted a specified disease, to the total population; expressed as either the *prevalence* of cases at a given time, or the *incidence* of new cases during a given period. II.C.

moron.   lay and legal, largely obsolete; synonym, someone who has mild *mental retardation.*

mortal.   1. liable to *death.* 2. causing death; fatal.

mortality.   death; the quality of being mortal. I.A.1.

mortality rate.   ratio of deaths to population during a given period in a specified area; synonym, death rate; compare *birth rate, morbid,* and *rate.*

Generally expressed as crude death rate, the number of deaths per 1000 population per year. More meaningful indices of mortality are age-specific death rate, the number of deaths per 100,000 population of a given age group such as *infant mortality rate;* death rate by cause of death, the number of deaths from a given disease or other cause per 100,000 population; or case fatality rate, the number of deaths due to a disease per 1000 population having contracted the disease. Other common rates include the maternal, neonatal, and prenatal mortality rates. *W. Petty* and *J. Graunt* pioneered the study of mortality rates. II.C.

moxibustion.   the application and burning on the skin of *moxa, herbal material used in Japan for therapeutic purposes.

The doctrine on which it is based is akin to *acupuncture,* the burning moxa substituting for the needle. Moxa is made with the down of dried leaves of *Artemisia,* or artificially from cotton saturated with niter. V.

M-team.   educational jargon, a multidisciplinary group organized to consider the needs of children with handicaps or other problems. II.

multidisciplinary team.   see *M-team.*

multiphasic screening.   combined use of a group or battery of *screening* tests as a *preventive* measure to attempt to identify any of the several *diseases* being sought for in an apparently healthy population. Such screening is now often part of a larger program of *health hazard appraisal.* V.A., VII.B.2.e.

multisource drug.   a *drug* available from more than one manufacturer or distributor, often under different *brand names.*

Limits on reimbursement are more likely to be feasible for multisource drugs than drugs available from only a single source. A drug may not be available from more than one source because it is protected by a patent, only one company has obtained Food and Drug Administration marketing approval, or the demand for it is such that only one supplier has entered the market. III.B.3.

Munchhausen syndrome.   (Baron K.F.H. von Munchhausen, eighteenth century German traveler, soldier, and teller of outrageous tales) a condition in which sufferers habitually attempt to hospitalize themselves with self-defined or self-induced pathology, yearning typically for a surgical remedy; synonym, *pathomimicry.*

This rare disorder has no definitive etiology or treatment; in the *Diagnostic and Statistical Manual of Mental Disorders* it is called a chronic *factitious* disorder with physical symptoms. II.B.2.

municipal waste.   see *solid waste.*

Murphy's law.   "if anything can go wrong, it will."

There are many medical corollaries, as the more *invasive* the *procedure,* the more likely the specimen is to be lost; all important decisions must be made with insufficient data; and Murphy runs the laboratory.

See *O'Shea's law.* VIII.B.3.

musicotherapy, music therapy. the use of music in *therapy* of disease, particularly *mental illness*. III.C., V.

mutagen. a physical or chemical agent, as heat, a radioactive element, ultraviolet radiation, or nitric acid, capable of inducing mutation by altering the structure of the DNA molecule.

Mutagens are said to be *mutagenic and their *mutagenicity measures their power or the frequency with which they cause mutations.

See *Ames test*. I.C.

mutation. a sudden alteration in a gene or the genotype of an individual. A *mutant is an individual with a mutation.

Mutations are unpredictable, fairly common, but rarely important. They are inheritable when they occur in a germ cell. The *mutation rate is the probability of mutation of a gene during the lifetime of an individual. I.A.1.

mutual benefit association. a fraternal or social organization or corporation organized for the relief of its members from specified *perils* or costs of *illness*.

Such associations pay *losses* with assessments on their members intended to liquidate specific losses rather than with fixed *premiums* payable in advance. IV.A.

mutual insurance company. an insurance company with no capital stock, owned by the policyholders; contrast, *stock insurance company*.

Trustees of the company are at risk for *losses,* operating *expenses* and *reserves* are the property of the policyholders, and profits are returned to them as dividends or reduced *premiums*. IV.B.

mutuality. "healthy relationships in which there is an awareness of each other's divergent needs and wishes and a willingness to accommodate to one another without loss of individuality, constriction, or fear" (*Pinney and Slipp, 1982*). I.B.1.

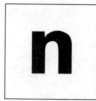

NAPCRG Process Classification. a hierarchical four-digit system for classifying and coding the *process* or content of episodes of care, as *encounters* or *visits*.

This process code records the site and duration of service, disposition, preventive and supportive services, *procedures,* drugs and pharmaceuticals, and x-ray, ultrasound, clinical laboratory, and other diagnostic procedures. It is more theoretically coherent and flexible than *Current Procedural Terminology.* Compatibility with the procedure axis of *SNOMED* is not attempted.

Read Tindall, Herbert L., et al., "The NAPCRG Process Classification for Primary Care" (*J Fam Pract,* 12(2): 309–18, 2/81). VII.

narcotic, narcotic drug. 1. any opiate derivative *drug,* natural or synthetic, which relieves pain (produces analgesia), alters mood, and produces *addiction.* 2. in the Comprehensive Drug Abuse Prevention and Control Act of 1970, any of the following *drugs,* whether produced directly or indirectly by extraction from substances of vegetable origin, independently by means of chemical synthesis, or by a combination of extraction and chemical synthesis: opium, coca leaves, and opiates; and a substance (and any compound, manufacture, salt, derivative, or preparation thereof) which is chemically identical with any of the substances referred to above.

The term is irregularly used as any sedative or analgesic or as any drug subject to special government control. Narcotics include heroin, morphine, meperidine, and *methadone.* They do not include marijuana, hallucinogens, amphetamines, or barbiturates. III.B.3.

narcotics officer (narc). slang, an agent of the Drug Enforcement Administration of the Department of Justice responsible for enforcing the Controlled Substances Act; loosely, any police officer concerned, at least at the moment, with enforcement of laws concerning the use and abuse of drugs. III.A.6., III.D.1.

National Board Examination. a standard national examination developed and administered by the National Board of Medical Examiners.

The examination has three parts: Part I tests knowledge of *basic sciences* and is ordinarily taken in the second year of medical school, part II tests *clinical sciences* and comes in the fourth year, and part III attempts to test clinical competence and is given in the internship year. Successful completion of the National Board is a requirement for licensure as a physician in some states and an acceptable alternative to the state's own medical examinations in other states.

See *Federation Licensing Examination.* III.A.1.

National Board of Medical Examiners (NBME). an organization which prepares and administers qualifying examinations of such high quality that state licensing boards and other legal agencies may grant successful candidates a license without further examination, see *Federation Licensing Examination* and *National Board Examination;* consults and cooperates with the examining boards of the states, medical schools, and other organizations concerned with the quality of medical education; assists medical *specialty boards* and societies in the measurement of clinical knowledge and competence for purposes of *certification;* and develops methods of *evaluating* such knowledge and competence.

The NBME was founded in 1915 and includes among its members the Federation of State Medical Boards of the United States, Council on Medical Education of the American Medical Association, Association of American Medical Colleges, American Hospital Association, Armed Services, United States Public Health Service, and Veterans Administration. Members at large are elected from among leaders in medicine throughout the United States.

See *CCME* and *LCME.* III.A.1.

National Center for Health Services Research (NCHSR). the administrative unit in the Department of Health and Human Services primarily responsible for doing and funding research, demonstrations, and evaluation in health care. III.D.1.

National Center for Health Statistics (NCHS). the administrative unit in the Department of Health and Human Services primarily responsible for operating and funding U.S. health and *vital statistics* programs.

NCHS operates some national surveys of health services, resources, and financing, as the National Ambulatory Care Survey, and guides and funds state and local statistical programs through the *Cooperative Health Statistics System.* III.D.1.

National Center for Toxicological Research. at Pine Bluff, Arkansas. See *megamouse experiments.* III.D.1.

national consensus standard. as defined in the *Occupational Safety and Health Act,* sec. 3(9), an *occupational safety and health standard* which (1) has been promulgated by a nationally recognized *standards* producing organization, as the *American National Standards Institute,* in a manner allowing affected parties to reach substantial agreement on the standard, (2) was formulated in a manner which afforded an opportunity for diverse views to be considered, and (3) has been designated as such a standard by the secretary of labor after consultation with appropriate federal agencies; synonym, American National Standard.

Most consensus standards have dealt with safety rather than health *hazards* and were adopted as interim standards early in OSHA's history. Standards are now more commonly developed by panels of *experts* or based on NIOSH *criteria documents.* VII.B.2.d.

National Death Index.   a central index of deaths for the United States, operated by the National Center for Health Statistics, to assist in identifying regional trends and environmental patterns in *mortality.* II.C.

National Environmental Policy Act.   U.S. law creating the *Council on Environmental Quality* and requiring *environmental impact statements.* VII.B.2.a.

National Formulary (NF).   a *compendium* of standards for certain *drugs* and preparations that are not included in the *United States Pharmacopeia.*

It is revised every five years and has been recognized as an official *pharmacopeia* since the Pure Food and Drugs Act of 1906. III.B.3.

National Health and Nutrition Examination Survey (HANES).   a program of physical examination and nutritional assessment of a *sample* of the U.S. population conducted by the *National Center for Health Statistics* as a coordinated part of its effort to assess the nation's *health status* and use of health services. II.C.

national health insurance (NHI).   1. a term still not defined in the United States. 2. a government program which finances, or assures financing for, health services for the entire population.

Some definitions also require that the covered services be uniform. NHI programs usually regulate but do not directly provide the services. By almost any definition, the U.S. federal income *tax credits* and *deductions* for medical expenses constitute NHI, although they are rarely thought of as such.

See *medical deduction* and *socialized medicine.* IV.D.

National Health Law Program (NHeLP).   a legal services backup center funded by the Legal Services Corporation to help poor people and their representatives with health law problems. III.B.1.

National Health Service (NHS).   1. in Great Britain, a government program providing health services for the entire population. 2. the agency in the British Ministry of Health responsible for administering the program.

The program was introduced in 1948. It provides inpatient and outpatient medical, dental, and nursing services; *drugs;* and *devices.* It is completely government financed and largely government owned and operated. See *health authority.* III.D.2.

national health service.   1. often synonymous, *national health insurance.* 2. properly, a government health program which directly operates a health system serving some or all of the population, as the British National Health Service.

See *social insurance* and *socialized medicine.* III.D.2.

National Health Service Corps (NHSC).   a program which places U.S. Public Health Service personnel in areas with a critical shortage of health personnel, see *medically underserved population,* to improve the delivery of health care in these areas.

The NHSC was established by the Emergency Health Personnel Act of 1970, P.L. 91-623. The NHSC has placed thousands of primary physicians,

dentists, and nurses in hundreds and hundreds of mainly rural communities.
See *Project U.S.A.* III.A., III.D.1.

National Health Survey. a continuing health survey by the National Center for Health Statistics which includes studies to determine the extent of illness and disability in the population of the United States, describe the use of health services by Americans, and gather related information.

The survey includes a continuing household interview survey of a *sample* of the U.S. population, surveys certain *medical records,* surveys a smaller sample of the population through health examination, and conducts related developmental and evaluative studies. II.C.

national institute. an institute operated by a national government. III.D.3.

National Institute of Occupational Safety and Health (NIOSH). the agency, administratively located since 1973 in the *Centers for Disease Control,* of the *DHHS* responsible for research and training in *occupational health,* developing and recommending *standards,* publishing lists of known toxins with their toxic *thresholds,* and evaluating *hazards.*

NIOSH originated in 1914 as the Office of Industrial Hygiene and Sanitation in the *Public Health Service.* The institute fulfills DHHS's responsibilities under the *Occupational Safety and Health Act* and the *Federal Coal Mine Health and Safety Act.* III.D.1., III.D.3., VII.B.2.d.

National Institutes of Health (NIH). the agency of the Department of Health and Human Services responsible for most of its medical *research* programs and related functions, including the *National Library of Medicine.*

The NIH is composed of individual research *institutes* whose division of the field of medicine is understandable only historically. III.D.3.

National Interns and Residents Matching Program (NIRMP). former name of the *National Residents Matching Program.*

National Library of Medicine (NLM). the part of the Department of Health and Human Services, administratively located within the National Institutes of Health, responsible for federal medical library programs, including *MEDLARS,* the regional medical library system authorized by the *PHS Act,* and the Lister Hill Medical Library in *Bethesda,* MD. III.C., III.D.1.

National Organization to Reform Marijuana Laws (NORML). an organization dedicated to the legalization of personal possession and use of marijuana. III.B.1.

National Reporting System for Family Planning Services (NRSFPS). a U.S. data system for *family planning* to which many *health departments* and *voluntary agencies* contribute data for federal publication and analysis. VII.B.3.b.

National Residents Matching Program (NRMP). the official system of obtaining first-year resident appointments in *graduate medical education,* used by U.S. hospitals and physicians and sponsored by their professional associations, including the Association of American Medical Colleges, American Medical Association, and American Board of Medical Specialties.

The rank-ordered program preferences of graduating medical students for first-year residency positions are computer matched with rank-ordered hospital preferences among graduating students. To participate in the program, hospitals and students agree not to offer or take positions outside the *match, as it is commonly known. Matching is on a *confidential* basis. III.A.1., III.B.1.

National Technical Information Service (NTIS). a repository and clearinghouse of reports, occasional publications, and other *fugitive literature,* usually available for sale as either text or microfiche. III.C.

natural. things, states, or events which occur in nature.

Nature's way is not necessarily good but is often better than people can do; thus it is a useful baseline for *evaluation* of *therapy.* I.A.1.

natural childbirth. any method of caring for childbirth in which the expectant mother, with father or friend as coach, is prepared with knowledge of labor and a regimen of exercises and then physically and emotionally supported through labor and delivery by physician and coach with as few drugs, as much self-control, and as little technical intervention as possible.

There are many variations in name and detail, all intended to balance excessive use of anesthesia, cesarean sections, and the like. I.A.1.

natural death act (NDA). a state law giving competent adults the right to make decisions concerning the use of life-sustaining treatment should they become terminally ill; sometimes known as a *living will* act.

Enacted in many states, but with varying scope and content, these acts generally require that decisions be made after a clear diagnosis has been made, when the patient is mentally competent and has been informed of the diagnosis and treatment alternatives, and before disease, pain, drugs, or other conditions alter the patient's judgmental capacity. The acts protect physicians and other providers from adverse civil, criminal, and professional consequences of complying with patient wishes. I.A.1., VIII.B.3.

natural food. food which does not contain synthetic or artificial ingredients and is not more than minimally processed.

This proposed (late 1980) FTC definition for regulation of *advertising* of natural foods said "minimal processing" was canning, bottling, and freezing food; baking bread; and peeling fruits and vegetables. The *FDA* does not apply similar regulation to *labeling* food as natural or, equally vague, *organic.* I.A.2.a.

natural history. the usual course of a disease, traditionally untreated, including average duration and severity, typical manifestations, and common complications.

The natural history is ordinarily characterized by following a large group of known cases for years. In modern medicine it is hard to find a series of untreated cases, because everything is treated, whether effective treatment is available or not. Therefore, the natural history becomes the typical progress of the disease with conventional management. Knowledge of the natural history is necessary for giving a *prognosis* and assessing therapy. II.

natural selection. the *genetic* process by which environmental factors favor or induce the survival and propagation of a particular genotype over others in a *population.*

Natural selection is the basis of Charles Darwin's (English naturalist, 1809–1882) theory of evolution and a major determinant of the genetic makeup of a population through elimination of genetic variation introduced by *mutation* and migration. Organisms produce variable progeny, with favorable variations accumulating by superior survival as generations pass.

The descendants thus diverge from the ancestors and remain adapted to changing living conditions. I.A.1.

naturopathy. a drugless, surgery-free system of *therapy* making use of physical forces such as air, light, water, diet, heat, and *massage* to improve health and treat a variety of diseases.

Much of the practice of naturopathy consists of *self-care,* learned through *health food* stores and magazines. Therapists are not subject to any particular educational requirements or regulation. Since their orientation is the creation of health, they leave the treatment of many diseases to *allopathic* physicians. In the United States in Seventh Day Adventist *sanatoriums* the two are practiced together. Naturopathy has no constant therapeutic content, and, like most *alternative medicine,* its practices, while sometimes effective, have rarely been subject to *random controlled trial.* V.

necessary. see *cause* and *need.*

necropsy. synonym, *autopsy.*

need. some thing or action which is essential, indispensable, or required or cannot be done or lived without; a condition marked by the lack or want of some such thing or action.

The presence or absence of needs should be measured by objective *criteria* or *standards.* Needs may or may not be perceived or expressed by the person in need and must be distinguished from *demands,* which are expressed desires whether needed or not. Like *appropriateness,* need is frequently and irregularly used in health care with respect to *health facilities* and services, see *certificate of need,* and people, see *medically needy.* It is important to specify the need being considered, by what criteria it is to be established, by whom (*provider, consumer,* or *third party*), and with what effect, as when payment for services by insurance is conditioned on their necessity. I.A.

neglect, negligence. the failure to exercise ordinary *care;* not doing something which a reasonable person, guided by the ordinary considerations which regulate human affairs, would do; the doing of something injurious to another which a prudent person would not do; the quality of being careless or negligent.

Negligence is not usually intentional, willful wrong typically being a crime. Negligence is the responsibility of the negligent party, creating a tort or wrong and making that party liable in civil law for damages resulting from the negligence. There are degrees of care and failure to exercise it, but not of negligence, which arises from any failure to exercise care. Negligence is the basis of *malpractice,* since one cannot ordinarily sue for bad results and injuries occurring despite good care. Neglect of children and incompetent adults by their *caretakers* and *self-neglect* are matters of social concern for the neglected, see *adult protective services,* and may be a source of civil or criminal action against the caretakers.

See *charitable immunity, contributory negligence,* and *locality rule.* V.D., VIII.B.3.

neighborhood health center. original name and synonym, *community health center.*

nematocide. see *pesticide*

neonatal mortality rate. the number of deaths reported of children under four weeks or one month of age per 1000 live births in a given area or program per year. *Early neonatal deaths are those occurring in the first week of life.
See *infant* and *perinatal mortality rates.* II.C

neonate. a newborn *infant;* specifically an infant in its first 28 days. I.A.1.

neoplasm. synonym, *cancer.*

nephrology. the *subspecialty* of *internal medicine* concerned with the kidneys. III.C.

net reproduction rate. see *birth rate.*

Network for Continuing Medical Education (NCME). an organization which produces and distributes videotaped *CME* programs. III.C.

neurological surgery. synonym, *neurosurgery.*

neurologist. a physician specializing by practice or education in neurology. Most neurologists also have some training in *psychiatry.* III.A.1.

neurology. the science and medical specialty devoted to the study and care of the brain and peripheral parts of the nervous system and their *organic* diseases; compare *psychiatry.* III.C.

neurosurgeon. a physician specializing by practice or education in neurosurgery. III.A.1.

neurosurgery. the science and surgical specialty devoted to the study and operative treatment of the central and peripheral nervous system. III.C.

new clear medicine. slang, *nuclear medicine* and nuclear diagnostic *radiology.* VIII.B.2.a.

new drug. a drug for which premarketing approval is required by the Federal Food, Drug, and Cosmetic Act; any drug which is not generally recognized, among experts qualified by scientific training and experience to evaluate the *safety* and *effectiveness* of drugs, as safe and effective for use under its prescribed conditions of use.
　　Since enactment of the Keefauver amendments to the Food, Drug, and Cosmetic Act in 1962, most new *prescription drugs* have been subject to the new drug application and premarket approval process. Most drugs marketed *over-the-counter* have not been through the new drug approval process because they were on the market before the law was passed.
　　See *GRAE* and *GRAS, not new,* and *"me too"* drugs. III.B.3.

new drug application (NDA). an application providing information demonstrating the *safety* and *effectiveness* of a new drug which must be approved by the FDA before the drug is marketed to the general public.
　　The NDA must include reports of animal and clinical investigations; a list of ingredients including the active drug and any vehicle, excipient, binder, filler, flavoring, and coloring; a description of manufacturing methods and *quality* control procedures; samples of the drug; and the proposed *labeling.* Approval of an NDA must be based on valid scientific evidence that the drug is safe and *adequate and well-controlled* clinical studies, as *random controlled trials,* demonstrating that it is effective for its intended, i.e., labeled, uses. NDA also commonly refers to the FDA's approval of an

application, the manufacturer's license to market the drug. See *investigational new drug.* III.B.3.

New Jersey rule. a ruling by the Supreme Court of New Jersey holding that *contingency fees* must be scheduled according to the size of the award, with the percentage of the award going to the claimant's lawyer declining as the size of the award increases.

Thus a lawyer might receive the traditional 50 percent of only a small settlement and as little as 10 percent of amounts recovered over $100,000. Several states have adopted variations of the New Jersey rule. V.D.

new problem. "the first presentation of a problem by a patient to a health care provider.

"This includes the first visit for a recurrence of a previously resolved problem, but excludes the presentation of a previously assessed problem to a different provider" (*NAPCRG, 1978*).

night hospital. a facility, usually part of a hospital, for nighttime *partial hospitalization* patients, often with mental illness, who spend the night in the hospital while holding jobs or attending school in the community. III.B.1.

Nightingale, Florence. British nurse, 1823–1910. She founded modern nursing, "helping the patient live," with the British Army in the Crimean War. Her experience and views were published in 1859 in her *Notes on Nursing.* III.A.2., VIII.A.1.

nocebo, nocebo effect. antonym, *placebo, placebo effect;* compare *iatrogenic.*
A term coined by Ivan Illich for the probably always present negative effects of medical care, as depersonalization, loss of autonomy, and *side effects.* VIII.D.

no code. an order not to attempt *cardiopulmonary resuscitation* in the event a patient with terminal illness suffers cardiac or respiratory arrest; the patient to whom the order applies. An irregular term with many synonyms.
In most situations people will automatically be resuscitated unless such an order has been written by the attending physician after discussion with the patient and family. Ambiguous halfway measures, as a brief or partial code, are to be discouraged. V.B.

noise. unwanted *sound.*
Sound is usually perceived as noise because it interferes with the perception of other sounds or has unpleasant, annoying, or traumatizing effects. Noise is also, by extension, unwanted disturbance resulting from an erratic or intermittent oscillation, as in electrical transmission. It is a *safety hazard* because *exposure* to excessive amounts produces temporary and permanent *deafness* and is an important source of *stress.* Occupational noise is regulated by the *Occupational Safety and Health Act,* and environmental noise by the Noise Control Act. I.C.2.

noise control. any effort to reduce or eliminate unwanted sound.
Noise control can be applied to the offending noise source or to the receiver. Among noise control methods applicable at the noise source are enclosure, installation of a noise muffler, lessening vibrations, and substituting quieter equipment. The least expensive method of lessening any noise at the receiving end is a pair of earplugs. I.C.2.

nomenclature. a classified system of names, as in the binomial nomenclature system of Linnaeus for plants and animals; compare *nosology.* VIII.C.

noninvasive. antonym, *invasive.*

nonparametric tests of significance. a statistical procedure which does not require assuming the data fit a *normal curve.*

These methods are often based on an analysis of ranks rather than on the distribution of the actual scores themselves and are used when data are not normally distributed. Widely used examples are the chi-square, Spearman rank order correlation, *median,* and Mann-Whitney U tests. VIII.D.

nonparticipating. see *participating*

nonparticipating insurance company. see *stock insurance company.*

nonproprietary name. synonym, *generic name.*

nonreplacement fee. the charge made by *blood banks* and programs to a patient who receives blood (or its products) which is not replaced by free donation to the bank by the patient or family and friends; synonym, replacement fee.

Sometimes the fee is not a charge but a requested contribution. Not all blood banks use such fees, and they do not exist in blood supply systems which are voluntary, as the one in Great Britain. VII.D.1.

non-service-connected (NSC) disability. in the Veterans Administration health care program, a disability which was not incurred or aggravated in the line of duty during active military service.

Care is available from the program for such disabilities on a bed-available basis after *service-connected disabilities* are taken care of. III.D.1.

norm. 1. a principle of right action, a standard of conduct or ethical value. 2. in statistics, synonym, *mean* or average.

The profound difference between these two common meanings is often obscured by considering the mean as right, as when the average number of appendixes removed by all surgeons in cases diagnosed preoperatively as appendicitis which are found diseased at pathology becomes the norm, or *standard,* for individual surgeon performance. VI.D., VII.D.2.

normal. 1. conforming to, constituting, or not deviating from an established or ideal norm, rule, type, or principle; functional, regular, average, common, *natural.* 2. in medicine, *healthy* or free of detectable disease; within a normal range, see *test.*

Family therapists avoid calling families normal or abnormal, preferring functional or dysfunctional. Besides, average is not necessarily healthy, and common and natural are not always best. Thus normal may not be good. II.

normal curve. the symmetrical, vaguely bell-shaped graph of the *normal distribution, the frequency distribution of many variable biologic measures, as height and *intelligence quotient,* in a population and of many random sample measurements.

The curve is specified mathematically by its *mean* and *standard deviation.* A and B are approximately normal curves with the same mean, although B is a little skewed and has a smaller standard deviation. VIII.D.

normal range. see *test.*

North American Primary Care Research Group (NAPCRG). a nonprofit, multidisciplinary organization founded in 1972 and dedicated to the development of *primary care.*

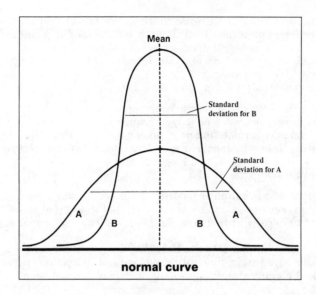

normal curve

It has sponsored the preparation of the *International Classification of Health Problems in Primary Care*, the *NAPCRG Process Classification*, and a fair glossary of primary care (*NAPCRG, 1978*). III.B.4., III.D.2, VII.D.2.

nosocomial. pertaining to a hospital; of disease caused or aggravated by hospital life. *Nosocomial infections are those acquired from hospitalization; failures of *barrier precautions.* II.B.1.a., III.B.1.

nosology. (Greek *nosos,* disease) the science of the classification of disease; a *nomenclature* of diseases. VIII.C.

nostrum. old-fashioned and irregular, a lay remedy, often secret or the work of a *quack;* a *panacea;* a *patent medicine,* an *over-the-counter* drug. V.B.

notch. a distinct discontinuity in *benefits* for individuals with slightly different incomes.

In public medical assistance programs, an additional dollar of *income* may mean a total loss of benefits. In Medicaid, families just below the income eligibility standard receive fully subsidized coverage while families with only slightly higher income who are just above eligibility standards receive no benefits. Substantial incentives for families to restrict their income in order to remain eligible may result. *Spenddown* provisions are used to compensate for notches. A notch may also occur when, without change in eligibility, *cost-sharing* requirements increase suddenly with a small change in income. IV.C.2., IV.D.

notice of proposed rulemaking (NPRM). an announcement in the *Federal Register* that an agency is going to make a *rule.*

The NPRM ordinarily provides a proposed text for the rule, an explanation, and a comment period. In urgent situations and during procedurally sloppy administrations, the NPRM often serves "de facto" as the rule it proposes. VIII.B.3.

notifiable.   pertaining to a *disease* which by law must be reported to federal, state, or local public health officials when *diagnosed*, as diphtheria, tuberculosis, and the venereal diseases; synonym, reportable.

Notifiable diseases are of public interest by reason of their infectiousness, severity, or frequency.

See *quarantine* and *registration.* VIII.C.

not new.   a drug for which premarketing approval by the Food and Drug Administration is not, or is no longer, required.

A drug may become "not new" upon a ruling by the FDA that the safeguards applicable to approved *new drugs,* as maintenance of records and submission of reports, are no longer required.

See *"me too" drug.* III.B.3.

nuclear magnetic resonance (NMR).   a method of imaging body tissues using the response or resonance of the nuclei of the atoms of one of the bodily elements, typically hydrogen or phosphorus, to externally applied magnetic fields.

This new window into the body, like *computed tomography,* promises enormous advances in diagnostic radiology and enormous expense. Nonionizing and noninvasive, it is presumptively, but has not been proved, safe. III.B.2.

nuclear medicine.   the science and specialty devoted to the study and use of radioisotopes in diagnosis and therapy.

See *radiology.* III.C.

nuclear winter.   the prolonged period of dreadful cold which will follow the *final epidemic,* nuclear war, because the clouds will prevent normal heating of the earth for months to years.

There will also be increased solar ultraviolet radiation from ozone depletion and persistent *radioactivity.* Even mutual deterrence seems unnecessary if any attack must be suicide for the aggressor.

Read the Scientific Committee on Problems of the Environment (SCOPE), *The Environmental Consequences of Nuclear War,* two volumes (New York: Wiley, 1985). I.C.1.

null hypothesis.   in statistics, the assumption that an observed difference, as between the means of two samples, is due to chance alone and not to a systematic cause or real difference.

The null hypothesis is conventionally considered incorrect if the method of sampling and observation is designed so that the probability, p, of obtaining a difference when no true difference exists is less than .05 (1 in 20, or 5 percent). It is common in science to form *hypotheses* in the negative; doing so makes them *falsifiable,* i.e., capable of being proved wrong. VIII.D.

nurse.   1. one who cares for another, ordinarily a woman looking after a child or *invalid.* 2. a person skilled or trained in caring for the sick, usually under the supervision of a physician; a person who provides nursing care.

In older definitions the nurse is always a woman under physician supervision. In law, she is a *professional* person licensed to practice nursing. There are many particular types of nurses whose names are reasonably descriptive of their special responsibilities, as charge or head nurse, private or private duty nurse, and school nurse.

See *clinical nurse specialist, P. and F. Fliedner, licensed practical nurse, F. Nightingale, patient care technician, public health nurse, registered nurse, visiting nurse,* and *L. Wald.* III.A.2.

nurse. 1. to suckle. 2. to care for, rear, nurture; to take charge of, watch over, and manage with care and economy. 3. to use carefully to conserve energy or avoid injury or pain. 4. to serve as a nurse.

By contrast, to doctor is more to educate and repair by intervention. Doctoring may be negative; nursing is rarely so. V.B.

nurse anesthetist. a *registered nurse* with special preparation who works under the supervision of an *anesthesiologist* in administering anesthetic agents to patients before and after surgical and obstetrical operations and other medical procedures. Certified registered nurse anesthetists are often known by the acronym CRNAs. III.A.2.

nurse midwife. a *registered nurse* with special preparation in the management and care of mothers and babies throughout the maternity cycle.

The American College of Nurse Midwives recognizes a nurse with appropriate training and experience as a *certified nurse midwife (CNM). Most midwives practice under physician supervision and follow *protocols* limited to care of normal pregnancy and labor. III.A.2.

nurse practitioner (NP). a *registered nurse* who has completed a program of study leading to competence in an expanded role; compare *physician assistant* (PA).

Nurse practitioners function under the supervision of a physician but not necessarily in the physician's presence. They are usually salaried rather than being reimbursed on a *fee-for-service* basis, although the supervising physician may receive fee-for-service reimbursement for their services. In addition to nurse anesthetists and midwives, nurse practitioners include *clinical nurse specialists* and others trained in *primary care,* oncology, or other specialty areas who work in either ambulatory or inpatient care. III.A.2.

nursery. 1. in a hospital, the room or area where newborns, and sometimes other infants, are cared for. 2. a place where children are temporarily cared for in the absence of their parents, usually without any particular educational effort; compare *day care.*

Nurseries have *bassinets* rather than beds and provide routine care for normal babies or intensive care for premature ones. Many hospitals have several rooms within the nursery which they rotate using to control potential *nosocomial* infections. III.B.1.

nurse's aide (NA). one who assists nurses in nonspecialized patient care tasks, as bathing, bed making, and feeding; old name for a female *patient care technician.* III.A.2.

nurse's station. the place within a *ward,* floor, or office of a health facility where the business of taking care of the patients is done. The charts, medications, telephones, and people who take care of the patients are usually located at the nurse's station. III.B.1.

nursing care. helping an individual, sick or well, in the performance of activities contributing to *health,* its recovery, or peaceful adaptation to *disability* and *death,* i.e., activities the individual would perform unaided if given the necessary strength, will, or knowledge.

This includes assisting patients in carrying out therapeutic plans initiated by physicians and assisting other *caretakers* in performing nursing functions and understanding patient needs. The specific content of nursing care varies in different countries and situations; note that, as defined, it is not given solely by nurses but also by many other health workers. See *kardex*. V.

nursing differential.   now repealed, a controversial add-on used in *Medicare*, originally 8.5 percent of routine *inpatient* nursing salary costs, added to the costs of such services to reflect the supposedly above average costs of providing routine inpatient nursing care to Medicare beneficiaries.

Medicare reimburses hospitals more by this amount for nursing services than do other insurance programs which cover the general population. There has always been controversy over the need for the differential. IV.C.1.

nursing home.   any of a wide range of inpatient health programs, other than hospitals, which provide various levels of personal and nursing care to people without personal or family ability to care for themselves.

People in nursing homes are principally old, retarded, schizophrenic, or in some similar way *incompetent*. The term includes freestanding institutions, or identifiable components of other health facilities, which provide nursing care and related services, personal care, and residential care. In the United States, and particularly with Medicare and Medicaid, nursing homes include *skilled nursing facilities* and *intermediate care facilities* but not *boarding homes*. III.B.1.

nursing intensity.   requirement for nursing care; jargon synonym, acuity.

A *nursing intensity index measures the amount of nursing time or effort a patient is likely to require. Nursing intensity correlates with, but should be distinguished from, *severity* of illness. III.A.2., V.B.

nursing procedure.   see *procedure*.

nursing service.   1. any specific *service* or activity performed by nurses. 2. the administrative unit in a hospital or other health program responsible for its nursing care.

Nursing services include bedside care, carrying out physician orders, attending to patients during procedures, health education, and the clinical services of nurse practitioners. VII.D.3.

nutrient.   1. affording nutrition. 2. a substance that affords nutrition; an organic or inorganic element or compound, including protein, fat, carbohydrate, vitamins, and minerals, constituting a nutritive element of *food* and used by a living organism through assimilation for heat or energy, growth or restoration, and physiologic activities.

See *deficiency disease* and *essential*. I.A.2.a.

nutrient budget.   the intake and output of biotic components or nutrients in an *ecosystem*. The *internal nutrient budget describes energy transfer through food within a *system*, and the *external nutrient budget applies to transfer between the system and its *environment*.

See *food chain*. I.C.

Nutri/System®.   a national business whose local franchises provide an organized program of *obesity* treatment which includes medical supervision, advice on diet and exercise, group support, refunds as rewards for successful sustained weight loss, and prepackaged foods to be used as the bulk of the diet; compare *Take Off Pounds Sensibly* and *Weight Watchers*. I.A.2.a., V.B.

nutrition. use of *food* by an organism to maintain life through digestion, assimilation, separation, elimination, and other complex physiologic processes; the act or process of nourishment; occasional synonym, dietetics.

See *diet* and *malnutrition*. I.A.2.a.

nutritionist. a specialist in nutrition; compare *dietician*. III.A.4.

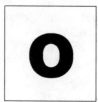

obesity. excess fat; body weight greater than required for physiologic purposes.

The numerous approaches to treating obesity testify to the relative ineffectiveness of all of them. Because it is so common, unhealthful, and considered ugly, so much money may be wasted treating it that some health insurance programs specifically exclude coverage for it.

See *bariatrics, fat doctor, malnutrition, Nutri/System®, Take Off Pounds Sensibly,* and *Weight Watchers.* I.A.1., II.B.2.

obligation. in the federal budget, the amount of an order placed, contract awarded, service *rendered,* or other commitment of federal *budget authority* made by a federal agency during a given period which will require *outlays* of federal funds during the same or a future period. VI.B.1.

objective. in health planning, a quantified statement of a desired future state or condition, with a stated deadline for achieving the objective, as development of an operational *health maintenance organization* by 1985.

Health systems agencies specified objectives, usually in their *annual implementation plans,* which would, when implemented, achieve their *goals.* See *budget* and *policy.* VI.A.

obstetrician. a physician specializing by practice or education in obstetrics; a specialist in obstetrics and gynecology who limits his or her practice to obstetrics. III.A.1.

obstetrics (OB). the study and care of women and their offspring during pregnancy, labor, and delivery, with continued care of women during the *puerperium;* the part of obstetrics and gynecology devoted to such study and care. See *O.W. Holmes* and *I.P. Semmelweiss.* III.C.

obstetrics and gynecology (OB-GYN). the science and surgical specialty devoted to the study and care of pregnancies, obstetrics, and women's sexual hormones and organs, gynecology.

Obstetrics and gynecology has subspecialties with *certificates of special competence* in gynecologic oncology, maternal and fetal medicine, and reproductive endocrinology. III.C.

occult. hidden or not evident, but usually suspected, as an occult malignancy known by manifestations or *metastases*. II.

occupancy rate. the average percentage of a facility's beds occupied. It may be institutionwide or specific for one *department* or service.

This common measure of inpatient health facility use equals total *patient days* as a percentage of *bed days* during a given period, usually a year. III.B.1.

occupation. an activity in which one engages regularly, usually for pay; one's work.

Work is important to health, and the inability to do work constitutes *disability*. In this context, benefits may depend on medical and other judgment respecting one's ability to work, or *work capacity,* and one's years of work and salary, or *work history.* I.B.2.c.

occupational air. the air in factories, offices, and other workplaces to which people are exposed in the course of their work.

It has special pollution problems, as *asbestos,* which may pollute occupational but rarely ambient air, and may be subject to both air pollution control and occupational health laws. Similar distinctions and problems exist for other kinds of pollution, as *occupational noise.* I.C.1.

occupational health. brief synonym, occupational safety and health.

Concern for the health of workers, and assuring a *healthful* workplace, is historically more recent than that for *safety,* although safety is certainly part of healthful work. Occupational illness presents different problems from injury because, while arising out of work, it may appear later and separately and be chronic rather than acute. VII.B.2.d.

occupational health services. *health care* services concerned with the physical, mental, and social well-being of people in relation to work and the work environment and with the adjustment of people to work and of work to people, see *ergonomics.*

The concern is thus more than the *safety* of the working place and includes health and job satisfaction. In the United States the principal federal law dealing with occupational health is the *Occupational Safety and Health Act.* III.B.2.d.

occupational injury and illness rate. see *industrial accident rate.*

occupational medicine (OM). the *specialty* of *preventive medicine* concerned with occupational safety and health.

It is a relatively new and untaught discipline, as yet finding little place in medical school curricula. Occupational medicine residencies are unusual for the fact that residents sometimes have to pay for the first two years of training rather than being paid, although the third year is typically salaried clinical training with a company. Many training costs are borne by employers. III.C.

occupational noise. see *noise* and *occupational air.*

occupational physician. synonym, *industrial physician.*

occupational safety and health. "the promotion and maintenance of the highest degree of physical, mental, and social well-being of workers in all occupations; the prevention among workers of departures from health caused by their working conditions; the protection of workers in their employment from risks resulting from factors adverse to health; the placing and maintenance of the worker in an occupational environment adapted to his physiologic and psychologic condition" (the accepted International Labor Organization and World Health Organization definition).

The inclusion of both safety and health in the name reflects the historically separate development of concern for the two. VII.B.2.d.

Occupational Safety and Health Act of 1970 (P.L.92-596, OSHA). the principal federal legislative authority for assuring the healthfulness and safety of work and workplaces and protecting workers from injury and disease.

The first comprehensive federal law, the act imposes on all employers engaged in interstate commerce a specific duty to comply with occupational *safety* and *health standards* promulgated by OSHA and a *general duty* to provide safe and healthful work for their employees. VII.B.2.d.

Occupational Safety and Health Administration (OSHA). the agency within the U.S. Department of Labor responsible for occupational safety and health and administering the authorities of the Occupational Safety and Health Act, other than those assigned to the *National Institute of Occupational Safety and Health.*

The agency's principal responsibilities include promulgating *rules,* setting *health* and *safety standards,* and overseeing enforcement, whether by direct federal effort or by relying on state enforcement programs. III.D.1., VII.B.2.d.

occupational safety and health standard. as defined in the *Occupational Safety and Health Act,* sec. 3(8), a *standard* which requires conditions, or the adoption or use of one or more practices, means, methods, operations, or processes, reasonably necessary or appropriate to provide safe or healthful employment and places of employment.

There are three types of standards: interim (initial) standards consisting of standards already adopted under other laws; *national consensus standards,* permanent standards; and *emergency temporary standards, which may be issued immediately upon the finding of grave danger to employees but must be followed within six months by an appropriate permanent standard. Standards are published as federal *rules* after consultation with heterogeneous advisory committees. Most standards to date have been safety, rather than health, related.

See *performance standard, specification standard, use permit system,* and *variance.* VII.B.2.d.

occupational therapist (OT). an individual trained in or practicing occupational therapy.

A therapist evaluates the *self-care,* work, and leisure skills of a client and plans and implements social and interpersonal activities to develop, restore, and/or maintain the client's ability to accomplish *activities of daily living* and necessary occupational tasks. About four-fifths of occupational therapists work in *hospitals,* others are employed in *home health* programs, *nursing homes, rehabilitation* centers, schools and camps for *handicapped* children, community health agencies, and educational and research institutions. At least four academic years of college education amd six months of fieldwork experience are required. People with a baccalaureate degree in a field other than occupational therapy may enroll in a postbaccalaureate program leading to a master's degree or certificate of *proficiency* in occupational therapy. III.A.4.

occupational therapy (OT). treatment by means of activity or occupation, especially creative activity or selected occupations, prescribed to promote recovery or *rehabilitation;* teaching of trades and arts as a means of rehabilitation of physically or mentally handicapped patients.

Occupational therapy is ordinarily done by an occupational therapist with supervision or orders from a *physiatrist* or other physician. OT has a primary purpose, such as the teaching of *activities of daily living* to people who cannot perform them. It also has an indirect purpose, since successful learning of new skills and work at any undertaking promote healing of almost anything. V.

office. a place where a service is supplied, as a physician's office.

The location and scope of physician office services are beyond the control of U.S. *health planning* programs but of concern because of the impact they have on the whole health system. III.B.1.

Office of Technology Assessment (OTA). an agency of the U.S. Congress, jointly created and run by the Senate and House of Representatives, which studies and advises the Congress on *technology,* including health technology. III.D.1.

office visit. see *visit.*

official drug. a *drug,* recognized by and conforming to the standards of the *United States Pharmacopeia* or the *National Formulary.* III.B.3.

official name. synonym, *established name.*

Old Age, Survivors, Disability and Health Insurance Program (OASDHI). a program administered by the Social Security Administration, DHHS, which provides monthly cash benefits to retired and disabled workers and their dependents and to survivors of insured workers and also provides health insurance benefits for persons aged 65 and over and for the *disabled* under age 65.

The health insurance component of OASDHI was enacted in 1965 and is known as *Medicare.* Commonly known as Social Security, the legislative authority for the program is found in the Social Security Act originally enacted in 1935. The program is an example of *social insurance.* I.A.2.c., IV.C.1.

oncology. the study and science of *cancer* or neoplastic growth; compare medical oncology. III.C.

ontologist. one who believes disease to have its own being and to invade the sick. Contrast, *physiologist, one who believes disease to be determined by the nature of the sick individual and understandable only in the context of the person's self, family, and environment.

Give the causes of at least some diseases, as influenza, to the ontologists, and give the illnesses to the physiologists. Hippocrates was a physiologist in this sense. II.B.1.a., III.C.

open-ended program. in the federal budget, an *entitlement* program for which eligibility requirements are determined by law, as *Medicaid.* Actual *obligations* and resultant outlays are limited only by the number of eligible people who seek benefits and the actual benefits received.

See *entitlement authority.* VI.B.1.

open enrollment. membership in a health maintenance organization (HMO) or health insurance program which is available to any, or to some ordinarily excluded, applicants. An *open enrollment period is a limited, as one month each year, period during which organizations open enrollment. Open enrollment periods may be used in the sale of either group or individual insurance and may be the only period of a year when insurance is available. Individuals perceived as high-risk, as by *preexisting condition,* may be subjected to high premiums or exclusions during open enrollment periods. III.B.1.

open panel.   see *panel.*

open season.   a period of open enrollment, especially in the *Federal Employees Health Benefits Program* and other employment-based health insurance programs which give people a choice of plans; an ordinarily annual period during which people may change plans fairly freely. IV.C.

open staff.   see *medical staff.*

operation.   1. the mode of action of anything. 2. any *procedure* done or performed, especially with instruments or by hand, compare *manipulation.* 3. in *surgery,* a procedure in which the method follows a definite routine. V.A., VII.B.3.a.

operational definition.   the meaning of a concept when specified in terms amenable to systematic observation and measurement, as temperature defined by a thermometer reading under standard conditions. VIII.B., VIII.D.

ophthalmologist.   a physician specializing by practice or education in ophthalmology; compare *optometrist* and *optician.*
    Ophthalmologists, as physicians, may prescribe drugs and perform surgery, which optometrists are rarely allowed to do by the states. Many programs, including Medicaid, require that legal determinations of *blindness* be made by *board certified* ophthalmologists. III.A.1.

ophthalmology.   the science and surgical specialty devoted to the study and care of the eye, its supporting structures, and their diseases; compare *optometry.* III.C.

opportunity cost.   in economics, the value that *resources* being used in a particular way would have if used in the best possible way or another specified alternative way.
    When opportunity costs exceed the value the resources have in the way they are being used, the difference represents lost opportunity to get value from the resources. An opportunity cost of devoting physician time to tertiary care is the value of devoting the same time to primary care. Opportunity costs are the appropriate cost concepts to consider when making decisions about resource allocation. Actual costs often, but not always, can be assumed to represent or be proportional to opportunity costs.
    See *marginal cost.* VIII.B.1.

optician (opt).   one who fits, supplies, and adjusts eyeglasses according to prescriptions written by *opthalmologists* or *optometrists* to correct optical or muscular visual defects. In some states opticians also fit contact lenses.
    Opticians do not examine the eyes or prescribe *treatment.* Qualification for licensure in states which require it usually includes successful completion of written, oral, and practical examinations. An apprenticeship or completion of a one- or two-year training program is often required. III.A.4.

optional service.   in *Medicaid,* a service which may be provided or covered by a state program in addition to the *required services* and, if provided, will be paid for by the federal government; compare *basic* and *supplemental services.*

The optional services states may offer are *prescribed drugs;* clinic services; *dental* services; eyeglasses; *hospice* care; private duty *nursing;* skilled *nursing facility services* for individuals under age 21; care for patients under age 21 in psychiatric hospitals; *intermediate care facility* services; prosthetic *devices; physical therapy* and related services; other *diagnostic, screening, preventive,* and *rehabilitation* services; optometry services; podiatry services; chiropractic services; care for persons age 65 or older in institutions for *mental diseases;* and care for patients age 65 or older in tuberculosis institutions. States may also offer any medical or other type of remedial care recognized under state law, furnished by licensed practitioners, and not specifically excluded from coverage by Medicaid. The exclusions are services for inmates of public nonmedical institutions, inpatient services in a mental institution for individuals over age 20 and under 65, and services for persons under age 65 in a tuberculosis institution. IV.C.2.

optometrist (DO, OD).   one trained in or practicing optometry; compare *ophthalmologist* and *optician.*

A doctor of optometry degree requires at least two years of preoptometry college education and four years of *professional* training in a school of optometry. The degree and an optometry board examination are required by all states for licensure to practice optometry. III.A.1.

optometry.   measurement of the visual powers; the art or science of examining the eye and related structures for defects and faults of refraction or focusing ability and prescribing corrective lenses or exercises.

Optometry does not generally treat diseases of the eye with drugs or surgery, the responsibility of *ophthalmology.* Optometry does compete vigorously with ophthalmology as a profession. III.C.

order.   an arrangement, direction, or command.

Physicians, and others, give orders to direct care. This is properly done by writing them unambiguously and legibly, one of the clinical arts. A *verbal order (VO) or *telephone order (TO) is usually written by the nurse receiving it and signed later. *Standing orders (SO) are often written in

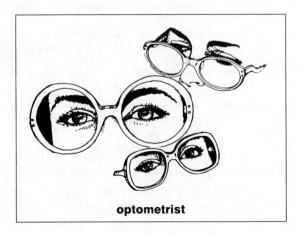

optometrist

nursing homes and other predictable situations for routine or recurrent problems. *Admitting orders for initiating inpatient care habitually specify the responsible admitting physician; the patient's problems, condition, diet, and activity; vital signs and other monitoring; investigations to be undertaken; and therapy. Current orders may be found in the patient's *kardex*. V.

orderly. one who assists nurses in simple patient care tasks, as bathing, bed making, and feeding; old name for a male *patient care technician*. III.A.2.

organic. 1. of or pertaining to living organisms or organs; having organs. 2. in chemistry, of or pertaining to compounds of carbon. 3. in medicine, of or pertaining to physical, as contrasted with mental, emotional, *psychosomatic,* or *functional* diseases or disorders. 4. of or pertaining to food grown and produced without the use of artificial fertilizers or *pesticides;* compare *natural.* 1. I.A., 2. II.B.1.a., 3. II.A., 4. I.A.2.a.

organophosphate. one of a group of *pesticide* chemicals containing phosphorus, as malathion and parathion, intended to control insects.

These compounds are short-lived and *biodegradable* and thus do not normally persist in the environment. Some, as parathion, are extremely toxic when initially applied; *exposure* to them interferes with the working of the nervous system, causing difficulty with motion, convulsions, and even death. Malathion, a common ingredient in household insecticides, is low in toxicity and relatively safe for humans and animals.

See *chlorinated hydrocarbon* and *dioxin.* I.C.

orgone. a vital energy held to pervade nature and to be accumulable for human use by sitting in a specially designed box, *the orgone accumulator.

Orgone was described by *Wilhelm Reich* in the 1930s. The accumulator was once as popular for treatment of whatever ails one (including cancer) as *Laetrile* has been for cancer. V.

orphan disease. one which affects fewer than 200,000 people in the United States. II.

orphan product. a *drug* or *device* which, although at least potentially useful, is unavailable because it has insufficient commercial potential, is not patentable, or lacks research priority. Some marketed products also have *orphan *indications,* for which they are not *labeled* because no one has conducted the necessary trials or submitted available data to support labeling for such indications.

Orphan products are used in treating orphan diseases and reach the U.S. market through a variety of special FDA programs, particularly those created by the Orphan Drug Act.

Read "Development of Orphan Products" (*FDA Drug Bull,* 13(1): 2–4, 3/83). III.B.2., III.B.3.

orthodontia, orthodontics. the part or *specialty* of dentistry concerned with the correction and prevention of irregularities and malocclusion of the teeth. V.

orthodontist. a dental specialist in orthodontics. V.

orthomolecular psychiatry, therapy. synonym, *megavitamin therapy.*

orthopedics, orthopedic surgery (Ortho). the science and surgical specialty devoted to the study and care of the bones, muscles, and joints, or the locomotor apparatus.

Orthopedics was originally devoted to the correction of deformities in children but now treats all ages with *orthoses* and *prostheses,* including casts, splints, and other *devices; manipulation;* and *operations.* III.C.

orthopedist. a physician specializing by practice or education in orthopedic surgery. III.A.1.

orthopsychiatry. the study and treatment of human behavior; preventive psychiatry, concerned especially with incipient mental and behavioral disorders in children and youth.

Its preventive and corrective efforts involve the collaboration of psychiatry, psychology, pediatrics, social services, and schools to promote healthy emotional growth and development. III.C.

orthoptic. pertaining to normal vision.

orthoptics. the science and practice of making vision right and efficient, particularly by correcting with exercise or training the visual axes of eyes not properly coordinated for binocular vision, as in amblyopia and strabismus. See *Bates methods.* III.C.

orthoptist. one trained in or practicing orthoptics, ordinarily with the supervision of an *ophthalmologist.*

The professional association, the American Orthoptic Council, administers a national board examination required for *certification.* To qualify for the exam a person needs at least two years of college and 15 months of training in a training center or 24 months of preceptorship, or apprenticeship. III.A.4.

orthosis (pl. orthoses). a medical *device* for supporting, shaping, or otherwise assisting the body. III.B.2.

orthotics. the science of making and using orthopedic appliances, from *orthosis, the straightening of a deformity. III.C.

orthotist. one trained in or practicing orthotics. III.A.4.

O'Shea's law. Murphy was an optimist.
See *Murphy's law.* VIII.B.3.

Osler, Sir William. Canadian physician in the United States and England, 1849–1919. During his years as professor of medicine at such influential universities as McGill, Pennsylvania, Johns Hopkins, and Oxford, Osler founded modern academic medicine, authored a great textbook, and was one of the greatest *clinicians.* III.A., VIII.A.1.

osteopath, osteopathic doctor or physician (OD, DO). one trained in or practicing osteopathy.

Osteopaths are licensed to perform medicine and surgery in all states, eligible for *graduate medical education* in either osteopathic or *allopathic* programs, reimbursed by Medicare and Medicaid, supported by health manpower legislation, and generally treated the same as allopathic physicians. III.A.1.

osteopathy. a school of healing based on the theory, propounded in 1874 by Andrew Taylor Still (U.S. physician), that the normal body, when in correct adjustment, is a vital mechanical organism naturally capable of making its own responses to and defense against *diseases,* infections, and other toxic conditions; medical science or practice based on osteopathic theory and therapy.

The body is seen as structurally and functionally coordinate and interdependent, with abnormality of either structure or function constituting

disease. The physician of this school seeks to correct any peculiar position of the joints or tissues or peculiarity of diet or environment which is a factor in destroying natural resistance with physical, hygienic, medicinal, and surgical measures. Osteopathy is now distinguished from *allopathy* principally by greater reliance on *manipulation*.
See *homeopathy* and *naturopathy*. III.C.

otolaryngologist. a physician specializing by practice or education in otolaryngology. III.A.1.

otolaryngology (ENT). the science and surgical *specialty* devoted to the study and care of the ear, nose, and throat and to surgery of the head and neck. See *audiology* and *speech therapy*. III.C.

outcome measure. a measure of medical care *quality* in which the standard of judgment is the attainment of a specified end result, or outcome.
To measure the effectiveness of a particular medical action in altering a disease's *natural history* is an outcome measure. Such measures are a proper way to assess the effectiveness and quality of medical care and are necessary for cost-benefit analyses. They are also more difficult than *input* and *process measures* and thus often are not done in comparing medical settings. *Random controlled trials* usually use outcome measures to compare the therapeutic effect of a new drug or medical procedure on a disease to its natural history without treatment or with treatment previously in use. VII.D.2., VIII.D.

outlay. in the federal budget, an actual expenditure of federal funds, as checks issued, interest accrued on the public debt, or payments, minus refunds and reimbursements. *Total budget outlays are the sum of outlays from *appropriations* and other funds in the budget universe minus offsetting receipts.
While *budget authority* is usually *obligated* in the fiscal year for which it is appropriated, it may be outlaid, once obligated, over several years. VI.B.1.

outlier. a hospital admission requiring either substantially more expense or a much longer *length of stay* than average.
Under *diagnosis related group* reimbursement, outliers are given exceptional treatment (subject to *peer review organization* review). II.B.1., IV.C.1., VII.C.5.

out-of-pocket cost, payment. one borne directly by a *patient* without benefit of *insurance*. Out-of-pocket costs include uninsured patient payments and those required by *cost-sharing* provisions. IV.A., B.

outpatient. a patient receiving *ambulatory care* at a hospital or other health facility without being admitted to the facility.
Outpatient ordinarily does not mean people receiving services from a physician's office or other program which does not also give inpatient care. *Outpatient care refers to care given outpatients, often in organized programs. VII.A.1.

outpatient department (OPD). the part, area, or administrative *department* of a hospital or other inpatient program which treats outpatients. It may or may not include the *emergency room*. III.B.1.

outpatient medical facility (OMF). as defined in the *Hill-Burton* program, a facility designed to provide a limited or full spectrum of health and medical services, including health education and maintenance, preventive services, diagnosis, treatment, and rehabilitation to outpatients. III.B.1.

outpatient surgery. minor *ambulatory surgery.*

output measure. any measure of productivity; variable, often a synonym for *process measure.* VII.D.2., VIII.D.

overhead. *costs* of doing business, as rent, insurance, or heating, not chargeable to a particular *good* or *service* produced or to a revenue-producing *cost center;* synonym, general and administrative costs. VII.D.1.

over-the-counter drug (OTC). a drug advertised and sold directly to the public without prescription, as aspirin; contrast *ethical drug.* III.B.3.

ovicide. see *pesticide.*

ownership disclosure. revelation by a health program of all ownership interests in the program.

By Medicare and Medicaid law, to help avoid fraud and abuse, a participating *skilled nursing facility* must supply ownership information to the state survey agency and an *intermediate care facility* must supply it to the state licensing agency. Complete information must be supplied on the identity of each person having a direct or indirect ownership interest of 10 percent or more in a facility, each officer and director of a corporation, and each partner in a partnership. IV.C.

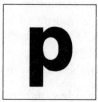

package insert. the *labeling* approved by the *Food and Drug Administration* for a drug product.

The labeling accompanies the product when shipped by the manufacturer to the pharmacist but for *ethical drugs* usually does not accompany the dispensed prescription. The package insert is directed at the prescribing professional, principally the physician, and states the appropriate uses of the drug, the mode of administration, dosage information, contraindications, and warnings. The legal effect of prescribing a drug in ways not described in the package insert is unclear.

See *compendium, patient package insert,* and *Physicians' Desk Reference.* III.B.3.

pain. 1. a local or diffuse unpleasant sensation, ranging from discomfort to agony, caused by stimulation of functionally specific peripheral nerve endings; a physiologic protective mechanism leading to evasive action. 2. acute mental or emotional distress or *suffering,* as grief or sudden *stress.* 3. trouble or care taken to assure a good result. 4. one that irks or annoys. I.A.1.

palliate. to abate or alleviate, without curing, the symptoms or *virulence* of a disease, as by *hospice* care. *palliation. the act or process of palliating. *palliative. something that palliates. V.B.

panacea. anything good for whatever ails you, see *Asclepius.* V.B.

Pan American Health Organization (PAHO). the regional part of the *World Health Organization* for North and South America. III.D.2.

pandemic. worldwide *epidemic,* as an influenza epidemic. VIII.C.

panel. a list of people, the group listed, as a research project's subjects, a panel of experts, or a list of physicians available to care for a patient; the patients cared for by a physician. Compare *list, registry,* and *practice.*

A *closed panel admits no additions; an *open one does. V.

PaperChase. a computer-based bibliographic retrieval system which permits users without previous training to search for authors' names, journals, title words, and *medical subject headings*, or any combination thereof, in a data base of 400,000 references from the National Library of Medicine.

Read Horowitz, Gary L., et al., "PaperChase: Self-service Bibliographic Retrieval" (*JAMA*, 250(18): 2494–99, 11/11/83). III.B.2., III.C.

Pap smear, test. (G.N. Papanicolaou, U.S. physician and anatomist, 1883–1962) the first and most famous example of *cytology;* a method of studying loose cells from the uterus and vagina for changes predictive or diagnostic of disease, particularly cancer. VII.B.1.

para. a woman who has given birth, live or still, for the number of times specified by a following numeral, as para I for a *prima para or *primi p. (primip) who has given birth once and para 2 or II for a *secundi para or *secunda; compare *parity*. I.A.1., VIII.C.

Paracelsus. Fully known as Philippus Theophrastus, Bombast of Hohenheim, Swiss physician, 1493–1541. He undertook to reconstruct medicine on a chemical basis. He exemplifies the Renaissance endeavor to overthrow the authority of *Galenic* medicine. His book on miners' diseases is the first monograph devoted to the *occupational health* problems of a specific group of workers. VII.B.2.c. and d., VIII.A.1.

paramedical personnel. *paraprofessionals* working in medicine, as nurses and *physician's assistants*, but irregularly includes *dental hygienists, medical technologists, nutritionists*, and receptionists.

See *allied health personnel*. III.A.4.

parameter. a characteristic element or factor; a *variable*, as a mean or variance, that describes a statistical *population;* a property whose values reflect or determine the character or behavior of something, as the temperature of the body.

Knowing which parameters of a disease to follow, and how often, is one of the clinical arts. VIII.D.

paraprofessional. pertaining to nonprofessional work, usually auxiliary to the work of a *professional;* one who does such work; compare *technician* and *allied health personnel*.

In *occupational health*, defined by the *National Institute for Occupational Safety and Health* as a junior college graduate with an associate degree in science, occupational health, and/or safety. III.A.4.

parasite. an organism that lives for all or part of its life on or in another, the *host*, at whose expense it obtains nourishment or other benefits necessary for its survival, ordinarily with detriment but not death to the host. *Ectoparasites *infest* by external attachment, *endoparasites by internal penetration.

See *pest*. I.A.1.

parasite index, rate. the percentage of individuals in a population hosting a parasite, as with malaria in the blood. III.C.

parasitism. the intimate association or union of two different organisms, a *parasite* and its *host*. II.B.1.a.

parasitoid. an organism resembling a parasite except that it normally kills the host. I.A.1.

parathion. an *organophosphate.*

Pare, Ambrose. French surgeon, 1510–1590. Famed as an army surgeon and court physician, Pare replaced boiling oil with simple dressings for open wounds and cautery with ligature for control of hemorrhage. III.C., VIII.A.1.

parens patriae. (Latin, father of the country; in England, the King; in the United States, the state) the constitutional power of the state of guardianship over those under disability, as to involuntarily *commit mentally ill* persons who are in need of care and treatment for their mental illness. II.B.2., VIII.B.3.

parental child. child relied on excessively or inappropriately for the care and rearing of siblings.

Such children are commonly, but not exclusively, found in single-parent families. Child parenting is not necessarily damaging as long as the parenting child is used only part time and is given adequate parenting and opportunity for age-appropriate activities. Otherwise, both the parenting child and the siblings may suffer. I.B.1.

parental consent. *consent* by a parent or legal guardian for a course of medical action proposed for a *child.*

The common law rule requiring parental consent for treating a *minor* has exceptions, as emergencies, *emancipated* and mature minors, and statutes in some states allowing treatment without parental knowledge of venereal disease, pregnancy, alcohol or drug abuse, and/or emotional problems. V.B., VIII.B.3.

parenting. preparing them to leave us.

Parents Anonymous. *self-help* organization, like *Alcoholics Anonymous,* primarily for parents who have battered their children.

They are made up of parents and a counseling professional who meet weekly to understand and support each other. II.B.2.

parity. the number of a woman's births, including live and *stillbirths* (pregnancies minus *abortions*); in *epidemiology,* sometimes refers only to live births; compare *gravidity* and *para.* A woman's obstetrical history is characterized by her gravidity, parity, abortions, stillbirths, and living children, abbreviated as $G_6P_4A_2S_1L_2$. I.A.1., VIII.C.

Park, William Hallock. U.S. bacteriologist, 1863–1939. The foremost exponent of applied bacteriology. He is best known for his work in diphtheria control, especially through immunization. However, his contributions to milk *sanitation* and control of tuberculosis, pneumonia, typhoid fever, scarlet fever, dysentery, and many other conditions made him an outstanding figure in *public health.* VII.B.2.e., VIII.A.1.

parsimony of diagnosis. the clinical principle that one should make as few diagnoses as possible, both to explain all presenting signs and symptoms consistently and to avoid overlabeling unexplained or inadequately understood problems.

Multiple, excess diagnoses are all likely to be wrong and receive excess treatment; premature ones not only are wrong, they halt the diagnostic search. V.A.

partial hospitalization. a formal program of care in a hospital or other setting on a less than full-time basis, involving services usually provided to inpatients. There are two principal types, *night hospitalization for patients who work or attend school during the day and *day hospitalization for people who require in-hospital diagnostic or treatment services but can safely spend nights and weekends at home.

Partial hospitalization programs for the mentally ill or incompetent may have little resemblance to a hospital; night hospitalization still allows the patient to work, and day hospitalization frees the person's *caretaker* to work. The distinction between partial hospitalization and *shelters* and *halfway houses* is irregular.

See *boarding home, day care, deinstitutionalization,* and *respite care.* V.B.

partial-service benefit. see *service benefit.*

participating. a physician who agrees to accept an insurance plan's established payment or *reasonable charge* for his or her services. A *nonparticipating physician may charge more than the insurance program's maximum allowable amount, the patient then being liable for the excess over the allowed amount.

This system developed as a way of providing the insured with specific services with no *out-of-pocket* costs. The term is used more loosely in *Medicare* and *Medicaid* for any physician who accepts reimbursement from either program, and more appropriately in Medicare for physicians who participate by accepting *assignment.* Any physician accepting Medicaid payments must accept them as payment in full. A health program is a participating *provider* when it meets the various requirements of, and accepts reimbursement from, a public or private health insurance program, see *conditions of participation.*

See *consumer participation* and *penetration.* IV.B.

participating insurance company. synonym, *mutual insurance company.*

particle. a small piece of solid or liquid matter. *particulate. composed of particles.

Finely divided solid or liquid particles dispersed or suspended in air produce fog, fumes, mist, *smog, smoke,* and spray. I.C.1.

passive smoking. see *smoking.*

Pasteur, Louis. French chemist, 1822–1895. Established the doctrine of the germ origin of disease. He studied the spoilage of beer and wine and diseases of silkworms and other animals, especially anthrax, chicken cholera, and rabies. Pasteur developed the idea of *immunization* against disease, which had first been suggested by *Jennerian* vaccination. VIII.A.1.

past medical history (PH, PMH). a traditional part of the medical *history* in which inquiry is made concerning medical events in the patient's life which have not been considered in describing the presenting *complaint.* While somewhat irregular in content, the past medical history ordinarily lists allergies, current problems, medications, diet and other pertinent health practices and habits, and past immunizations, illnesses, hospitalizations, and surgeries. V.A.

pastoral counseling. therapy by *ministers* for people with personal and family problems.

Many clergy are well trained by seminaries in psychologic theory and practice; others just do it. V.B.

patent medicine. an *over-the-counter* preparation, ordinarily with a trade secret formula; a nostrum.

An old-fashioned term since federal regulation of *labeling* of *drugs* has practically eliminated the old extravagant, unproven therapeutic claims and much of the secrecy. V.B.

pathogen.   an agent capable of producing disease, usually applied to living agents; compare *fomite.* *pathogenesis. the origin and course of development of disease; compare *natural history.* *pathogenic. producing or capable of producing disease; pertaining to pathogenesis. *pathogenicity. ability or capacity to produce disease. I.A.1., II.

pathognomic, pathognomonic.   a *symptom, sign,* or clinical presentation solely and specifically *associated* with a disease, enabling its recognition and differentiation from other diseases. II.A.

pathologist.   a physician specializing by practice or education in pathology. Most pathologists are *hospital-based physicians.* III.A.1.

pathology.   1. an abnormality of structure or function produced by disease, particularly one recognized in the *laboratory* at *autopsy;* by extension, the disease producing the abnormality, and abnormality of mental, family, or social function. 2. a department, laboratory, or *service* in a hospital or other health program providing pathology services, including autopsies, *blood banking, cytologic* services, laboratory testing, *microbiology,* and analysis of tissue obtained by surgery or biopsy. 3. the science and specialty devoted to pathology and the causes, processes, and effects of disease.

Pathology has subspecialties with separate residencies in blood banking, dermatopathology, *forensic* pathology, and neuropathology and with certificates of special competence in chemical pathology, hematology, and medical microbiology.

See *Armed Forces Institute of Pathology* and *Rudolph Virchow.* 1. II.B.1, 2. III.B.1, 3. III.C.

pathomimicry.   synonym, *Munchhausen syndrome.*

pathosis (pl. pathoses).   diseased condition, abnormality, or finding suggestive of disease; perhaps dental, see *endodontics.* II.A.

patient (PT).   one who receives health care; compare *consumer.*

The North American Primary Care Research Group defines a patient as a person who receives or contracts for professional advice or services from a health care provider.

> *temporary or transient patient. patient who receives one or more services from the practice but who usually receives his/her health care elsewhere. *registered patient. patient who has contracted for ongoing health care from a practice (excludes former, temporary, or transient patient). *former patient. patient (excluding temporary or transient) who has previously been registered but who is no longer considered (by the practice or by personal determination) to be part of the practice population and is removed from the *register.* For practices registering by families: *active patient. a registered patient who has received services from the practice at least one time and who belongs to a family, one member of which has received services within the last two years. *inactive patient. a registered patient who has received services from the practice at least one time, but neither he nor she nor any members of his/her family have received services within the last two years. For practices not registering by families: *visiting patient. a registered patient who has received ser-

vices from the practice at least one time in the last two years; this includes attending patients. *attending patient. a registered patient who has personally received services from the practice in the past year. *nonvisiting patient. a registered patient who has received no services from the practice within the last two years (*NAPCRG*, *1978*).

See *activated patient, identified patient, inpatient, outpatient, private patient, profile,* and *service patient.* VII.A.1.

patient care technician (PCT). one who assists nurses in nonspecialized patient care tasks, as bathing, bed making, and feeding.

A new, nonsexist name for nurse's aides and orderlies which also reflects their more formal training and responsibilities than was historically the case. The bottom rung on the nursing ladder below *licensed practical nurse.* III.A.2.

patient days. the number of *inpatients* in a health facility at a specified time of day, as midnight.

See *occupancy rate.* VII.C.5.

patient dumping. see *dumping.*

Patient Management Categories (PMCs). a system for grouping patients according to their admitting diagnoses and other *morbidities.*

This computerized system using the *Uniform Hospital Discharge Data Set* was developed by Blue Cross of Western Pennsylvania for use in reimbursement and is an alternative to the *diagnosis related groups.* For each of the 800 categories an optimal "treatment path" is specified upon which predicted costs are based.

See *severity.* II.B.1, IV.C.1.

patient medication information (PMI). see *patient package insert.*

patient mix. the numbers and types of patients served by a hospital or other health program.

Patients may be classified by their homes, see *patient origin study,* socioeconomic characteristics, diagnoses, see *case mix,* or *severity* of illness. Knowledge of a program's patient mix may be important for comparative planning and reimbursement purposes.

See *scope of services.* III.B.1.

patient origin study. a study, as by a health program or health planning agency, to determine the geographic distribution of the homes of patients served by one or more health programs. Such studies help define *catchment* and *medical trade areas* and are used in locating and planning the development of new services. VI.A., VIII.D.

patient package insert (PPI). *labeling* or other information in plain English concerning a prescription drug intended for patient use; synonym, patient medication information (PMI); compare *package insert.*

The FDA requires such inserts for a few drugs, as birth control pills, but not most, having been opposed in doing so by physicians, pharmacists, and manufacturers. The American Medical Association and others make information available for some common drugs for optional dispensing by physicians. III.B.3.

payroll deduction. an amount withheld from an employee's earnings to finance a *benefit,* whether a *payroll tax,* as the Social Security tax, or a required payment for a benefit, as a group health insurance premium. IV.A.

payroll tax. a tax *liability* imposed on an employer or employee, related to the amount of the company payroll or individual pay, the revenues from which are used to finance a specific *benefit,* as Social Security.

Payroll taxes which do not apply to all earnings, as the Social Security tax, or are the same absolute amount for each employee, as a health insurance premium, are *regressive.* IV.C.

pearl. commonly, any useful bit of *clinical* knowledge; properly, a clinical observation that pairs two apparently unassociated phenomena, as Hippocrates' "Eunuchs do not take the gout." III.C.

Peckham Experiment. a British project during the 1920s and 1930s in which Pearse and Crocker sought to maximize the health of families by helping them achieve full potential physical and social function.

Families, rather than their individual members, were seen as the human organism and were genuinely the unit with which the project was concerned. For a small weekly fee, families joined a health center that provided a swimming pool and exercise facilities, social activities, and an initial and periodic "health overhaul." This focus on families and *health maintenance* was so far ahead of its time that its time has yet to come, although family physicians in health maintenance organizations may begin to approach it.

Read Pearse, I.H., and L.H. Crocker, *The Peckham Experiment* (London: George Allen & Unwin, Ltd., 1943). I.B.1., III.C.

pediatrician. a physician specializing by practice or education in pediatrics. III.A.1.

pediatrics. the science and specialty devoted to the study and care of children.

Pediatrics is concerned with the growth and development of the *child* through adolescence and with the prevention and treatment of defects, diseases, and injuries of children. It is one of the *primary care* specialties. Its subspecialties with separate residencies are pediatric allergy and pediatric cardiology, and with *certificates of special competence* are neonatal-perinatal medicine, pediatric endocrinology, pediatric hematooncology, and pediatric nephrology. III.C.

pedorthics. the art and science concerned with nonsurgical treatment of conditions of the feet. *pedorthist. one educated or certified in or practicing pedorthics.

Pedorthics may make *podiatry* redundant, since orthopedists are available to do surgery, the thing that a podiatrist but not a pedorthist can do. Pedorthists tend to dispense widgets, as fancy heel cups, rather than services but at their best will fix your aching feet easily. III.C., IV.A.4.

peer review. evaluation by practicing physicians or other professionals of the *effectiveness* and *efficiency* of the services of their colleagues. Peer review has become nearly synonymous with the activities of *peer review organizations.*

Peer review is advocated as the best form of *quality* control for medical services because it is said that only a physician's peers can judge the physician's work. It has been criticized for inherent conflict of interest, since physicians will not properly judge those who judge them, and for not adequately reflecting patient needs and point of view. VI.D.2.

peer review organization (PRO). an organization with which the *Medicare* program and hospitals contract for quality and *utilization review* of services covered by the program.

The Tax Equity and Fiscal Responsibility Act of 1982, P.L. 97-248, phased out *professional standards review organizations,* replacing them with PROs in 1983 as *diagnosis related group*–based prospective payment was introduced. PROs differ from PSROs by virtue of funding from the Medicare trust funds independent of the appropriations process; less physician control, although most will still be physician organizations; and concern for appropriateness of admissions, DRG validation, and *outliers* rather than for excess use. III.B.1., VI.D.2.

pelotherapy. treatment of disease by earth or mud; specifically, treatment by mud baths. V.B.

penetrance. probability or frequency of manifestation of an inherited trait in an individual carrying it. Penetrance depends on the total genotype and environmental factors. I.A.1.

penetration. in marketing insurance or health maintenance organizations, the percentage of possible *subscribers* who have contracted for *benefits* or subscribed; synonym, participation; compare *saturation.* III.B.1., IV.B.

per diem cost. *cost* per day; hospital or other inpatient institutional costs for a day of care.

Hospitals *charge* for services with a per diem rate derived by dividing total costs by the number of inpatient days of care given. Such per diem costs are averages and do not reflect the true cost for each patient. This means patients who use few services, as at the end of a long stay, subsidize those who use many, as on the day of admission. This creates an incentive to prolong stays and has led to payment for whole stays or diagnoses, see *diagnosis related group.* VII.D.1.

performance standard. a *standard* which specifies how *safe* or *healthful* something must be or how well a job must be done, but not how to achieve the specified objective; contrast *specification standard.*

For example, rather than specifying that a guardrail be 42 inches high and be made of 3-inch steel tubing, a standard could allow any guardrail that kept a 200-pound, 2-foot cube from falling. Performance standards may be used by states as *occupational safety and health standards.* They are more flexible and require few variances but are hard to enforce. VI.D., VII.D.2.

performance status. ability to function; compare *health status.*

People with similar cancers often respond variably to treatment according to their performance status. This makes optimization of performance status a general goal of treatment and requires *controlling* for it in testing new treatment. II.A.2.c.

peril. in insurance, a cause of possible *loss,* as an accident, death, sickness, fire, or burglary; compare *hazard.* I.C., IV.B.

perinatal mortality. death during the late prenatal period, birth process, and early *neonatal* period; usually measured as the *perinatal mortality rate: the number of perinatal deaths per 1000 *live births* in a given area or program and time period.

The *late prenatal period is variously defined as beginning after the 28th week of gestation or when the fetus reaches 1000 grams. *Stillbirths* are counted with deaths of live births. II.C.

periodic interim payment (PIP). in *Medicare* and some other payment programs, a regular payment made by a *carrier* to a hospital, home health agency, or skilled nursing facility which approximates anticipated revenues, is adjusted periodically to conform to actual revenues, and is constant enough to assure predictable cash flow. Medicare PIPs were eliminated by Congress in 1987 for most providers. IV.C.1.

periodontics. the science and dental specialty devoted to prevention and treatment of *periodontal disease, disease of the gums and other supporting tissues of the teeth. III.C.

periodontist. a dentist specializing by education or practice in periodontics; slang, a gum farmer. III.A.3.

period prevalence. a measure of the total number of cases of a disease known to have existed at any time during a specified period; the sum of *point prevalence* and *incidence*. VIII.C.

permissible concentration. new official synonym, *threshold limit value.*

persistence. retention by *pollutants* of their toxic strength.
Persistence varies from hours for some bacteria to thousands of years for radioactive materials. It is determined by their resistance to *biodegradation,* dilution, removal, or elimination by the organism or environment and by their transfer from one organism to another through *trophic* levels. I.C.

persistency. in *insurance,* the rate at which policies written in a given line of insurance or for *members* of a given *group* are maintained in force until completion of the terms of the policies. IV.B.

persistent pesticide. a *pesticide* that will be present in the environment for longer than one growing season or one year after application. I.C.

personal health service. any health service provided to a specific individual; contrast *community health, consultation and education service, environmental health service, health education,* and *public health;* compare *basic health services.*
Personal health services are those which constitute *medical care* and include most medical, dental, hospital, and nursing home services. The concern is disease and individual health rather than healthful environments and lifestyles or populations. VII.B.3.

personal insurance. synonym, *individual insurance.*

personal physician. an individual's primary or principal doctor.
A personal physician ordinarily provides *primary care* on a *continuous* basis but is not necessarily a *family physician* or *specialist.* A good personal physician assumes responsibility for *comprehensive* care of the individual, coordinating the efforts of other providers in light of his or her knowledge of the patient as a whole.
See *private patient.* III.A.1.

pest. 1. an annoying, destructive, or *infectious* organism; ordinarily, visible organisms detrimental to human activity, as weeds or predators; often, large numbers of such organisms, as a cockroach or rat pest. 2. a plague; pestilence; historically, any major epidemic. 3. bubonic plague.
See *infestation* and *parasite.* I.A.1.

pest control. use of techniques for destruction of pests or inhibition of their growth and reproduction.

Chemical control techniques rely on the use of pesticides; physical control on use of physical agents, as temperature, humidity, electric shock, or radioactivity; biologic control on use of biologic means, as parasites, predators, or sterile males (through chemical or radiation sterilization); and cultural control on use of people, as to swat flies. I.A.1., I.C.

pesticide. an agent, ordinarily chemical, used to control pests. This includes *insecticides for use against harmful insects; *herbicides for weed control; *fungicides for control of plant diseases; *rodenticides for killing rats, mice, etc.; *germicides used in disinfectant products; and algaecides, slimicides, nematocides, bactericides, molluscicides, ovicides, and virucides.

Pesticides are chemicals whose toxicity, mobility, *persistence,* and cumulative effect may result in damage to other than the target species, beyond the area of application, and after the application period. Pesticides can contaminate water, air, or soil; accumulate in people, animals, and the environment, particularly if misused; and interfere with the reproductive processes of predatory birds and other animals.

See *Federal Insecticide, Fungicide, and Rodenticide Act.* I.A.2.a., I.C.

petition for modification of abatement (PMA). see *abatement period.*

Petty, William, and Graunt, John. British civil servants, 1623–1689 and 1620–1674, respectively. They applied numerical methods to the study of social and health problems in community life. Petty developed the idea of a statistical approach to problems of health and welfare, and his friend Graunt undertook to apply this approach specifically to such matters as births, disease *prevalence,* and deaths. The results of these studies were published by Graunt in 1662 as *Natural and Political Observations upon the Bills of Mortality.* II.C., VIII.A.1.

pharmaceutical. see *drug.*

pharmacist (DP, PD, Pharm.D.). a *professional* person qualified by education and authorized by law, as by *license,* to practice pharmacy.

See *apothecary* and *druggist.* III.A.4.

pharmacopeia, pharmacopia, pharmacopoeia (P, PH, pharm). 1. a list of drugs, usually with descriptions, formulas for their preparation, dosage forms, and standards for testing identity, purity, and strength; synonym, compendium. 2. a collection or stock of drugs.

The Federal Food, Drug, and Cosmetic Act recognizes three: the United States Pharmacopeia, the National Formulary, and the Homeopathic Pharmacopeia of the United States, and any supplements to any of them.

See *formulary* and *Physicians' Desk Reference.* III.B.3.

pharmacy. 1. the science, art, and practice of preparing, dispensing, and giving appropriate instruction in the use of *drugs.* 2. a place where pharmacy is practiced.

Pharmacy is an ancient profession, historically including clinical practice by the pharmacist and still requiring special training.

Pharos, The. the great lighthouse at Alexandria and, since 1938, the quarterly publication of the *Alpha Omega Alpha Honor Medical Society.* III.B.1.

phenylketonuria (PKU). a hereditary (autosomal recessive) disorder characterized by lack of phenylalanine hydroxylase (an enzyme), phenylketones in the urine, and *mental retardation* in untreated cases.

The ability to detect phenylketones in the urine shortly after birth and prevent retardation by diet made this the first disease for which all newborns were *screened*. Its rarity gives the effort low cost benefit, but the precedent for other screening efforts, as for cretinism or congenital hypothyroidism, is important. II.B.2.

phlebotomy. the opening of a vein for the purpose of letting blood.

This ancient therapeutic practice is rarely used, its practice now belonging to *phlebotomy technicians or phlebotomists, as they are called at the Clinical Center of the National Institutes of Health, who draw blood for diagnostic and other investigative purposes in their phlebotomy room. III.A.4.

physiatrics. synonym, *physical medicine and rehabilitation.*

physiatrist. a physician specializing by practice or education in physical medicine and rehabilitation. III.A.1.

physical. 1. pertaining to nature, the body, or material things. 2. informal synonym, *physical examination.*

physical diagnosis. diagnosis by physical examination rather than by history taking or laboratory testing. V.A.

physical examination (PE, Px). the study and observation, often aided by instruments, of a patient's body using inspection, palpation, percussion, auscultation, and measurement.

A *history* and physical, combined with appropriate *laboratory* work, constitute a complete *check up.*

See *gundeck physical* and *liability exam.* V.A.

physical fitness. see *fit.*

physical medicine (PM, Phys Med). synonym, *physical medicine and rehabilitation.*

physical medicine and rehabilitation (PM&R). the science and specialty devoted to the education, repair, and maintenance of bodies damaged by disease or injury.

Physical medicine is practiced by physiatrists, physical, occupational, and speech therapists, and other disciplines. III.C.

physical therapist (PT). an individual trained or licensed in or practicing physical therapy.

A license is required to practice physical therapy in all states. Licensure requires a baccalaureate degree or certificate from an approved school of physical therapy and, usually, passing a state board examination. III.A.4.

physical therapy (PT). treatment of disease and injury by physical means, as cold and heat, electricity, exercise, light, massage, and water; synonym, physiotherapy.

Physical therapy uses understanding of biomechanical and neurophysiologic principles and experience with assistive *devices* to relieve pain, restore maximum function, and prevent unnecessary disability.

See *activities of daily living* and *rehabilitation.* III.C., VII.B.3.b.

physician. a professional person skilled in the art of healing; one duly authorized, as by license, to treat disease; a *doctor* of *medicine.*

See *allopathic* and *osteopathic physician, bedside manner,* and *profile.* III.A.1.

physician assistant (PA). a trained and licensed (when necessary) or otherwise *credentialed* individual who performs tasks which might otherwise be performed by physicians, under the direction of a supervising physician; synonym, physician extender; contrast *barefoot doctor, feldsher, medical assistant,* and *nurse practitioner.*

U.S. physician assistants originated as paramedics trained by the military as medical corpsmen and pharmacists' mates and later further trained in medical schools to assist physicians in civilian health services, see *Medex.* Physician assistants are usually salaried rather than reimbursed on a *fee-for-service* basis, although supervising physicians may receive fee-for-service payment for their services. There are many synonyms for, similar occupations to, and national variations of physician assistants, making detailed definition difficult. III.A.4.

physician extender. synonym, *physician assistant.*

physician office. see *office.*

physician-patient privilege. the statutory prohibition of disclosure without the patient's consent in court or other legal proceedings of information given by a patient in confidence to a physician or other health professional. Special privileges sometimes also exist for communications with psychotherapists and the clergy.

Federal rules of evidence leave questions of privilege to individual courts where state law does not govern. The physician-patient privilege usually applies only in judicial proceedings and belongs to the patient, not the provider. The privilege is recognized in neither common nor military law and has many statutory exceptions where it does exist.

See *therapeutic privilege* and *separation program number.* VIII.B.3.

physicians' and surgeons' professional liability insurance. synonym, *malpractice insurance.*

physician's assistant. variant, physician assistant.

***Physicians' Desk Reference* (PDR).** an annual *compendium* of information concerning drugs, primarily *prescription* and *diagnostic* products, which is widely used as a reference document by physicians, other health workers, and patients.

The information included is the *labeling,* or *package insert,* required by the Food and Drug Administration for each drug and covers indications, effects, dosages, administration, and relevant warnings, hazards, contraindications, side effects, and precautions. The PDR is distributed free or at a reduced cost to many physicians and other providers through the patronage of the drug manufacturers, which have paid by the column inch for having information on their products included. It is the only readily available source of identifying photographs of drugs. The drugs are listed by *brand name* for each manufacturer, and are indexed by manufacturer, brand name, drug classification, and *generic name.*

See *American Hospital Formulary Service* and *formulary.* III.B.3.

Physicians for Social Responsibility (PSR). an organization, primarily of physicians, dedicated to professional and public education on the medical hazards of nuclear weapons and nuclear war, the *final epidemic.* III.B.4.

Physicians for the Twenty-first Century. the report of the Panel on the Graduate Professional Education of the Physician and College Preparation for Medicine, known as *The GPEP Report (Washington, DC 20036: Association of American Medical Colleges (One Dupont Circle, N.W.), 1984, or J Med Educ,* 11/84, part 2). Five conclusions and 27 recommendations on modern medical education. III.A.1.

physician shortage area. an area with an inadequate *supply* of physicians; an area having a physician to population ratio less than some standard; compare *medically underserved area.*
      What is considered a shortage varies with era, country, and the nature of the health system in which the physician functions. II.C., III.A.1.

Physician's Recognition Award. an American Medical Association *certification* of completion of acceptable *continuing medical education* recorded with the AMA by physicians; a good example of a growing number of such registration programs. III.C.

physiologist. see *ontologist.*

physiotherapy. synonym, *physical therapy.*

Piaget, Jean. Swiss *psychologist,* 1896–. Noted for his theoretical concepts of and research on the mental development of children. I.A.2., III.C., VIII.A.1.

Pinel, Philippe. French physician, 1746–1826. The father of modern psychiatry. During the French Revolution, he struck the shackles from the mental patients at the Salpetriere Hospital in Paris. Pinel profoundly influenced the handling of mentally ill patients by approaching them from a naturalistic rather than theological viewpoint. III.C., VIII.A.1.

ping-ponging. passing a patient from one physician to another in a health program for unnecessary cursory examinations so that the program can charge the patient's *third party* for a visit to each physician. The term originated in venereal disease control programs, but the practice has persisted in *Medicaid mills.* IV.C.2.

pink lady. slang, a member of a hospital or other health program's volunteer service or *auxiliary,* derived from the uniforms they wear, which are often pink, pink-striped, or decorated in pink to distinguish them from nurses; synonym, *candy striper, from the pink-striped version. III.A.4., VIII.B.2.a.

placebo (ADT, meaning "any damn thing"). an inactive or inert substance or procedure, as an injection of sugar water, given to please or gratify a patient or physician or given to controls in a *random controlled trial* to conceal who is actually receiving the experimental substance or procedure being tried; compare *demand characteristic.*
      The placebo should be indistinguishable from the experimental substance, an *active placebo being one which has its recognizable *side effects.* Where experimental therapy is indistinguishable from established therapy, the latter may be used as the placebo for the former. An *attention placebo controls for the effect of simply paying attention to subjects, see *Hawthorne effect,* by paying similar attention to controls. VIII.D.

placebo effect. either therapeutic or *side effects* following use of a placebo; by extension, the nonspecific results of any treatment, usually mediated by the patient's expectation of improvement, as the placebo effect of psychotherapy; compare *Hawthorne effect.*

All therapy has a placebo effect, often surprisingly large or its only effect. Placebo effects are generally positive, compare *nocebo.* VIII.D.

plague. 1. any severe *contagious epidemic* disease; an outbreak of a serious affliction, as a plague of locusts. 2. a disease of rodents due to the bacterium *Yersinia pestis,* transmitted to humans through the bite of infected fleas or by inhalation. The human disease has three forms, septicemic, pneumonic, and the famous bubonic plague. VIII.C.

planned parenthood. synonymous early euphemism for *family planning.* I.B.1.

Planned Parenthood Association. a local planned parenthood program; the national association of such programs.

These programs raise funds for research, public education, and other activities designed to make *birth control* available and *family planning* possible. III.B.4., VII.B.3.b.

planning. the act or process of designing desired future states described in a plan by *goals* and *objectives,* defining and selecting among alternative means of achieving these states, conducting activities necessary to the designing, as data gathering and analysis, and conducting activities needed to implement a plan.

There are many different types of planning, including: *long-range or *perspective (covering 15 or more years); *midrange or *strategic (5 to15 years); *short-term or *tactical (1 to 3 years, see *budget); categorical* or com- *prehensive health planning;* *normative (based on *norms* or *standards* with a legal basis; and *inductive or *deductive (used when the planning is done locally and consolidated and used at state and federal levels, *bubbled up, or vice versa, *trickled down, respectively). Further defined by its primary user, as hospital planning or corporate planning; geographic area of concern, as the *Regional Medical Program* or neighborhood planning, urban planning, or state planning; or its functional concern, as *health facilities* or *health manpower* planning. The extent to which planning is responsible by definition for implementation of plans is variable, as is its relation to *management.*

See *health planning* and *policy.* VI.A.

plastic surgeon. a physician specializing by practice or education in plastic surgery. III.A.1.

plastic surgery (PS). the science and surgical specialty devoted to the study and care of defects and deformities, principally by operative repair with transplantation or refashioning of tissue; compare *cosmetic surgery.* III.C.

play therapy. use of play in treatment of disease, particularly with children since they communicate with play rather than talk.

Play therapy is often available to hospitalized children to deal with both the boredom and the emotional impact of hospitalization. Family therapy emphasizes its use with adults who may change more, and enjoy changing more, when playing than when working on the problem. III.C., V.

playing God. making nontechnical, moral, or valuative decisions, usually describing only decisions by physicians to limit in some way the use of available medical *technology* rather than to undertake its full use; more generally, provider behavior which is unreasonably authoritarian.The pejorative connotation is warranted only when the decision involved is not properly the physician's, because the patient or the patient's family is capable and desirous of making it or because law or common practice reserves it for someone else. V.

pneumoconiosis. disease of the lung caused by inhalation of dust or *particles*, especially mineral dusts, as *asbestosis, bagassosis, black lung, brown lung,* and *silicosis*.

These are occupational diseases sharing a common pathology and *natural history,* e.g., a delayed slow death. There are differences between the pure pneumoconioses which resist inhalation, although they are substantially the same, and the chronic obstructive diseases which resist exhalation, as smoker's disease, asthma, and emphysema. The latter are not usually occupational but often coexist. One year in the mines and 30 years of smoking will get you black lung benefits. II.B.2.

podiatrist. a professional educated in or practicing podiatry, the care of feet.

A podiatrist performs surgical and other operative procedures, prescribes corrective devices, and prescribes and administers drugs and physical therapy. *Medicare* regulations state that a doctor of podiatry is considered a "physician," but only with respect to functions the doctor is legally authorized to perform by the state in which he or she is licensed. III.A.4.

podiatry. the science and care of the human foot in health and disease; synonym, chiropody. III.C.

point prevalence. the frequency of a disease at a designated point or moment in time; compare *prevalence.* VIII.C.

poison. a substance harmful or fatal to an *exposed* organism, often in small or unrecognized amounts; anything destructive or harmful to the health or success of an individual, business, or endeavor; compare *threshold limit value, toxic substance,* and *toxin.* I.C.

poison control center (PCC). a program concerned with prevention of poisoning and assisting victims of poisoning.

The heart of most centers is a well-advertised telephone number, often answered by *house staff* in a local emergency room, equipped with *toxicology* texts and files listing ingredients of common household and industrial products, who provide patients and professionals with advice on management of poisonings. III.B.11., VII.C.2.

police power. 1. authority conferred by the American constitutional system on the individual states to adopt and enforce laws securing the health, among other things, of the state and its citizens. 2. in psychiatry, the constitutional power of the state to involuntarily *commit* mentally ill persons in order to prevent harm, ordinarily physical, to the self or others. 1. VIII.C., 2. III.B.2.

police surgeon. a physician trained in *forensic medicine* whose expertise is called upon to provide information for documentation and later presentation in legal matters, whether of concern to criminal or to civil courts, and who examines living persons as well as performing autopsies; compare *coroner* and *medical examiner.*

The position, virtually unknown in the United States, has been long established in European, British Commonwealth, and Asian countries as well as in Mexico and other parts of Latin America. Except for medical examiners seeing patients for *disability* determinations, regular physician use by governments in legal matters concerning the living, as the rape victim or homicidal maniac, is limited in the United States. III.A.1., III.D.2., VIII.B.3.

policy. 1. a course of action adopted and pursued by a government, party, statesman, or other individual or organization; any course of action adopted as proper, advantageous, or expedient. 2. synonym, *insurance policy.*

The term is sometimes used to describe any stated position on matters at issue, as an organization's policy statement on *national health insurance,* whether or not any action is expected. The Congress makes policy by writing legislation and conducting oversight activities. In the executive branch of the federal government, policies interpret or enlarge upon *rules* (regulations) and may be referred to as *guidelines. Guidelines or policies bear the same relationship to rules as rules do to law, except that, unlike rules, they do not have the force of law. VI.A.

pollutant. something which pollutes; an introduced physical, chemical, or biologic agent, generally resulting from human activity, which reduces the quality of the *environment,* makes a resource unfit for some purpose, or endangers a living organism.

See *criteria pollutant.* I.C.

Pollutant Standard Index (PSI). a federally recommended *air quality index.*

The five *criteria pollutants* are included in the PSI, with the concentration of each being expressed by an index value between 0 and 500. These index values are associated with descriptors of the air quality and its health effects and appropriate cautionary statements. Index values of 300 represent air quality poor enough to warrant warning the public; the health effects are described as "very unhealthful," and elderly persons with heart or lung disease are cautioned to stay indoors and reduce physical activity. The *criterion* for each criteria pollutant is given an index value of 100. The index number is derived from scientific information on the health-related, significant-harm concentrations of each pollutant. The highest index value for each pollutant may be reported, or at the least, the highest single index value among all of the pollutants is reported. The public is thereby apprised of the worst air pollutant in the area surveyed. Precautionary statements and general health effects are publicized when the health-effect descriptor is either "unhealthful," "very unhealthful," or "hazardous." I.C.1.

pollute. make physically impure or unclean; befoul, taint; compare *contaminate.* I.C.

polluter. one who pollutes; a producer of pollutants.

Since most efforts to control pollution are directed at polluters, it is worth noting their variety: individuals, corporations, or governments; and *sources* as mobile as automobiles or as stationary as power plants. Polluters often are not responsible for the costs of the pollution.

See *social cost.* I.C.

pollution. the act or process of defiling or rendering impure; the state of being polluted with matter or energy whose nature, location, or quantity produces undesired effects. I.C.

polychlorinated biphenyl (PCB). any biphenyl molecule with chlorine atoms attached; any *pesticide* with polychlorinated biphenyl residues; any such compound used in manufacture, as of plastics.

In the environment, PCBs exhibit many of the same characteristics as DDT and may therefore be confused with it. PCBs are toxic to aquatic life, *persist* in the environment for long periods of time, and are biologically accumulative. I.C.5.

pool.   see *insurance pool.*

poor.   see *poverty.*

population.   1. a group of people, organisms, or things, having some quality or characteristic in common, usually occupying a particular area. 2. in *demography*, the *whole number* of people inhabiting a specific area at a given period. 3. in *ecology*, a group of organisms of a *biome* sharing a common gene pool. 4. in statistics, the group of all individuals or events theoretically available for observation from which *samples* are taken for statistical measurement.

See *control* and *profile.* I.B., VIII.C.

population pyramid.   a graphic representation of the age structure of a population.

Usually each five-year age group is represented by a horizontal bar with females on the right and males on the left of a central line. Different countries have distinctly different pyramids determined by birth rates, longevity, wars, living standards, epidemiology, medical care, and the like. I.B., VIII.C.

portability.   of insurance *coverage,* the ability of the covered individual to carry or continue the coverage when changing job, location, or other important status.

Group insurance often depends on continued membership in the group, typically by continued employment. Insurance which cannot be continued when leaving the group lacks portability. IV.B.

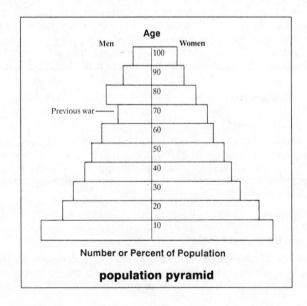

population pyramid

positron emission tomography (PET). a technique for producing colored contour images of the brain by mapping areas of high and low neural activity. Studies of the brain using this technique, and the images produced, are known as *PET scans.

This quite safe technique depends on the measurement of gamma ray emissions from a series of *tomographs* of the brain. These emissions result from the annihilation of short-lived positrons when circulating positron-labeled glucose, given as the source, is used by the brain. The emissions are supposed to correlate with the level of metabolic activity of each brain area.

See *CAT scan, NMR,* and *tomography.* V.A.

post, *postmortem.* literally, anything after death; synonym, *autopsy.* II.B.1.

potable. drinkable; fit for drinking or cooking by virtue of both *safety* and aesthetic acceptability.

Safety is a medical consideration; aesthetics requires clarity, acceptable taste, and lack of odor. I.C.5.

potable water standard. a *standard* of potability; commonly, as in Great Britain, a biochemical oxygen content of 20 parts per million (ppm) or suspended solids, as dirt and microorganisms, of less than 30 ppm. I.C.5.

poverty. lack or relative lack of money, *income, resources,* goods, or means of subsistence; privation, want, scarcity, death, feebleness.

The sick get poor and the poor get sick, but the connection is hard to define, as is poverty itself. There is no single national definition.

See *index* and *means test.* I.A.2.c.

poverty area. an urban or rural geographic area with a high proportion of low-income families.

Typically, average income is used to define a poverty area, but other indicators, as housing conditions, illegitimate birth rates, and incidence of juvenile delinquency, are sometimes added to define geographic areas with poverty-associated conditions. Such areas may be designated for research or demographic purposes or may be eligible for additional or special services. I.B.2.

practical nurse. a *nurse* who is skilled in the care of the sick but is not a graduate of a formal program of nursing education or is not licensed; compare *registered nurse, licensed practical nurse,* and *patient care technician.*

Practical nurses with no formal education are now uncommon; most have been to a hospital or vocational nursing school and are licensed. III.A.3.

practice. 1. exercise oneself in a profession, skill, or such for instruction, improvement, or acquisition of discipline and proficiency. 2. use one's knowledge of an art or profession as a way of life. 3. collectively, the patients of a physician or other practitioner, a *panel.*

Practicing medicine is applying the principles of medicine and serving as a physician in the diagnosis and treatment of disease. *Group, independent, private,* and *solo practices* are among the many ways of doing it. Practices are classified by the North American Primary Care Research Group according to the personnel involved (solo or group), their geographic location (central city, urban, suburban, small city, or rural), and their main source of income (fee for service, prepaid, or capitation). V.

practice effect. the modification, ordinarily improvement, in task performance as a result of repeated trials or training in the task; compare *Hawthorne effect* and *placebo*. VIII.D.

practice management. the knowledge and skills needed for effective *management* of a *practice* and of the physician's personal estate; the use of such knowlege and skills.

These business skills are barely covered in a physician's *undergraduate medical education,* which generally covers little of the economic, ethical, legal, or social forms of medicine, since its clinical content is so vast. They are required in a *family medicine* residency curriculum by the *American Board of Family Practice.* V., VI.C.

practice privilege. synonym, *staff privilege.*

practice register. a "listing of all *registered* patients in a practice" (*NAPCRG, 1978*).

See *age-sex register.* V.

pratique. the bill of health given to an incoming vessel by a health officer of a port, traditionally after *quarantine*. VII.B.2.e.

preadmission certification. see *admission certification.*

preclinical. 1. occurring prior to the period in a disease in which recognized symptoms or signs make diagnosis possible; compare *clinical* and *subclinical*. 2. pertaining to medical studies undertaken before the study of patients, traditionally the first two years of medical school; compare *basic* and *clinical sciences*. 1. II., 2. III.C.

predictive value. a measure of a *test*'s ability to predict actual results.

It is distinguished from *sensitivity* and *specificity* and varies with the *prevalence* of the condition being tested for in the population being tested. VIII.D.

preexisting condition. an *injury* occurring, *disease* contracted, or physical condition which existed prior to the issuance of a health insurance policy, ordinarily one which results in an *exclusion* from coverage under the policy for costs resulting from the condition. IV.B.

preferred provider organization (PPO). an organized group of providers which contracts with a *third-party payer, self-insured* industry, or union trust fund to sell health services to a defined group of patients at preferential *fee-for-service* rates.

A PPO may be a group of physicians, a hospital, or another organization. It is not a *health maintenance organization* since it is paid on a fee-for-service basis. It lowers charges in return for prompt payment, regular volume, and the inherent competitive advantage. Insured individuals may see the doctor of their choice but forfeit *first-dollar coverage* and face *cost sharing* if they do not use PPO services. A new name for an old form of competition in which the provider receives volume, the payer gets a discount, and the patient is *locked in* only because the benefits are passed to him or her.

Read de Lissovoy, Greg, et al., "Preferred Provider Organizations: Today's Models and Tomorrow's Prospects" (*Inquiry*, 23(1): 7–15, Spring/86). III.B.1.

premature birth. see *abortion* and *birth*.

premium. money or other considerations paid by an *insured* person or policyholder (or on his or her behalf) to an *insurer* or *third party* for insurance coverage under an *insurance policy.*

The premium is based on the actuarial value of the *benefits* provided by the policy plus a *loading* for administrative costs, *profit*, and the like. Premium amounts for employment-related insurance are often shared by employers and employees, see *contributory* insurance. Some of the premiums paid by employees are tax-deductible, see *medical deduction.* Premiums paid by employers are nontaxable *income* for employees. Premiums are paid for coverage whether benefits are actually used or not and should not be confused with *cost sharing,* which occurs only when benefits are used. IV.B.

prepaid. of a practice which "receives an advance payment to provide specified health services to a particular patient during a specified time period" *(NAPCRG, 1978).* IV.A.

prepaid group practice. a formal association of three or more physicians which provides a defined set of services to people for a specified time period in return for a fixed periodic prepayment made in advance of the use of the service; compare *group practice, health maintenance organization,* and *medical foundation.* III.B.1., V.

prepaid health plan (PHP). 1. a contract between an *insurer* and a *subscriber* or group of subscribers in which the PHP undertakes to provide a specified set of health *benefits* in return for a periodic *premium.* 2. in the 1970s, an organizational entity in California which provided services to beneficiaries of MediCal, California's *Medicaid* program.

The MediCal Reform Program of 1971 allowed MediCal administrators to contract with groups of medical providers to supply specified services on a prepaid per capita basis. One of many efforts in California and elsewhere to improve or control Medicaid programs, the PHPs were the subject of much controversy regarding the *cost* and *quality* of their services, see *skimming* and *skimping.* III.B.1., IV.C.2.

prepayment. inconsistently used: 1. synonym, *insurance.* 2. of or pertaining to financing programs such as insurance which are not *at risk* as *Blue Cross plans.* 3. any payment ahead of time to a provider for anticipated services, as an expectant mother paying in advance for maternity care. 4. of or pertaining to payment to organizations, as *health maintenance organizations,* prepaid group practices, and medical foundations, which, unlike an insurance company, take responsibility for arranging for and providing needed services as well as paying for them. IV.B.

prescribe. write an order for *therapy* and give instructions concerning its use. V.B.

prescription (Ps) (Rx). a written direction or *order* for the preparation and administration of a *drug* or other therapy.

A prescription properly specifies the drug or treatment to be given, the form and quantity to be dispensed, refills if needed, the schedule and amounts to be used, the method of administration, and any other needed instructions. Prescriptions for drugs are filled by *pharmacists;* for *devices,* by *orthotists;* and for therapy, as physical therapy, by the appropriate therapist. III.B.2., III.B.3., V.B.

prescription drug. a drug available to the public only upon prescription. The availability of such a drug is limited because the drug is considered dangerous if used without a physician's supervision.
See *ethical* and *over-the-counter drugs.* III.B.3.

presenting complaint. synonym, *chief complaint.*

preservative. an *additive* used to prevent or retard spoilage or decay or other chemical or physical change, as in a medicine or food product. I.A.2.a.

president's budget. in the federal *budget,* the budget for a particular *fiscal year,* specifying proposed *budget authority, obligations,* and *outlays* and transmitted to the Congress by the president in accordance with the amended Budget and Accounting Act of 1921.

Some elements of the budget, as the estimates for the legislative and judicial branches, are included without review by the Office of Management and Budget or approval by the president. The budget is submitted in January for the fiscal year beginning during the calendar year.
See *congressional budget.* VI.B.1.

prevailing charge. a *charge* which falls within the range of charges most frequently used in a *locality* for a particular medical service or *procedure;* the top of the range of charges which a *carrier* using prevailing charges in reimbursement will accept as *reasonable* for a given service without special justification.

Current Medicare *rules* make the limit on an area's prevailing charge the seventy-fifth percentile of the *customary charges* for the service by physicians in a given area. For example, if customary charges for an appendectomy in a locality were distributed so that 25 percent of the services were given by physicians whose customary charge was $250, 25 percent by physicians who charged $300, 25 percent by physicians who charged $350, and 25 percent by physicians who charged over $350, then the prevailing charge would be $350, since this is the level that would cover at least 75 percent of the cases.
See *actual charge* and *fractionation.* IV.C.1., VII.D.1.

prevalence. frequency of occurrence. *prevalence rate. the number of cases of a disease present at a specified time (*point prevalence, compare *period prevalence*) in a population or area per 1000 or 100,000 people.

Such rates measure *morbidity* at a moment in time, as the number of cases of hemophilia in the country on the first of the year. The prevalence of arthritis is high relative to its *incidence.* Prevalence equals incidence times average case duration. VIII.C.

preventative. affected synonym, preventive.

preventive medicine. the science and specialty devoted to the study and application of means of maintaining a *healthful* environment, *health maintenance,* and reducing or eliminating disease, disability, and their consequences; compare *community medicine, environmental health, epidemiology, family planning, health education, occupational health, public health,* and *social medicine.*

Preventive medicine includes any activity intended to prevent illness, as by immunization, or to eliminate *hazards,* as failure to use seat belts; to produce early detection of disease, as by Pap smears; or to inhibit deterioration of health, as by exercise. It is the only specialty whose practitioners do not have a name, as pediatrician or physiatrist. It has *subspecialties* in aerospace medicine, general preventive medicine, occupational medicine, and public health. Prevention is irregularly and ambitiously, but not helpfully, divided into: *primary prevention. measures to create healthful environments, societies, and families; improve the quality of life; and reduce the incidence of disease in a population. This corresponds roughly to the traditional concept of prevention. *secondary prevention. measures to reduce the prevalence of disease in a population by shortening its course and duration. This takes in some treatment. *tertiary prevention. measures to reduce the prevalence of chronic *disability, relapses,* and recidivism in a population by minimizing functional impairment consequent to disease. This extends prevention into *rehabilitation.*

See *consultation* and *education services.* III.C., VII.2.c.

PriCare. short commercial synonym, *International Classification of Health Problems in Primary Care.*

price. synonym, *charge.*

Drugs, devices, and other things have prices; *services* have charges, at least in medicine. VII.D.1.

price elasticity. see *elasticity.*

primary care. *medical care* and *services* at the point when a person first seeks assistance from the health care system, for the simpler and more common illnesses, and which takes ongoing responsibility for the recipient's *health maintenance* and illnesses.

Note the conflicts among the three parts of the definition: ongoing responsibility is not simple to practice, nor is first contact care, and first contact may be for a complex problem. Primary care may be *comprehensive* when responsible for overall coordination of care of the patient's health problems, whether biologic, behavioral, or social. Effective use of *consultants* and community resources is an important part of primary care. It may be provided by physicians or other personnel, as family *nurse clinicians.*

See *family physician* and *personal physician, general practice, primary health care,* and *secondary* and *tertiary care.* V.

primary diagnosis. the most important problem in a particular context, whether the first diagnosis made; the most emergent, serious, or expensive; the one requiring admission to a hospital, the *admitting diagnosis; or the final diagnosis of the admitting problem, the *discharge diagnosis; compare *principal diagnosis.* II.B.1.

primary gain. the relief from emotional conflict and freedom from anxiety derived by a patient from mental defense mechanisms or from symptoms or illness used to deal with unresolved emotional, familial, or other conflicts; contrast *secondary gain.*

The patient is ordinarily unconscious of the use of the mechanism, the symptoms or illness, the conflicts, and the gain, although the patient knows he or she is sick. Whatever the illness, the patient may not recover until the conflicts are dealt with in some other way. II.A.1.

primary health care. synonym, *primary care.*

Defined by the World Health Organization as "essential health care based on practical, scientifically sound, and socially acceptable methods and technology made universally accessible to individuals and families in the community through their full participation and at a cost that the community and country can afford to maintain at every stage of their development in the spirit of self-reliance and self-determination. It forms an integral part both of the country's health system, of which it is the central function and main focus, and of the overall social and economic development of the community. It is the first level of contact of individuals, the family and community with the national health system bringing health care as close as possible to where people live and work, and constitutes the first element of a continuing health care process" (*Primary Health Care.* Report of the International Conference on Primary Health Care, Alma-Ata, USSR, 6–12 September, 1978. Geneva: World Health Organization, 1978. pp. 3–4). V.

primary payer. the insurer obligated to pay *losses* prior to any liability of other, *secondary insurers.

Medicare is a primary payer with respect to Medicaid but secondary to liability insurance, workmen's compensation, and any private group coverage. For a person eligible under both programs, Medicaid pays only benefits not covered by Medicare, or after Medicare benefits are exhausted.

See *duplication* and *coordination of benefits.* IV.B.

primary prevention.   see *preventive medicine.*

primum non nocere.   (Latin, first do no harm) the ancient clinical precept urging practitioners always to avoid making matters worse.

It is claimed that only in this century have patients had a better than even chance of benefiting from an encounter with a physician. Yet as medicine becomes more effective, it also becomes more dangerous. Not hurting people remains difficult. V.B.

principal diagnosis.   the condition established after study to be chiefly responsible for admission of a patient to a hospital; the diagnosis, thus defined, which determines the *diagnosis related group* for a case, although actual payment is affected by other factors, including the patient's age and sex, secondary diagnoses, and the applicable *DRG rate* and *weight;* compare *primary diagnosis.* II.B.1, IV.C.1., V.A.

prior authorization.   a requirement imposed by a *third party,* under some systems of *utilization review,* that a *provider* justify for a *peer review* committee, insurance company representative, or state agent the need for delivering a particular service to a patient before actually providing the service in order to receive reimbursement.

Prior authorization is typically required for expensive nonemergency services, as an *elective* hospital stay, see *preadmission certification,* or for services particularly likely to be overused or *abused* (many state Medicaid programs require prior authorization of dental services). IV.C.2., VII.D.2.

prior determination.   similar to *prior authorization* but less restrictive in that payment will be made without prior authorization, provided the services are later approved as needed.

Providers who want to be assured of payment seek prior determination rather than risk later disapproval. VII.D.2.

private corporation (PC, p.c.).   a legal entity which buys and sells the services of an individual.

Many physicians incorporate themselves for tax purposes and added protection from malpractice. The initials p.c. after a physician's name mean one is dealing with that physician as a thing, not additional academic accomplishment. III.A.1., III.B.1.

private duty. of a nurse, caring for a single patient, either in the home or a hospital, typically in the direct employ of the patient or the patient's family.
See *registry*. III.A.2.

private nurse. a nurse doing private duty. III.A.2.

private patient (PP). a patient whose care is the responsibility of an identifiable individual physician or other *professional* paid directly by the patient or the patient's *third party* for services to the patient. The physician is a *personal physician*, and the patient is his or her private patient.

Private patients are contrasted with *service patients*, whose care is the responsibility of a health program and staff paid by the program; see *house staff*. The program, rather than the individual practitioner, is paid for the care. The distinction is important to third-party payers, including *Medicare*, because situations arise in which payment is made to both a program and an individual practitioner for the same services; see *teaching physician*. It occasionally refers to a patient occupying a room in an institution by himself or herself, a private room. VIII.A.1.

private physician (PP). a *personal physician;* a physician in *independent practice;* the physician of a private patient. IV.A.1.

private practice (PP). *practice* in which the practitioner and his or her practice are free of external *policy* control; ordinarily the practitioner is self-employed or salaried by a partnership in which he or she is a partner with similar practitioners. Sometimes wrongly synonymous with *fee-for-service* practice (the practitioner may sell services by another method, as *capitation*) or *solo practice* (*group practice* may be private).

Physicians practice in many different settings, and there is no agreement about which constitute private practice. Regulation, which does exert external control, is not generally felt to make all practice public. The opposite of private practice is not necessarily public, in the sense of employment by the government. Practitioners salaried by private hospitals are not usually thought to be in private practice. (The author thought this a difficult concept to define, but the 13-year-old son of a physician got it started by saying, "That's easy. Practice of your own, charging what you want.") V.

privilege. a special right, benefit, immunity, power, or exemption, as *physician-patient, staff,* and *therapeutic privileges.*

*Privileged communications, which common law will not permit or require to be divulged, are those occurring in *confidential* or *fiduciary* relations, as between physician and patient, client and attorney, or husband and wife. VIII.B.3.

proband. the individual or *index case* who is the starting or focal point for a genogram or pedigree. I.B.1.

probationary period. see *waiting period.*

problem. a source of perplexity, vexation, or current or potential trouble.
People seek care for problems they perceive, the profound differences between patient and *caregiver* perceptions of the same person's problems being a major subtlety in health care. So is the labeling of problems; it is better to use informal, specific patient labels than formal, general ones and not to use ones which diagnose undiagnosed problems.

The North American Primary Care Research Group uses the following definition: "a provider-determined assessment of anything that concerns the patient, the provider, or both. Problems should be recorded at the level of specificity determined at the time of that particular visit" (*NAPCRG, 1978*).

See *International Classification of Health Problems in Primary Care.* II.A.1.

problem contact.   an episode of care for a single problem. A visit which deals with several problems constitutes several problem contacts. VII.

problem index.   "a compilation of lists of patients by problem or diagnosis; synonyms, diagnostic index, disease index, *E-book,* and morbidity index" (*NAPCRG, 1978*); any system for identifying patients in a practice with particular problems. VII.C.

problem list.   a list of a patient's problems kept at the beginning of a *problem-oriented medical record.*

The list serves as an index to the record and a guide to the patient's care. It may separate active and inactive or permanent, temporary, and resolved problems. VII.D.

problem of living.   economic, family, or other difficulty, other than a disease, for which a person seeks help from a health care program or provider.

Problems of living often present as illness, real or psychosomatic, which may itself require treatment. Adolescents fighting with parents and parents who cannot afford food who seek care, with or without symptoms, have problems of living. Family physicians and some others care for such problems. Others refer to *social workers, ministers,* or other resources or simply do not help.

See *medical model.* I.A.2., II.A.1.

problem-oriented medical record (POMR).   a *medical record* in which the information and conclusions are formally organized under specific patient problems rather than by source of information (history and physical, laboratory, and so forth), as was traditionally done.* The Problem-Oriented Medical Information System (PROMIS) is a computerized POMR.

The POMR was developed by Lawrence Weed (U.S. physician) and his coworkers in the early 1960s and is now widely used in medical practice, although often in modified or relaxed form. *Progress notes* in a POMR should be *SOAPed, i.e., formally organized to show separately for each problem appropriate Subjective and Objective information, Assessment, and Plan of diagnosis and treatment. Weed's focus on the problems patients present encourages *comprehensive,* orderly, and reliable care, although its concern for form is sometimes time-consuming. VII.D.

procedure.   a way of doing something; the thing done; compare *service.* In nursing, *procedure manuals contain complete descriptions of how to do specialized tasks for which nurses are responsible.

See *Current Procedural Terminology.* VII.

process measure.   an indicator of the quality of medical care which documents the content or means of care used for various *populations* or *diagnoses,* as the percentage of cases of strep throat which are cultured before treatment.

Such measures do not measure the outcomes of care. They do reflect the use of diagnostic and treatment methods which are thought to be *ef-*

fective. They do indicate conformity with *standards* established by peer groups or with expectations formulated by leaders in the profession.

See *input, output measures, NAPCRG Process Classification,* and *Professional Activity Study.* VII.D.2.

proctologist. a physician specializing by practice or education in *colon and rectal surgery.* III.A.1.

proctology. synonym, *colon and rectal surgery.*

productivity screen. a minimum or maximum rate of production considered appropriate in a given situation.

Third-party payers sometimes screen payments to providers to identify program abuse, such as *family ganging,* which is revealed by excess productivity. *Community health centers* are required to pass minimum productivity screens to receive continued funding. VII.B.3.

profession. 1. a learned calling. 2. the whole body of people engaged in such a calling.

Professions ordinarily have specialized knowledge, skills, and methods; require formal education in such knowledge and skills as well as the scientific, historical, and scholarly principles underlying them; maintain high standards of achievement and conduct by force of professional associations and concerted opinion; grant membership only upon examination and achievement of *certification* or *licensure;* have a code of ethics, as the *Hippocratic oath,* and technical standards; and commit their members to continued study and public service. Professionals function with autonomy and authority since they alone have the expertise to make decisions in their disciplines. Medicine is the prototype health profession. The term is irregularly and casually used since all health occupations aspire to being professions. III.A.

professional. of or pertaining to a profession or to the ethical or technical standards of a profession.

See *bedside manner.* III.A.

Professional Activity Study (PAS). a computerized *medical record* information system purchased by hospitals from the *Commission on Professional and Hospital Activities* (CPHA).

Information flows into the system through a *discharge abstract* completed by the hospital medical records *department* on every discharged patient. The patient information is displayed back to the hospital in a series of monthly, semiannual, and annual reports which compare such things as average *lengths of stay,* number and types of tests used, and *autopsy* rates for given diagnostic conditions with those of other hospitals of similar size and scope of services (good examples of *process measures*). III.B.1.

professional association. an organization responsible for furthering the interests and development of a profession, enforcing its ethics and standards, and representing its members.

Such associations are sometimes called colleges or societies and sometimes represent groups with common interests other than a true profession. III.A.

professional component. the part of a service, and of its charge, provided by the responsible physician. The **hospital* or *technical component* is the part of the service, and charge, provided by the health facility in which the service is performed using the facility's equipment and personnel.

The two components are often charged for separately, which is why patients often complain of being billed twice for laboratory and radiology services. VII.D.1.

professional courtesy. caring for fellow health professionals for free or at a reduced charge.

Traditionally physicians and some professional colleagues such as nurses have not charged each other for their care because they knew each other and would someday themselves need care. Professional courtesy is now usually a fee discount rather than free care and, as with other courtesies, is disappearing as society fragments and *competition* overwhelms *charity*. IV.A.

professional liability. the obligation of professional providers or their insurers to pay for damages resulting from their acts of omission or commission in treating patients.

The term is preferred by some providers to *malpractice* because it does not necessarily imply *negligence*. It also better covers the obligations of all professionals, including lawyers, architects, and other health professionals, to their clients. V.D.

professional liability insurance. synonym, *malpractice insurance.*

professional standards review organization (PSRO). a physician-sponsored organization responsible for comprehensive and ongoing review of services provided by the *Medicare, Medicaid,* and *maternal and child health* programs.

The requirement for establishment of PSROs was added by the Social Security amendments of 1972, P.L. 92-603, to the Social Security Act as part B of title XI. PSRO areas were defined throughout the country. The review was to determine for reimbursement purposes in these programs whether services were medically necessary; provided in accordance with professional *criteria, norms,* and *standards;* and in the case of institutional services, given in an *appropriate* setting. PSROs have since been replaced by *peer review organizations.* III.B.1., VI.D.2.

proficiency testing. assessment of technical knowledge and skills related to the performance requirements of a specific job, whether such knowledge and skills were acquired through formal or informal means; compare *equivalency testing.* III.A.

profile. 1. an outline or presentation of the distinctive features of something. 2. a graph, curve, or other schema presenting quantitatively or descriptively the chief characteristics of something, as an organ, process, or person.

*Patient profiles list all the services provided to a particular patient during a specified period of time. *Physician profiles are statistical summaries of the patterns of practice of individual physicians. *Population profiles characterize a specific population's *health status* or use of medical care. *Diagnostic profiles are physician, hospital, or population profiles of experience with a specific condition or diagnosis. VI.D., VIII.D.

profit. the gain made by the sale of a *good* or *service* after deducting the value of the labor, materials, rents, interest on *capital,* and other expenses involved in production of the good or service.

Economists define profit as return to or on capital investment and distinguish *normal (competitive) profit and *excessive (more than competitive) profit. Profit in the sense of a profit-making or *proprietary* institution is present when any of the net earnings of the institution inure to the benefit of any individual. Profit is hard to define operationally or in detail, and unreasonable or excessive profit even more so. Reasonable profit on investments must vary with the *risks* involved in the investments. Profit bears a close relationship to the balance of *supply* and *demand,* being a measure of unmet demand. VIII.B.1.

prognosis. the act or art of foretelling the course of a disease; the probability of survival and recovery from a disease, anticipated from knowledge of its *natural history* and special features of the case in question.

Predicting the future, one of the clinical arts, requires conscious effort, practice, and judgment. An intelligent prognosis is as important and difficult a part of the assessment of many problems as is a *diagnosis.*

See *hanging crepe.* II.B.3.

program review team. an interdisciplinary team which conducts *medical review* of *skilled nursing* facilities and *intermediate care facilities* as one of the *conditions of participation* in the Medicare and Medicaid programs. IV.C.2., VI.D.2.

progress note. a written description in the *medical record* of an *encounter,* the evolution of a patient's problems, and their diagnosis and treatment.

See *problem-oriented medical record.* VII.D.

progressive patient care. an inpatient care system in which patients are grouped in units depending on their need for care and degree of illness rather than by consideration of diagnosis or medical specialty.

There are three conventional levels or stages of progressive patient care: *intensive care,* needed for critically ill patients; *intermediate care,* intermediate between intensive and minimal care; and minimal care or *self-care,* which seems self-explanatory. Except for the development of *intensive care units,* the concept of progressive patient care has had little impact on the organization of hospitals, which still separate medical, surgical, pediatric, and other specialties' patients. The levels of care defined in this context are particular to it; this intermediate care is not the same as the level of care available in an *intermediate care facility.* VII.C.5.

progressive tax. a tax which takes an increasing proportion of *income* as income rises, as the federal personal income tax; compare *regressive tax* and *proportional tax.* Incremental increases in taxable income are subject to an increased *marginal tax rate.* IV.C.

project grant. a grant of federal funds to a public or private agency or organization for a specified purpose authorized by law, as development of an *emergency medical services system* or operation of a *community health center.*

The making of project grants is usually discretionary with the Department of Health and Human Services. Applicants are chosen on the basis of merit, often competitively, and the amount of the grant is based on need (the estimated cost of achieving the purpose), all of which contrasts with the usual practice with *formula grants.* IV.C.

Project Hope. an international medical *charity* founded and run by William B. Walsh (U.S. physician).

The project's principal original instrument was a hospital ship, the *U.S.S. Hope,* that visited the ports of poorer nations, providing medical and surgical care and training local health workers. The organization has since enlarged and diversified its activities. III.B.4.

Project U.S.A. an American Medical Association program which finds and places physicians as *locum tenentes* for *solo* practitioners, as in the *National Health Service Corps.* III.A.1., III.D.1.

prolotherapy. the rehabilitation of an incompetent structure, as a ligament or tendon, by the induced proliferation of new cells.

Injecting the attachments of ligaments and tendons to produce fibrous tissue in order to stabilize a joint is used mainly in treating chronic head, neck, and low back pain. Its *efficacy* has not been established by *random controlled trials,* nor has it become part of established medical practice, although its proponents report an 80 percent success rate. V.B.

prophylaxis. measures controlling *exposure* to *hazards* and preventing the development or spread of disease; *preventive medicine.* The adjectival form, *prophylactic, has become slang for a condom.

proportional tax. a tax which takes a constant proportion of *income* as income changes. The social security *payroll tax* is proportional up to the limit on income to which it applies; compare *progressive tax* and *regressive tax.* IV.C.

propositus. synonym, *proband.*

proprietary. *profit*-making; owned and operated for the purpose of making profit, whether or not made. III.B., VIII.B.1.

proprietary hospital. a hospital operated for the purpose of making a *profit* for its owners.

Proprietary hospitals were traditionally owned by physicians for the care of their own and others' patients. Most are now investor-owned corporations, some of which own national chains of hospitals. Such hospitals ordinarily offer only profitable services, as surgery and psychiatry, rather than what the community needs; see *green screen.* III.B.1.

proprietary name. synonym, *brand name.*

prospective medicine. medical care concerned with predicting and improving people's future health through *health hazard appraisal,* lifestyle modifications, and such individual *health maintenance* rather than through *public health* or other group approaches. VII.B.3.b.

Prospective Payment Assessment Commission (ProPAC, PROPAC). a committee which advises the secretary of the Department of Health and Human Services on Medicare's *diagnosis related group*–based prospective payment system.

The commission is required by the Social Security Amendments of 1983 (P.L. 98-21). Its members are appointed by the director of the Office of Technology Assessment. The commission's main responsibilities include recommending an appropriate annual percentage change in DRG payments; recommending needed changes in the DRG classification system and individual DRG weights; collecting and evaluating data on medical practices, patterns, and technology; and reporting on its activities. III.D.1., IV.C.2.

prospective payment system (PPS). 1. any method of financing medical care which pays for services before they occur, as *capitation.* 2. the Medicare system based on *diagnosis related groups* paying for hospital care. IV.C.1.

prospective reimbursement. any method of paying hospitals or other health programs in which amounts or rates of payment are established in advance and the programs are paid these amounts regardless of the costs they actually incur.

These systems of reimbursement are designed to introduce a degree of constraint on charge or cost increases by setting limits on amounts paid during future periods. Some systems provide incentives for improved *efficiency* by sharing savings with institutions that perform at lower than anticipated costs. Prospective reimbursement contrasts with traditional methods of payment in which institutions are reimbursed for *reasonable costs* incurred on a *retrospective* basis.

See *diagnosis related group* and *section 222.* IV.A., VI.C.1.

prospective study. a *study* planned to observe events that have not yet occurred; compare a *retrospective study,* which examines events which have already occurred. VIII.D.

prospective trial. an experiment based on data or events which occur subsequent in time to the initiation of the investigation; compare *cohort study* and *random controlled trial.*

Prospective trials take time, even decades, to develop large enough populations and usable results but are likely to be particularly meaningful because they can be properly designed and *controlled* at the outset. VIII.D.

prosthesis (pl. prostheses). replacement or substitute; an artificial substitute for a missing part, as a denture, eye, or leg; compare *medical device* and *orthosis.* III.B.2.

prosthetics. the branch of surgery, art, and science concerned with prostheses. III.C.

prosthetist. one who makes prostheses. A *CPO* is a *certified* prosthetist and *orthotist.* III.A.4.

prosthodontics. the dental specialty, science, and practice of replacement of missing dental and oral structures; synonyms, prosthetic dentistry and prosthodontia. III.C.

prosthodontist. a dentist who specializes in prosthodontics. III.A.3.

protective action level. an *exposure* of a human organ to a radioactive substance defined by the Nuclear Regulatory Commission as large enough that measures should be taken to save the organ from further exposure.

Thyroid exposure to radioactive *iodine* greater than 25 rem should require administration of potassium iodine to protect the thyroid. I.C.

protective services. see *adult protective services.*

protocol. 1. an official account of a proceeding, especially the original notes or records of an autopsy, case, or experiment; a *protocol statement is a basic observational sentence that reports uninterpreted results of observations and provides the basis for scientific confirmation. 2. the outline or plan of a scientific or medical experiment or procedure. 3. a guide to diagnosis and treatment of a problem, as one used by a physician to guide the practice of a *physician assistant* or *nurse.* V., VIII.D.

provider. an individual or program giving *health care.* For *Medicare* usage, see *institutional provider* and *supplier.*

Providers must sometimes be distinguished from *consumers,* as when requiring consumer representation in a health program. For these purposes, health planning law elaborately defines the term in section 1531(3) of the *Public Health Service Act* to include *direct providers, individuals whose primary current activity is the provision of health care to individuals, e.g., a physician, dentist, nurse, podiatrist, or physician assistant; or the administration of facilities or institutions in which such care is given, e.g., a hospital, long-term care facility, outpatient facility, or health maintenance organization, and *indirect providers, individuals who receive (directly or through a spouse) more than one-tenth of their income from the provision of health care, or research or instruction in health care, or from producing or supplying drugs, devices, or other items used in health care, research, or instruction; who hold a *fiduciary* relation with any entity engaged in the provision of health care, or research or instruction in health care; who are engaged in issuing *health insurance;* or who are members of the immediate family of anybody otherwise defined as a provider. III., VI.A.

Provider Reimbursement Review Board (PRRB). an advisory group to the secretary of the Department of Health and Human Services on payment of providers by the *Medicare* program, on disputes between providers and intermediaries, and on related issues. IV.C.1.

prudent buyer principle. the principle that *Medicare, Medicaid,* and other payers should not reimburse providers more than *reasonable cost* because any excess would be more than a cost-conscious or prudent buyer would expect to pay.

An organization that does not seek the customary discount on bulk purchases could, through the operation of this principle, be reimbursed for less than its full costs by Medicare because it has been an imprudent buyer. Similarly, Medicaid programs should as prudent buyers seek to buy the cheapest physician services available. IV.C.

psychiatric diagnosis. a medical mugging; see *Diagnostic and Statistical Manual.* II.B.2., VIII.B.2.

psychiatric nurse. a *nurse* employed in a psychiatric setting or one who has special training and experience in the management of psychiatric patients. The designation is sometimes limited to nurses with a master's degree in psychiatric nursing. III.A.2.

psychiatric social worker. a *social worker* employed in a psychiatric setting or one who has special training and experience in the management of psychiatric patients. Sometimes limited to social workers with a master's or higher degree in psychiatric social work. Some engage in *independent practice.* III.A.4.

psychiatrist. a physician specializing by practice or education in psychiatry; a chiropractor with tired hands.

Most psychiatrists also have some training in *neurology.* III.A.1., VIII.B.2.b.

psychiatry (Psy). the science and specialty devoted to the study and care of mental and emotional disorders and, by extension, of many behavioral, personal adjustment, and family problems.

Psychiatry has a subspecialty, child psychiatry, and several specialized areas, including administration, *community psychiatry,* consultation and liaison, *forensic* or legal psychiatry, mental retardation, and *psychoanalysis.*

See *community mental health center, mental health, P. Pinel, psychology,* and *W. Tuke.* III.C.

psychic surgery. surgery in which the offending cancer, spirit, or agent is removed by psychic power rather than conventional surgical intervention. There are many forms of psychic or spiritual healing, all equally likely to maximize *placebo effect* and suspect as to their real efficacy. V.

psychoanalysis. a theory of the *psychology* of human development and behavior, a method of research, and a system of *psychotherapy* originally developed by *Sigmund Freud.*
Through analysis of free associations and interpretation of dreams, emotions and behavior are traced to the influence of repressed instinctual drives and defenses against them in the unconscious. Psychoanalytic treatment seeks to eliminate or diminish the undesirable effects of unconscious conflicts by making the patient aware of their existence, origin, and inappropriate expression in current emotions and behavior. The theorem and the body of data developed with it concern the conflict between infantile instinctual striving and family or social demand and the way the conflict affects emotional growth, character development, and the formation of disorders of character and emotional function. III.C.

psychoanalyst. a person, usually a psychiatrist, who has had training in psychoanalysis and who employs the techniques of psychoanalytic theory. Lay analysts were fairly common prior to the early 1950s. III.A.1.

psychoanalytic family therapy. *family therapy,* rooted in traditional individually oriented psychoanalytic theory and practice, which "establish[es] a collaborative working alliance to explore the relationship of individual and interpersonal factors in the current relationships, providing insight into genetic and unconscious factors from past conflicts and helping the members to function more freely and authentically in terms of emotions and thoughts" (*Pinney and Slipp, 1982*).
Change comes by working through old conflicts that influence current relationships. In more directive family therapy, change comes from outside by solving problems, teaching skills, and manipulating the family power and communication structure or through paradoxical prescriptions. Change from growth developing within family members is believed to produce greater and more permanent personality strength and individuation. V.

psychologist. an individual trained or licensed in psychology; one who practices psychology.
Psychologists are ordinarily trained at the master's or doctoral level. A *licensed psychologist must generally have a doctoral degree from an accredited program and two years of supervised work experience. Ordinarily only *clinical psychologists* need be licensed. III.A.4.

psychology. 1. the science and profession of the mind and its functions, including memory, perception, sensation, sleep, and thought, and of the *behavior* of people and other organisms in relation to their *environments.* 2. the psychologic or mental activity characteristic of a person, group, or situation, as the psychology of surgeons or the psychology of dying. 3. therapy of *mental illness* using psychologic principles and training.
There are many kinds and branches of psychology, typically named after their principal concerns, as criminal or educational psychology. *Clinical* and *experimental psychology* form two major branches, mainly because training separates psychologists into those with and those without clinical skills. III.C.

psychometrics. the measurement of mental and psychologic abilities, potentials, and performance; frequently applied specifically to the measurement of *intelligence.* V.A.

psychosomatic. of or pertaining to the mind-body interaction and conditions involving both mind and body; compare *functional* and *organic.* *Psychosomatic medicine studies *psychosomatic illnesses, physical ailments, as asthma and ulcers, with significant emotional as well as other causes. II.B.1.a.

psychosurgery. surgery on the brain done with the intent of changing a patient's personality, thought, emotions, or behavior rather than for treatment of a physical disease.

Psychosurgery is irregularly used and defined: occasionally including all surgery done on the brain, sometimes including surgery done for relief of intractable pain, Parkinson's disease, or psychomotor epilepsy, and rarely being extended to include alteration of the brain by physical means other than surgery, as electrical stimulation or direct application of drugs to brain tissue. The definition is also variable in places where psychosurgery is subject to special regulation because of controversy arising from its use and permanence and the difficulty of obtaining *informed consent.* III.C., V.B.

psychotherapy. treatment of any disease or problem, particularly one of the mind or person, by psychologic means, as by communication with the person or *psychoanalysis* rather than by drugs, surgery, or other physical means.

Psychotherapy is done by physicians and many others in many forms usually involving an explicit or implicit contract between therapist and client to work in some prescribed way to relieve psychic or emotional symptoms, resolve *problems of living,* or encourage the client's self-growth. III.C., V.B.

psychotropic. mind-altering, affecting the psyche; pertaining to any substance or drug which affects mental function, behavior, or experience. III.B.3.

public accountability. see *accountable.*

public cleansing. British, *sanitation.* I.C.4.

public health (PH). 1. the state of *health* of a *population,* as of a state or a particular community. 2. the art and science dealing with the protection and improvement of community health by organized community effort, including *preventive medicine, health education, communicable disease* control, and application of the *sanitary* and social sciences. 3. a subspecialty of preventive medicine.

Public health activities are ineffective when undertaken on an individual basis and do not typically include direct *personal health services.* Immunizations; *quarantine; occupational health;* assurance of the healthfulness of air, water, and food; and *epidemiology* are recognized public health activities.

See *G. deBaillou, E. Chadwick, T.H. Park, Rhazes,* and *T. Sydenham.* VII.B.2.e.

public health nurse. a nurse working for a *public health* program who assists in safeguarding the health of people at home or in public health *clinics;* synonym, community health nurse.

Many but not all public health nurses are *registered nurses* and work as *visiting nurses*. III.A.2.

Public Health Service (PHS).   see *United States Public Health Service.*

Public Health Service Act (PHS Act).   one of the principal acts of Congress providing legislative authority for federal health activities, 42 U.S.C. 201-300.

Originally enacted July 1, 1944, and sometimes referred to as the *Act of July 1, the PHS Act was, when enacted, a complete codification of all accumulated federal public health laws. Since then many of the acts written concerning health matters have actually been amendments to the PHS Act, revising, extending, or adding new authority to it, as the Health Maintenance Organization Act of 1973, P.L. 93-222, which added a new title XIII. A compilation of the PHS Act, as amended, and of related acts is published for public use by the Committee on Interstate and Foreign Commerce of the U.S. House of Representatives. Generally the act contains authority for *public health* programs, *biomedical research, health manpower* training, *family planning, emergency medical services, HMOs,* regulation of drinking water supplies, and *health planning* and resources development.

See *quotes* and *Social Security Act.* VII.B.2.e., VIII.B.3.

public law (P.L.).   an act of Congress.

The acts, including those affecting health and health care, are numbered in order of their enactment by each Congress and are often, quite meaninglessly, known by these numbers. Thus, P.L. 93-222, the Health Maintenance Organization Act of 1973, was the two hundred twenty-second law enacted by the Ninety-third Congress (a new Congress is convened in each odd-numbered year, the One Hundredth convening in 1987). VIII.B.3.

public patient.   synonym, *service patient;* antonym, *private patient.*

puerperal.   pertaining to, caused by, or following childbirth. II.

pulmonary medicine.   the *subspecialty* of *internal medicine* concerned with the lungs.

See *black lung* and *smoke.* III.C.

pure research.   see *research.*

pusher.   an illicit peddler of narcotics, *scheduled drugs,* or other illegal drugs. III.A.4., IV.B.3.

pyramid system.   the practice in some medical and surgical *residencies* of having fewer residents in each succeeding year of training.

This uncommon system assures a small group of high-quality senior residents but is hard on residents who are dropped. III.A.1.

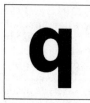

q-sort. a personality assessment technique, introduced in 1953, in which the subject, or someone who observes the subject, indicates the degree to which a standardized set of descriptive statements actually describes the subject by sorting the statements in specified piles. V.A.

quack. a pretender to medical skill, a medical charlatan; short for quacksalver, a mountebank peddling his or her own salves and medicines. V.

qualification. meeting *standards* for program eligibility, licensure, reimbursement, or other benefits. Thus a qualified educational program meets *accreditation* standards, a health maintenance organization qualified for the benefit of mandated *dual choice* under section 1310 of the Public Health Service Act meets the standards imposed by the act, and a provider qualified for reimbursement by an insurance program meets its *conditions of participation.* III.B.1., VII.D.2.

quality. 1. nature, kind, property, or character; an essential or particular attribute or capacity. 2. degree of excellence, grade, or caliber.

Quality is a recurrent important concern in health care but is vague and meaningless without careful specification of the object of consideration, as a service or provider; the attributes being considered, as competence, humanity, *need, acceptability, appropriateness, inputs,* structure, *process,* or *outcomes;* and the measurement methods and *standards, criteria,* and *norms* being used.

See *effectiveness, efficacy,* and *efficiency; medical, peer,* and *utilization review; tissue committee;* and *peer* and *professional standards review organizations.* Read Donabedian, Avedis, *Explorations in Quality Assessment and Monitoring,* three vols. (Ann Arbor, Mich: Health Administration Press, 1985). VII.D.2.

quality assurance. an organized program of activities intended to assure the *quality* of care provided in a defined medical setting or program; compare *evaluation*.

Such programs must include educational and other components intended to remedy identified deficiencies in quality as well as the components needed to identify such deficiencies, as *peer* or *utilization review,* and assess the program's *effectiveness.* A program which identifies quality deficiencies and responds only with negative sanctions, as denial of reimbursement, is not considered a quality assurance program, although the latter may include use of such sanctions. Quality assurance is required of *health maintenance organizations* and other health programs assisted under the authority of the *PHS Act,* see section 1301(c)(8). VI.D.2, VII.D.2.

Quality Assurance Program for Medical Care in the Hospital (QAP). a program developed by the American Hospital Association in the 1970s for use by hospital administrations and medical staffs in development of a hospital program to assure the quality of the hospital's services. III.B.1.

quality of life. a real concept and recurrent phrase without definition. The *Baby Doe* debate produced the suggestion that for a newborn the potential quality of life is defined by the infant's biologic, familial, and social endowments.

Good quality life is characterized by the presence of a predominantly contented consciousness. I.A.1.

quality review study (QRS, QRSs). *medical review* of the *appropriateness* and quality of *services* and *procedures* provided for specified diagnoses or problems.

QRSs are done by peer review organizations (PROs) and required by PROs of *delegated* health programs. They require identifying a problem, developing *criteria* specifying adequate quality of care, examining records to identify deficiencies, designing educational programs or sanctions to correct the deficiencies, and rechecking for improvement. VI.D.2.

quantitative variable. an object of observation which varies in manner or degree in such a way that it may be measured. VIII.D.

quarantine. 1. limitation of freedom of movement of *susceptible* persons or animals exposed to a *communicable* disease in order to prevent spread of the disease. 2. the place of detention of such persons or animals. 3. the act of detaining vessels or travelers suspected of having communicable diseases at ports or other places for inspection or disinfection; see *pratique.*

Quarantine traditionally was for 40 days in nonspecific situations or for the longest usual *incubation period* of the disease in question.

See *barrier precautions.* VII.B.2.e.

Quarterly Cumulative Index Medicus (QCIM). an accumulated *Index Medicus* published quarterly. III.C.

quid pro quo. anything required in return for another thing of like value.

Used during consideration of health personnel legislation in the 1960s to refer to requirements of health professional schools set as conditions of their receiving federal *capitation* payments. III.A.

quotes. material in an act of Congress which amends another earlier act and is therefore placed in quotes. Material which does not and creates new freestanding legislative authority is not in quotes. Thus material amending another law, as the Public Health Service Act, is said to be "in the quotes." The fact that many laws amend older more basic statutes is the source of much confusion about which law and enactment date apply. VIII.B.3.

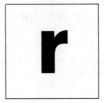

rad. the unit for measurement of absorbed *dose* of any ionizing radiation; energy absorption of 100 ergs per gram (0.01 joule per kilogram) by an irradiated organism or material.

Originally an acronym for radiation absorbed dose, rad has become the word itself. Occasionally, casually, short for radiation or radiology. I.C.3.

radiation. 1. emission and propagation of energy in the form of particles, as electrons and alpha and beta particles, or waves, as light, sound, and x-rays. 2. of *pain* or other sensation experienced in a remote part of the body because of stimulation, injury, or illness of another part, as heart attacks which produce radiating pain in the (normal) left arm. 1. I.C.3., 2. II.A.1.

radiation absorbed dose. see *rad*.

radiation exposure. total quantity of ionizing radiation received and measured at a given point, measured in rads or roentgens. I.C.3.

radiation injury. damage to cells of living organisms caused by ionizing radiation.

The effect is proportional to the intensity of the radioactivity and appears in a variety of forms, particularly burns, tumors, and cancer. It can be incremental, genetic, immediate, or delayed. Long-lived radioactive isotopes may persist through links in the *food chain,* and concentration may occur in ingested or inhaled substances, air and water in particular, and in individual organisms (after *Brace, 1977).* I.C.3., II.B.1.a.

radiation sickness syndrome. illness from *exposure* to radiation, as in radiotherapy or by explosion of an atomic bomb, characterized progressively by fatigue, vomiting, loss of teeth and hair, depression of blood formation, convulsions, and death. The exact form of the sickness will depend on the nature of the exposure. I.C.3., II.B.2.

radiation standard. a regulation concerning *exposure* to or permissible concentrations, transportation, or other aspects of radioactive material. I.C.3.

367

radiation therapy. synonym, *therapeutic radiology;* see *radiology.*

radical. 1. belonging to or relating to a root. 2. going to the root, or attacking the cause, of a disease, especially by extreme, extensive, or dangerous rather than conservative measures. V.B.

radioactive. pertaining to or possessing *radioactivity.*

radioactive fallout. particles of radioactive contaminant emitted into the atmosphere by a nuclear or thermonuclear explosion and descending to the earth's surface by gravity or precipitation (after *Brace, 1977*). I.C.1., I.C.3.

radioactive half-life. average time needed for the radioactivity of material to be reduced to half its intensity by radioactive decay and biologic elimination.

See *half-life.* I.C.3.

radioactive waste. a useless material, by-product, or leftover which has radioactivity.

These *wastes* are common in medicine, pose special *hazards* to health, and are difficult to dispose of because of their longevity and the special handling they require. They are separated into low-level and high-level wastes and into various types, as absorbed liquids. *Drain dumping* such wastes may be particularly hazardous and is only occasionally legal. I.C.3., I.C.4.

radioactivity. emission and transmission of ionizing radiation by spontaneous disintegration of an unstable atomic nucleus. By extension, the ability of certain substances, *radioactive materials, to emit this radiation, and the radiation itself. I.C.3.

radiography. the practice or act of making radiographs, or pictures made with x-rays. I.C.3., III.C.

radioisotope. a radioactive form of an element which is stable, whether occurring naturally or prepared by bombarding an element with atomic particles.

Radioisotopes are used as sources of radiation for diagnostic and therapeutic purposes. For example, small amounts of ^{131}I and ^{133}I, radioisotopes of iodine, will be taken up by the thyroid gland and reveal their image on x-ray, a thyroid scan. Larger amounts will damage the gland and are used as treatment for the overproductive or hyperthyroid state. I.C.3.

radiologic technician, technologist. an individual who maintains and safely uses equipment and supplies in diagnosis and treatment using x-rays, fluoroscopy, ultrasound, and other techniques of radiology; synonym, radiographer.

Radiologic technology programs are conducted by hospitals and medical schools and by community colleges with hospital *affiliations.* Programs are open to high school graduates, although a few require one or two years of college or graduation from a school of nursing. The length of the training varies from a minimum of two years in a hospital radiology *department* or an associate degree from a community college with hospital affiliation to a four-year university course. III.A.4.

radiologist (R). a physician specializing by practice or education in *radiology.*

Most radiologists are *hospital-based* physicians. III.A.1.

radiology (R, Rad, Radiol). the science and specialties, derived primarily from nuclear physics and medicine, devoted to the principles and methods of radioactivity, the properties and application of ionizing radiation, and their use in medicine for the diagnosis and treatment of disease.

Radiology is divided into three specialties: *diagnostic radiology, the traditional use of exposure to ionizing radiation to diagnose disease; *nuclear radiology or diagnostic (nuclear) radiology, concerned with the use of radioactive isotopes for diagnostic imaging of the body; and *therapeutic radiology or radiotherapy, which uses either form of radiation in treating disease.

See *nuclear medicine* and *x-ray technologist*. III.C.

radionuclide.   a nucleus, or particular isotope of an element, that is radio-active, as of ^{131}I and ^{133}I. I.C.3.

radiotherapist.   a physician specializing by practice or education in thera-peutic *radiology*. III.A.1.

radiotherapy (RT).   synonym, therapeutic radiology; see *radiology*.

Ramazzini, Bernardino.   Italian physician, 1633–1714. His volume, *De Morbis Artificium Diatriba,* was the first full-scale treatise on *occupational health*. Originally published in 1700, it remained the fundamental text for this branch of preventive medicine until the nineteenth century. VII.B.2.d., VIII.A.1.

ranch hander, Ranch Hand Study.   see *Agent Orange*.

Rand Health Insurance Experiment.   the only *controlled* trial of the effects of *cost sharing* on *health status* and the use of health services; compare the *Framingham Heart Study*.

This decade-long nationwide experiment, conducted in the late 1970s and early 1980s by the Rand Corporation, has produced a series of signif-icant substantive conclusions, as people insured without cost sharing will be healthier than those with it, and has made major methodological con-tributions in health economics and *health services research*. IV.B., VIII.D.

random.   see *volunteer bias, correlation*.

random controlled trial (RCT).   a *prospective* study of the effects of a par-ticular drug, procedure, or treatment in which subjects (human or animal) are assigned randomly to either of two groups, experimental and *control*. The experimental group receives the drug or procedure while the control group does not.

Random controlled trials also are often conducted as *double-blind stud-ies*. Differences in the fates of the subjects in the two groups are usually validly attributable to the treatment under study, with *bias* and the ef-fects of other variables being eliminated by the randomization. VIII.D.

random sample.   a *sample* or group of subjects selected in such a way that each member of the *population* from which the sample is chosen has an equal and independent probability of being chosen. VIII.D.

rape.   intimate sexual contact by a male with a female, without her valid *con-sent,* by compulsion through deceit, violence, or threats; synonyms, first-degree rape and ravishment. Compare *battery*.

Laws vary as to whether contact with or penetration of the female gen-italia is required, as to whether rape can occur between husband and wife, and as to the degree of force and resistance required. In some laws a woman who is psychologically or physically incapable of resisting the male is pre-sumed not to have given valid consent; compare *statutory rape*. VIII.B.3.

rate. in epidemiology, the quantity or degree of something, measured as a ratio to a unit of another thing, as the *birth rate* or *death rate;* the number of events occurring in a study *population* divided by the size of the study population.

Rates per 100 or per 1000 are typical, but this may change to 10,000 or 100,000 as the frequency of the event decreases. For some rates the denominator refers to providers rather than patients, as the number of patients seen per provider. Rates may have any of the following numerators: problems, encounters or services, patients, or families, and any of the following denominators: provider, team, practice, study population, registered practice population, or area population.

See *age-specific rate* and *denominator problem.* VIII.C.

rate. in *insurance,* the price of insurance. IV.B.

rating. in insurance, the process of determining rate or price of insurance for individuals, groups, or classes of risks. IV.B.

ratio. synonym, *rate.*

Reach for Recovery. a *self-help* group of and for women who have had a mastectomy, surgical removal of the breast, as treatment of breast cancer.

Mastectomies, particularly older radical versions, interfere with use of the arm, hence the concern for reaching. Volunteers from the organization support women with breast cancer before and after surgery, teaching exercises which facilitate recovery, demonstrating the use of breast prostheses, and giving instruction about living with the disease and its scars. II.B.2.

reaction. 1. a chemical change or interaction; a response to stimulus. 2. in medicine, a negative, deleterious, or damaging effect (whether or not expected) of treatment, most commonly a drug reaction, as contrasted with a positive effect.

See *iatrogenic* and *side effect.* III.B.3., V.B.

reader bias. see *bias*

reasonable charge. 1. for a specific *service* covered by *Medicare,* the lower of the *customary charge* by a particular *physician* for the service and the *prevailing charge* by physicians in the *locality* for the service. Medicare reimbursement is based on the lower of the *reasonable* and *actual charges.* 2. any charge payable by an *insurance* program determined in a similar fashion.

For example, suppose the prevailing charge for a fistulectomy is $100 and Dr. A's actual charge is $75, although he customarily charges $80. Dr. B's actual charge is her customary charge of $85, Dr. C's is his customary charge of $125, and Dr. D's is $100, although she customarily charges $80, with no special circumstances in any case. Then the reasonable charge for Dr. A would be $75, since the reasonable charge cannot exceed the actual charge even if it is lower than his customary charge and below the prevailing charge for the locality. The reasonable charge for Dr. B would be $85, because her customary charge is lower than the prevailing charge. The reasonable charge for Dr. C would be $100, the prevailing charge for his locality. The reasonable charge for Dr. D would be $80, because that is her customary charge, which is lower than the actual charge in this particular case. The reasonable charge cannot exceed the customary charge in the absence of special circumstances, even if the actual charge of $100 is the same as the prevailing charge.

See *comparability provision* and *section 224*. IV.C.1., VII.D.1.

reasonable cost. 1. the amount which a *third party* or other payer using *cost-related reimbursement* will actually reimburse. 2. in M*edicare,* a *cost* incurred in delivering health services, excluding any part of such incurred cost found to be unnecessary for the efficient delivery of needed health services, section 1861 of the Social Security Act.

Original Medicare law stipulated that, except for certain *deductible* and *coinsurance* amounts that must be paid by beneficiaries, payments to hospitals would be made on the basis of the reasonable cost of providing covered services. Regulations required that cost be apportioned between Medicare beneficiaries and other hospital patients so that neither group subsidizes the costs of the other. Items or elements of cost, both *direct* and *indirect,* which regulations specify as reimbursable are known as *allowable costs.*

See *section 223.* IV.C,1., VII.D.1.

recidivism. tendency to relapse into a previous condition or mode of behavior; repetition of criminal or delinquent acts; repeated readmission to a mental hospital, prison, or other institution because of recurrent difficulty. The person involved is a *recidivist. I.A.2., II.B.2.

recipient. see *beneficiary.*

reciprocity. in *licensure* of health personnel, recognition by one state of the licenses of a second state when the latter state extends the same recognition to licenses of the former.

Licensing requirements in the two states usually must be equivalent before formal or informal reciprocal agreements are made. Reciprocity is often used interchangeably with *endorsement.* However, licensure by endorsement requires only that the qualifications of the licensee or the standards required for licensure in the original licensing state be deemed equivalent to the licensure requirements of the state in which licensure is being sought, not that the two states have a reciprocal arrangement. VII.D.2.

recision. alternative spelling of *rescission.*

recognized hazard. in occupational health, a *hazard* of common knowledge or general recognition in the industry in which it occurs, detectable by means of the senses or by generally known and accepted tests which make its presence known.

The *general duty clause* of the *Occupational Safety and Health Act* requires employers to provide a workplace free of recognized hazards and thus makes them liable for damages arising from such hazards. VII.B.2.d.

recombinant DNA. see *genetic engineering.*

recommended dietary allowance (RDA). an estimate made by the Food and Nutrition Board of the National Research Council, National Academy of Sciences, of the amount of an *essential* nutrient that each healthy person in the United States must consume daily in order to have reasonable assurance that his or her physiologic needs will be met.

The ninth edition of the recommendations in 1979 gave recommended allowances by age and sex for protein, energy, three fat-soluble vitamins, seven water-soluble vitamins, and six minerals. Safe and adequate daily intake ranges are also given for three vitamins, six trace elements, and three electrolytes for which a range is a more appropriate recommendation. The allowances apply to what people actually eat rather than to their food supply, allowing for loss of nutrients when food is processed or prepared. They are the basis for nutrition labeling of food and planning the diet of large populations, as the armed forces. Older, slightly different versions, the *minimum daily requirements, are now obsolete.

Read *Recommended Dietary Allowances,* ninth ed. (Washington: National Academy of Sciences, 1980.) I.A.2.a.

reconstituted family.   synonym, blended family; see *family.*

record.   see *medical record.*

recordable injury.   in occupational health, an *injury* which results in medical treatment, loss of consciousness, restriction of work or motion, or transfer to another job.

The *Occupational Safety and Health Act,* section (2)(6)(12), requires employers to maintain record-keeping systems for recordable injuries and worker *exposure* to toxic or physically harmful substances regulated by *standards.* They are to be available to inspectors and employees and provide data for the Occupational Safety and Health Administration's *industrial accident rates.* II.B.1.a.

recovery room (RR).   an area, *nurse's station,* or department of a hospital where patients are treated during initial recovery from general anesthesia and surgery, typically for the first two to six hours after surgery during full recovery of consciousness and stabilization of vital signs. III.B.1.

recreation therapy.   use of music, theater, games, and such activities in *therapy* to provide relaxation and outlets for self-expression, particularly of bad feelings; an adjuvant to *psychotherapy.* III.C., V.

recrudescence.   increase or recurrence of an illness, particularly after apparent improvement or brief *remission;* compare *relapse.* II.B.3.

recurring clause.   a provision in a health *insurance* policy, specifying a period of time, as a month, during which recurrence of a condition is considered a continuation of a prior period of disability or hospital confinement rather than a separate *spell of illness.* IV.B.

Redbook.   see *Drug Topics Red Book.*

Red Crescent.   Islamic equivalent of Red Cross.

Red Cross (RC).   1. a red Greek cross on a white background adopted by the Geneva convention of 1864 as the emblem to identify noncombat installations, vehicles, and personnel ministering to the sick and wounded in war; now used as the emblem of the International Red Cross and its affiliates in disaster relief and other humanitarian services as well as war. 2. the International Red Cross or one of its affiliates. III.B.1.

Reed, Walter.   U.S. Army physician, 1851–1902. He demonstrated the transmission of yellow fever by its mosquito *vector, Aëdes aegypti,* and thus was able to protect the army from it in Cuba in 1902 and make possible the completion of the Panama Canal. VIII.A.1., VIII.C.

refer. send or direct for treatment, information, or decision, usually when the referring source is not prepared or qualified to provide the needed service.

In contrast with *consultation,* referral involves a delegation or passing of responsibility for patient care to another practitioner or program. The referring source may or may not follow up to ensure that services are received. V.A.

reference. used or usable as a *standard* for measuring, as a *reference drug of known potency used in the assay of a sample of the same drug of unknown strength, or a *reference laboratory which provides standard specimens and verifies results for other laboratories as well as doing complex and infrequent tests. III.B.1., III.B.3.

reflexology. synonym, *Ingham Reflex Method of Compression Therapy.*

regimen. whatever the doctor ordered; a systematic plan, as of diet and exercise, physical and other therapy, and drugs and devices, designed to improve and maintain health or treat illness.

A useful term for a whole program of therapy for all of an individual's problems. V.B.

region. a naturally differentiated area within a larger whole. *regional. of or pertaining to such an area. *regionalism. development of political, theoretical, social, or other systems on the basis of such areas.

While there are regions of the body and other things, one is typically referring to geographic areas. Although boundaries are usually somewhat arbitrary, they reflect geographic barriers, travel and trade patterns, and historic cultural areas. Regions are usually not coincident with political boundaries, typically being larger than cities and counties and smaller than states in the United States. Since neither patients nor pollution respects political or other boundaries, many environmental and health programs are organized on a regional basis following the natural boundaries of the flow of the people, services, or pollutants with which they are concerned.

See *catchment area, health service area, locality,* and *medical trade area.* VI.A.

regional health authority (RHA). see *health authority.*

Regional Medical Program (RMP). a program of federal support for regional organizations, called regional medical programs, which sought to improve care for *heart disease, cancer, strokes,* and related diseases.

The legislative authority, created by P.L. 89-239, is found in title IX of the Public Health Service Act. The programs were heavily oriented toward initiating and improving *continuing medical education,* nursing services, and intensive care units. Some features of the RMP were combined into the health planning program authorized by the National Health Planning and Development Act, P.L. 93-641 (see *health systems agency*), and, without further federal support, the programs disappeared about 1975. RMP was a good example of a *categorical* program. VI.A.

register. see *registry.*

registered nurse (RN). a nurse who has graduated from a formal program of nursing education, as a *diploma school,* or completed an *associate degree* or *baccalaureate program* and been licensed by an appropriate state authority.

Registered nurses are the most highly educated of nurses with the widest scope of responsibility, including, at least potentially, all aspects of nursing care.

See *graduate nurse, licensed practical nurse, nurse anesthetist, nurse practitioner,* and *patient care technician.* IV.A.2.

registrar. 1. an individual responsible for a registry or registration; a custodian of records. 2. in British hospitals, a junior or resident specialist, the first assistant to a consultant physician or surgeon. 1. III.A.6., 2. III.A.1.

registration. 1. the act of recording, as of marriages, deaths, or *notifiable* diseases. 2. a document certifying a registration. 3. the process by which qualified individuals are listed on an official roster maintained by a governmental or nongovernmental agency, see *registry.*

Standards for registration may include successful completion of a written examination given by the registry, membership in the *professional* association maintaining the registry, and education and experience, as graduation from an approved program or equivalent experience. Registration is a form of *credentialing,* similar to *certification.* III.A.

registration number.   see *Drug Enforcement Administration number.*

registry. 1. a list of people, the group listed, as nurses available for *private duty;* those who have indicated, as by contracting for membership, that they use or rely upon a given health professional or program (whose registry it is) for the services that the program provides; patients with a particular disease, as a cancer registry. 2. the organization or place which keeps the list.

Panel is preferred to registry with respect to an individual practitioner's patients.

See *catchment area, enrollment, registration,* and *roster.* III.B.1.

reglementation.   the legal restriction or regulation of prostitution, as by compulsory medical inspection. I.B.4.

regression.   a trend or shift toward a *mean* or toward a lower or less perfect state, as of function or differentiation; progressive decline in size, severity, or intensity of a manifestation of disease, as in tumor regression after irradiation.

In psychology, regression is reversion to earlier developmental levels in response to *stress* or suggestion. In statistics, it is a functional relationship between correlated *variables,* often empirically derived, which allows prediction of the value of one variable from the values of others. When a series of events has a *normal distribution,* the one following an extreme one will usually *regress to the mean, or be closer to average. Thus punishment of a poor effort will appear to produce a better effort the next time. Rewarding a good try seems to lead to worse performance, although it can be shown empirically that positive reinforcement is actually better pedagogy. II.A.2., VIII.D.

regressive tax.   a tax which takes a decreasing proportion of *income* as income rises, as a sales tax and the Social Security *payroll tax* on earning above the maximum to which the tax applies; contrast *progressive tax.* The payroll tax takes a constant percentage of income up to the maximum wage and thus is a *proportional tax* to that level.

See *marginal tax rate.* IV.C.

regulation.   1. the act of controlling, the condition of being regulated. 2. an authoritative rule or principle dealing with details of procedure, especially one intended to promote safety and efficiency. 3. a *rule* or order having force of law issued by an executive authority of a government, usually with power delegated by constitution or law.

Regulation includes intervention of government in health care or health *insurance* to control entry or change the behavior of any participant in the marketplace through specification of rules for the participants. This does not usually include programs which seek to change behavior through financing mechanisms or incentives or to private *accreditation* programs, although they may be relied upon by government regulatory programs, as is the *Joint Commission on Accreditation of Hospitals* under *Medicare*. Regulatory programs of rules may be described in terms of their purpose, for example, to control *charges;* who is regulated, *hospitals;* who regulates, state government; and method, prospective rate review.

See *certification, registration, licensure, certificate of need,* and *peer review organization.* VI.D.

rehabilitate. to recreate former capacity; the action, methods, or process of restoring *disabled* people to maximum functioning, independence, and adjustment and of preventing relapse or recurrence of illness; compare *tertiary prevention.*

Rehabilitation develops residual capacities with prescribed training and combined use of many different methods and professional workers. These may include educational, medical, occupational, physical, social, speech, and *vocational rehabilitation.*

See *activities of daily living, habilitation,* and *physiatry.* V.B.

Reich, Wilhelm. German psychoanalyst, 1897–1957. Noted for his concept of **orgone,* a vital primal raw material energy permeating space and accounting for the functions of life, including sexual libido. Reich, who immigrated to the United States in 1939, wrote profusely and gave his name to many interesting ideas but lived controversially at the boundary of sanity and charlatanism. *Reichian therapy or *vegeto-therapy,* supplemented with *orgone* therapy, was developed by Reich and never independently established. III.C., V.

reinsurance. the practice of one insurance company buying *insurance* from a second company to protect itself against part or all of the *losses* it might incur in the process of honoring policyholders' *claims.* The original company is called the **ceding company, and the second is the *assuming company or reinsurer.

Reinsurance may be sought by the ceding company to protect itself against losses in individual cases beyond a ceiling amount, where competition requires it to offer coverage in excess of these amounts; to offer protection against catastrophic losses in a certain line of insurance, as aviation accident or polio insurance; or to protect against mistakes in *rating* and *underwriting* in entering a new line of insurance. IV.3.

reinsurance reserve. in insurance, a *reserve* or theoretical amount which is the difference between the present value of the total insurance and the present value of the future premiums on the insurance; synonym, reinsurance fund. It constitutes the amount for which another insurance company could afford to take over the insurance. IV.B.

relapse. return or recurrence of an illness after apparent recovery or *remission;* compare *recrudescence.* II.B.3.

relative risk. the ratio of the *risk* of developing the same disease in two different populations, as smokers having a greater relative risk of developing lung cancer than do nonsmokers.

If someone with red hair were twice as likely to be allergic to penicillin than the general population, that person would have a relative risk of 2.0; if equally likely, then 1.0; and if only half as likely, 0.5. Relative risk may be large even when real risks are small. If two groups each have the small chance of developing a disease of 10 and 1 in a thousand, respectively, then the first has a relative risk of 10 compared with the second. VIII.C.

relative value unit (RVU). a number representing the resources needed to provide a service; a measure of the comparative cost of a service or procedure, ordinarily taking into account the time, skill, and overhead cost required for the service.

The RVU for a given service is the ratio of its costs or required resources to those of an arbitrary "base" service which is given the RVU of 1. Thus, if the base service were a routine office visit and a family therapy session were six times as "costly," the office visit RVU would be 1 and the therapy session's would be 6. IV.

relative value scale, schedule (RVS). a coded list of physician or other professional services using relative value units which indicate the comparative resource requirements or costs of the services.

The scales do not consider the services' relative *cost-effectiveness,* the relative need or demand for them, or their importance to people's health. The units in most scales are actually based on median charges by the physicians. Appropriate conversion factors are used to translate the abstract units in the scale to dollar fees for each service. Given individual and local variation in practice, the relative value scale can be used voluntarily as a guide to physicians in establishing *fees for service,* and to insurance carriers and government agencies in determining reimbursement. An early and important example is the scale prepared and revised periodically by the California Medical Association, the CRVS, which includes independent scales for medicine, anesthesia, surgery, radiology, and pathology. Relative value scales, originally written by surgeons, contain biases favoring certain specialties, as surgery over family practice, and types of services, as highly technical or specialized over cognitive.

See *fractionation.* IV.

relaxation response. deceleration of bodily functions elicited by *meditative* techniques. This deceleration, opposite to the fight or flight response elicited by *stress,* helps with the fatigue, anxiety, and tension produced by stress. I.A.1.

reliability. 1. probability that an instrument or process will perform its intended function satisfactorily and without failure, for a specified period under defined conditions of use, maintenance, and environment; degree of accuracy expected of a measurement or other data. 2. in research, the reproducibility of an experimental result, as how closely a second measurement agrees with a first, whether or not correct; contrast *validity.*

There are several types of reliability: *test-retest reliability, the correlation between separate tests of a number of subjects; *split-half reliability, the correlation within a single test of two similar parts of the test; and *inter-rater reliability, the agreement between different individuals scoring the same procedure or observations. VIII.

Relman doctrine. "transfers of patients are justified only when intended to provide better care," an ethical principle articulated by Arnold S. Relman (U.S. physician and editor) in the early 1980s.

The point is that *dumping* patients is inappropriate, i.e., that transferring patients just because they are poor is an abdication of *professional* and *charitable* responsibility.

Read Bryan, J.E., "View from the Hill" (*Am Fam Physician,* 32(3): 257, 9/85). V.D.

remarried family (REM family). synonym, blended or reconstituted family, see *family.*

remedy. 1. anything used in *treatment* of a disease. 2. something that corrects or counteracts an evil. 3. the legal means to recover a right or prevent or obtain redress for a wrong.

These three medical, spiritual, and legal meanings are often properly combined in primitive cultures and at nonmolecular levels of the *biopsychosocial model* of illness. They are also frequently confused, as when drugs are used to treat wrongs. V.B.

remission. abatement or subsidence of an illness, the period of diminution thereof; compare *recrudescence* and *relapse.*

The ability of some diseases, as arthritis, leukemia, and multiple sclerosis, to disappear completely, spontaneously or with treatment, makes assessment of therapy and definition of cure difficult. Cure is ordinarily arbitrarily considered to occur in remitting diseases after five disease-free years. II.B.3.

render. something you do to pig fat; ugly synonym, provide or give, common in health care. VIII.B.

renovation. synonym, *modernization.*

replacement fee. see *nonreplacement fee.*

reportable. synonym, *notifiable.*

reproduction rate. see *birth rate.*

request for proposal (RFP). a formal government or private request for bidders on a contract specifying the work to be done by the contractor.

The acronym is common because much government health work, particularly training and evaluation activities, is done by contract. RFPs are published in such conventional forums as the *Commerce and Business Daily* to assure all parties the opportunity to bid. IV.C., IV.C.

required service. a service which must be offered by a health program in order to meet some external requirement or standard; compare *basic health service.*

The *Medicaid* required services are hospital services; laboratory and x-ray services; skilled nursing facility services for individuals over 20; early and periodic screening, diagnosis, and treatment services for individuals under 21; family planning services; physicians' services; and home health care services for all persons eligible for skilled nursing facility services. Within these requirements, states may determine the scope and extent of benefits, as by limiting covered hospital care to 30 days a year. States may offer additional services in their Medicaid programs, called *optional services* because they are offered at the option of the state. IV.C.2.

rescission, recision. 1. in the federal *budget,* enacted legislation canceling *budget authority* previously provided by Congress. Unless Congress approves a rescission within 45 days of continuous session, the proposed budget authority in question must be made available for obligation. 2. in insurance, cancellation, with repayment of premiums, of a policy. 1. VI.B.1., 2. IV.B.

research. careful, diligent search for new facts and their correct understanding; or for practical application of such facts and understanding.

Several types of research are distinguished by their nature and concern: *pure and *applied research (roughly, before and after the above semicolon, respectively), *biomedical research,* and *health services research.*

See *epidemiology, national institute,* and *study.* VIII.D.

reserves. money or its equivalent kept on hand or set aside to meet specified or anticipated liabilities; a balance sheet account set up to show the liabilities faced by an insurance company under outstanding *insurance policies.*

Reserves help show as true a picture as possible of the financial condition of the organization by permitting conversion of disbursements from a paid to an accrual basis. Companies set the amount of reserves according to their own estimates, state laws, and recommendations of supervisory officials and national organizations. Regulatory agencies can accept the reserves or refuse them as inadequate or excessive. All reserves, while estimated, are obligated amounts. There are many particular types, typically named for their purpose, as catastrophic and initial reserves, which fall into four classes: reserves for known liabilities not yet paid; reserves for losses incurred but unreported; reserves for future benefits; and other reserves for special purposes, as *contingency reserves* for unforeseen circumstances.

See *reinsurance reserve.* IV.B.

reservoir. 1. a place where something is kept in store. 2. an organism or host in which a *parasite* that causes disease in other organisms lives and multiplies without damaging its host; broadly, a noneconomic organism within which a *pathogen* of economic or medical importance flourishes; a colony or group of organisms, as virulent bacteria, that persists when the general population of the organism declines and that serves as a breeding nucleus, as a reservoir population of mosquitoes missed by control operations; compare *fomite* and *vector.* 3. an artificial lake or other place where water is collected and kept in quantity for later domestic or industrial use.

The reservoirs for tuberculosis include humans and cows. For rickettsia, the agent of typhus, lice and fleas, and the rats carrying them are reservoirs.

See *J. Howard.* 1. VIII.C., 2. I.A.1, 3. I.C.5.

residency. a prolonged, as one or more complete years, period of on-the-job training which may either be a part of a formal educational program or be undertaken separately after completion of a formal program, often a requirement for *credentialing.*

In medicine, dentistry, podiatry, and some other health professions, residencies are the principal part of *graduate medical education,* beginning either after graduation, increasingly, or after *internship,* traditionally, lasting two to seven years, and providing *specialty* training. Most physicians now take residencies. Although not required for *licensure,* a residency is commonly needed to obtain hospital *staff privileges* and other entry into practice. Residencies are needed for *board eligibility*. See *flexible residency* and *pyramid system*. III.A.

Residency Assistance Program (RAP). a program of services to residencies in *family medicine*.

It has written guidelines for residency curricula, facilities, and staffing and provides consultation and assistance to programs in meeting the guidelines. The RAP guidelines have had a major influence on the content and nature of family medicine, particularly as they have converged with the *Essentials*. III.C.

residency review committee (RRC). one of the committees appointed by the *Accreditation Council for Graduate Medical Education;* responsible for ascertaining whether residencies in a particular specialty, as family medicine, are in compliance with the general requirements for all residencies, the *Essentials* or requirements particular to the specialty, and otherwise accreditable. III., III.C.

residential care. assistance for residents of a nonmedical facility with *activities of daily living,* as meals, housekeeping, and laundry; synonym, *domiciliary care*.

Such care is provided in *boarding homes* and *life care communities,* sometimes known as *residential care facilities. VII.C.5.b.

residual substance. a trace of a chemical used in agricultural processes, as a pesticide or veterinary drug, remaining in its original form or a metabolized form on or in food, and potentially capable of causing harmful effects in exposed living organisms. I.A.2.a.

res ipsa loquitur. (literally, "the thing speaks for itself") in *malpractice,* the tort law doctrine that when a proven *injury* occurs to a plaintiff in a situation under the sole and exclusive control of the defendant and where such injury would not normally occur if the one in control had used due care, there is a rebuttable presumption that the defendant is *negligent,* as in the classic case of the surgeon who leaves a sponge in the abdomen. V.D.

resistance. 1. opposition to force or external stimulus; lack of sensitivity or response. 2. native or acquired *immunity*. 3. physiologic or psychologic processes or means by which an organism or a population becomes progressively insensitized to the effects of an environmental factor, a toxic or polluting substance or agent, or a treatment. I.A.1.

resources. 1. generally, new or reserve sources of support or supply; available means; computable wealth; immediate and possible sources of revenue. 2. in economics, the basic inputs or component parts of an economy, as land, labor, *capital,* and entrepreneurial ability. 3. in health, synonym, *health resources.* 4. in *welfare* programs, sources of support available to an individual in addition to the individual's regular earned or unearned income.

Resources refer to an individual's wealth or property, including cash savings, investments, home and other real estate, and automobiles or assets which could be converted to cash if necessary. Programs for the *poor* usually limit total resources an individual or family may have and still be eligible. Most existing resource tests exempt a home of reasonable value on the basis that it would not be right to require selling a home to qualify for benefits. The key thing about economic resources, and the basis of much of economics, is that they are limited, even scarce, and cost money. See *opportunity cost*. 1. III., 2. VIII.B.1., 3. III., 4. IV.C.2.

respiratory therapist. a technician trained in *respiratory therapy*. III.A.4.

respiratory therapy. the care of breathing, the lungs and related structures, and of people with lung disease.

Smoking and pneumoconioses, see *black lung*, combined with incredibly sophisticated technology for assessing and supporting the lungs have created large new populations of patients and therapists living with chronic lung disease, all in preference to effective prevention of the causes. V.

respite care. temporary substitute *care* for frail or *disabled* adults, as in a nursing home or hospital; compare *day care* and *partial hospitalization*.

Respite care allows *caretakers* to maintain normal routines and provides relief from the stresses and responsibilities of providing constant care for dependents. Such an *alternative to long-term care* is not routinely covered by programs which pay for long-term care, as Medicaid, but may be available from *community mental health centers* or *hospices*. It appears as *holiday relief care in *ICD-9-CM*. V.B., VII.C.2.

respondeat superior. (Latin, "let the master answer") in *malpractice,* a vicarious *liability* in which an employer may be held liable for the wrongful acts of an employee even though the employer's conduct may be without fault.

Before liability predicated on *respondeat superior* may be imposed upon an employer, it is necessary that a master-servant or controlling relationship exist between the employer and employee and that the wrongful act of the employee occur within the scope of employment. The doctrine of *respondeat superior* does not relieve the original wrongdoer, the employee, of liability for wrongful acts. V.D.

responsibility accounting. an accounting system in which costs are allocated to and reports prepared for *cost centers,* with the objective of controlling costs by assigning responsibility for specific costs to individual managers. VI.C.1.

retention, retention rate. synonym, *risk charge*.

retrospective reimbursement. payment after the fact, the traditional method of reimbursement; payment of *providers* by a *third-party carrier* for *costs* or *charges* actually incurred by *subscribers* in a previous time period; contrast *prospective reimbursement*. IV.A.

retrospective study. a study designed to observe events that have already occurred; contrast *prospective study,* which observes events as they occur. III.D.

retrospectoscope. slang, an instrument for viewing the past, hindsight, as "now that we can see through the retrospectoscope, we know we should have admitted him to the ICU instead of the ECU." A play on the names of the many fiber-optic scopes now used diagnostically in medicine. II.B.3., VIII.B.2.a.

review. look over or examine with a view to amendment or improvement; compare *evaluation* and *quality*.

See *admission certification, concurrent review, medical review,* and *peer review*. VI.D.

reviewed literature. scientific and clinical *medical literature,* particularly journal articles, which is subjected to peer review prior to publication; contrast *throwaway literature.*

An article submitted is forwarded for critical review to two or more experts in its subject matter. Authors are ordinarily given an opportunity to make appropriate changes. The process is variably anonymous. Most research is published in reviewed literature. Most journals indexed in *Index Medicus* are reviewed.

See *Inglefinger rule.* III.C.

review of symptoms, review of systems (ROS). a traditional part of the medical *history,* in which a patient is asked if he or she has suffered any of a regular list of common or important *symptoms* even though the patient has made no *complaint* of them. The inquiry, variable among examiners, is usually organized by body system, starting with the head and proceeding to the feet, hence review of systems. V.A.

Rhazes. Persian physician, 860–932. He studied and taught in Baghdad, Palestine, Egypt, Spain, and other cities of the eastern caliphate. His most important contribution to public health was the differentiation of smallpox from measles and other rashes. VII.B.2.e., VIII.A.1.

rheumatology. the *subspecialty* of *internal medicine* concerned with the joints. III.C.

rider. a legal document which modifies the protection of an *insurance policy,* either expanding or decreasing its *benefits* or adding or *excluding* certain conditions from the policy's coverage. IV.B.

right to treatment. the legal doctrine that a facility or program is legally obligated to provide adequate treatment for an individual when it has assumed responsibility for that individual's care.

Failure to provide treatment may represent *negligence,* may require discharge if the patient was involuntarily *committed,* and in public facilities may lead to court required and supervised improvements in services. The doctrine is easily confused with the hypothetical "right to health care" advocated by those who believe government should assure health services for all citizens, see *national health service.* III.B.1., VIII.B.3.

risk. 1. any chance of *loss;* the probability that loss will occur. 2. in insurance, the individual or property insured by an insurance policy against loss from *peril* or *hazard;* short for amount at risk, the value of potential loss.

See *acceptable risk, assigned risk, at risk, attributable risk, insurable risk,* and *relative risk.* IV.B.

risk charge. the fraction of a *premium* which goes to generate or replenish *surpluses* which a *carrier* must develop to protect against the possibility of excessive *losses* under its policies; synonyms, retention, retention rate. *Profits,* if any, on the sale of insurance are also taken from the surpluses developed using risk charges. IV.B.

risk factor. anything which adds to an individual's *risk* of suffering a disease or condition.

Such a factor may be the history or presence of a specific disease, continued *exposure* to a hazardous occupation or habit, or the presence of an abnormal finding on physical or laboratory examination. Risk factors for

heart attacks include a family history of heart attacks, sedentary job and lifestyle, smoking, high blood fats, and hypertension.
See *at risk* and *behavioral risk factor*. VIII.C.

Robens Report.   the report of the British Parliamentary Committee on Safety and Health at Work, *Report of the Committee, 1970–1972* (London, 1972), so called because the committee was headed by Lord Robens.
The report emphasizes self-regulation by employers in standard setting and enforcement and simplification and unification of Great Britain's large, fragmented body of law on occupational safety and health. VI.B.2.d.

Robert Wood Johnson Foundation (RWJ).   a private, nonprofit *charity* endowed by Robert Wood Johnson, U.S. manufacturer of Band-Aids and other medical products, devoted to the improvement of health services, as by funding demonstration and pilot projects, training programs, and studies of health services. III.B.4.

rodenticide.   see *pesticide*.

Roemer's law.   (Milton Roemer, U.S. physician) a bed built is a bed filled.
The demand for hospital and nursing home services is nearly inexhaustible and even generated by providers, who have many incentives to be busy. Thus, when additional beds are built because existing ones are fully occupied, the new beds will also be filled in all but the most extreme situations. III.B.1., VI.A., VIII.B.3.

roentgen, rontgen (r).   (W.C. Röntgen, German physicist, 1845–1923) 1. the international unit of x-rays and gamma radiation; the quantity of either radiation which results in associated corpuscular emission or ionization of one electrostatic unit of electrical charge, positive or negative, per cubic centimeter of air under standard conditions. 2. of or pertaining to x-rays. I.C.3., III.C.

Röntgen, Wilhelm Conrad.   German physicist, 1845–1923. He discovered rontgen or x-rays and initiated their medical use. VII.A.1.

rolfing.   see *structural integration*.

room.   a part of a health facility, whether a simple chamber or a *department*, as an emergency room. III.B.1.

Ross, Ronald.   Indian army physician, 1857–1923. In 1897 he solved the riddle of malaria by discovering the malarial parasite in the stomach of the anopheles mosquito. Later he developed methods of mosquito control and carried on campaigns for this purpose. VIII.A.1., VIII.C.

roster.   a list of patients served by a given health professional or program; compare *catchment area* and *panel*.
The roster may be derived from a *registry* or list of *encounters,* but the listing of an individual on a provider's roster does not imply any ongoing relationship between the provider and the individual. III.B.1., V.

rotation.   a period of service in a *specialty* or on a hospital *service* during medical school, where it is also known as a *clerkship,* or during *internship* or *residency*. III.A.

round, rounds.   1. a series of professional calls on patients by a doctor or nurse, typically in a hospital or nursing home or in the patients' homes on a regular schedule or circuit, as in making work or morning rounds. 2. by extension, a review of patients for teaching purposes, as *attending* or teaching rounds. V.

rule. in the executive branch of the federal government, an agency statement of general or particular applicability and future effect designed to implement, interpret, or prescribe law or *policy* or to describe the organization, procedure, or practice requirements of an agency; synonym, *regulation*.

Rules are published in the *Federal Register*. The process of writing a rule is a *rulemaking. A rule, once adopted in accordance with the procedures specified in the Administrative Procedure Act (Title V, U.S.C.), has the force of law.

See *notice of proposed rulemaking*. VIII.B.3.

rule out. to exclude or eliminate something, particularly a diagnostic possibility. Thus a negative throat culture rules out a streptococcal sore throat. V.A.

rural. of, relating to, or characteristic of living in the country or engaging in agriculture; contrast *suburban* and *urban*. I.B.2.

rural health care. health services and programs for people living in rural areas, as the *Frontier Nursing Service*.

Rural populations are often old, isolated, and poor, while resources are limited and stretched over great distances. VII.C.2.

Rural Health Initiative (RHI). a federal program, begun in 1972, of grants and special Medicare and Medicaid provisions for support of *primary care* programs in rural areas.

The program supports community health services for all, regardless of income, in areas historically characterized by inadequate access to health services. Rural is defined as "any area not in a *standard metropolitan statistical area*." The program is now part of the *community health center* program authorized by section 330 of the *Public Health Service Act*. III.B.1.

Rush, Benjamin. U.S. physician, politician, and reformer, 1745–1813. A signer of the Declaration of Independence, author of the first American book on *psychiatry*, published in 1812, and thus known as the father of American psychiatry. He was a champion of free schools and religious toleration, an opponent of the abuse of alcohol and tobacco, and a pioneer of *occupational therapy*. II.B.2., III.C., VIII.A.1.

Ryan's law. anyone making three consecutive correct guesses is established as an expert. VIII.B.2.b., VIII.B.3.

safe. free of *hazard* or *risk* of harm, *injury,* or danger. I.C.

safe house. a secret place providing temporary shelter and protection for *battered* women and their children who are justly afraid of harmful pursuit by their spouses.

    These havens are now to be found in most U.S. cities through social agencies such as community mental health centers and provide help in making a new start. V.III.B.1., I.B.1.

safety. 1. the condition of being safe. 2. any method or device used with equipment or procedures to reduce their *hazards* or *risks.* 3. knowledge of or skill in ways of avoiding accident or disease, as in safety engineering.

    Safety in medicine is a relative concept which must be balanced against the benefits or *effectiveness* of a drug or procedure. Treatment known to cause injury or disease when used is not thought of as unsafe if the benefits are expected to exceed the damage. The Federal Food, Drug, and Cosmetic Act requires a demonstration of safety for drugs marketed for human use. No similar requirement exists for most other medical procedures. I.C.

safety engineer. a safety *professional* with an engineering degree, the degree itself being in *safety* or *occupational health.* III.A.5.

safety hazard. in occupational safety and health, a *hazard* to worker safety, as things in the work environment which can cause burns, electrical shock, cuts, bruises, sprains, broken bones, or the loss of limbs, eyesight, or hearing.

    There is no consistent distinction between safety and *health hazards,* although with safety the harm is usually immediate or violent, is usually associated with industrial equipment or the physical environment, and often involves a task requiring care and training. Safety professionals treat safety as all-encompassing and including health, but their concern is more with the explosive nature of chemicals than with their toxicology, and with the effects of noise on hearing rather than as a stressor and cause of disease. I.C., VII.B.2.d.

safety inspector. see *inspector.*

safety professional. in *occupational health* as defined by the *National Institute of Occupational Safety and Health,* a person with at least a baccalaureate degree in engineering, science, or occupational health and/or safety; compare *professional, paraprofessional,* and *technician.* III.A.5., VII.B.2.d.

same-day surgery. synonym, major *ambulatory surgery.*

sample. a specimen, example, or instance; a representative portion of a whole, a small part taken as an example of the quality or character of the whole; a part of a *population* used for investigation and comparing properties.

There are many types of sample: *instantaneous sample, one done at a moment in time; *integrated sample, one taken over an entire period of time, as of *occupational air* collected over an entire shift; and *interval sample, one taken at several moments over a period of time, as hourly during a shift.

See *random sample.* VIII.C., VIII.D.

sampling error. mistaken or false result due to chance, as when the result obtained in a *sample* differs from that which would have been obtained if the entire *population* had been studied; contrast *systematic error.*

*Type I, or alpha, sampling error occurs when a true *null hypothesis* is rejected; an apparent but not *valid* difference between sample and population is found. A *type II, or beta, error is made when the null hypothesis is false but is not rejected; real differences are not discovered. VIII.D.

sanatorium. irregular and old-fashioned, an establishment or *hospital* for care of people with *chronic disease,* especially *alcoholism,* tuberculosis, or *mental illness;* an establishment providing therapy by natural agents, as light, diet, and exercise; an establishment offering rest and recuperation for convalescents.

See *Christian Science.* III.B.1.

sanitarian. a person skilled in sanitation and public health, ordinarily with a baccalaureate or master's degree and often with registration or licensure; occasionally, casually, a garbage collector or janitor. III.A.5.

sanitary. of or pertaining to health, the restoration or maintenance of health, or the absence of any agent injurious to health. I.C.

sanitary code. a municipal code which delineates methods of sewage disposal, solid waste disposal, and more recently, air and water pollution prevention and control.

These codes are primarily based on public health and hygiene considerations. Regrettably, there is no uniform sanitary code, so hygienic considerations often vary with the locality. I.C.

sanitary engineering. the branch of civil engineering concerned with the design, construction, and operation of structures and *systems,* particularly for water and *wastes,* for ensuring the healthfulness of a community's environment. III.C.

sanitary landfilling. a method of solid waste disposal on land in which the waste is spread in thin layers, compacted to the smallest practical volume, and covered with soil at the end of each working day. I.C.4.

sanitary sewer. a *sewer* that carries only domestic or commercial sewage. Storm water runoff is carried in a separate system, a *storm sewer.* I.C.4.

sanitation. 1. the act or process of securing a sanitary or healthful condition. 2. the application of measures and techniques for control of all the factors in people's physical environment that exercise a deleterious effect on physical development, health, and survival.

Most municipal sanitation departments are mainly concerned with the collection, haulage, and disposal of refuse and solid wastes. Sanitation is, however, also concerned with food safety, pollution, noise, and radiation. See *W. Farr, health officer, public health,* and *sewage.* I.C., I.C.4.

sanity. soundness of mind; contrast *mental health* and *illness.* I.A.2.

saturation. in marketing *insurance* or *health maintenance organizations,* the point at which further *penetration* is improbable or excessively costly. III.B.1., IV.B.

scan. 1. to image or observe systematically, especially by subjecting something, as an area or volume, to a series of partial observations, views, or slices by a sensory organ or device. 2. the observation, or record of it, made by such an organ or device.

Modern *diagnostic radiology* with *tomograms,* radioisotopic imaging, and *computed tomography,* whose products are known as scans, as a brain scan or CT scan, has given this lovely old word new use. It has traditionally meant either a cursory, hasty look through or a systematic, thorough scrutiny. III.C., V.A.

scapegoat. a person bearing the blame for others' fault; compare *blaming the victim.*

Scapegoating is common in families; children, for instance, often bear the blame for inadequate parental disciplining skills. The scapegoat, unlike the *identified patient,* may be conscious of his or her plight, not sick, and not presented to the family physician. Scapegoat applies to "the family member seen as bad or sick. The scapegoat, when a child, serves to displace aggression away from conflict between the parents, thereby preserving the marital relationship" (*Pinney and Slipp, 1982*). I.B.1.

scarcity area. an area lacking an adequate *supply* of a particular type of health service, as physician services, or of all health services; compare *medically underserved area.* II.C.

schedule A. the list of occupations which the Department of Labor considers to be in short supply throughout the United States for purposes of *labor certification.* All occupations listed on schedule A are generally health occupations, but some health occupations, as dentists, are not listed. III.A.

scheduled benefit payment. a *workmen's compensation* or insurance benefit, as for an *impairment,* which is determined by a standard list or schedule of amounts for specified losses, as $5000 for loss of a foot or $15,000 for an arm lost at the shoulder; synonym, allocated benefit, compare *fixed, indemnity,* and *unscheduled benefit.*

Scheduled payments have been variable among states and subject to criticism for their arbitrariness and failure to consider the *disability* resulting from the impairment. Some *permanent partial disability benefits that continue indefinitely at a rate less than total disability are also scheduled, as when loss of a foot automatically earns a permanent partial benefit at 10 percent of total disability benefits. The benefit in insurance is the lesser of the actual charge for the service and the amount specified in the policy's *schedule of benefits or list of payable amounts. IV.B.2., VIII.B.2.d.

scheduled drug. a drug included by the *Drug Enforcement Administration* in one of its six schedules, i.e., groups of *controlled substances*. III.B.3.

schism. describes a family situation in which "the parents live in a chronic state of severe discord and fail to achieve complementarity of needs."

"Because of this, there is undercutting of a spouse's worth and a tendency to compete for and form alliances with the children, thereby breaching generational boundaries" (*Pinney and Slipp, 1982*). Such families may lack role reciprocity, have excessive attachment to parental homes, and produce schizophrenic children, typically daughters; compare *skew*. I.B.1.

Scientology. a religious movement begun in 1952 which teaches immortality and reincarnation and claims a sure psychotherapeutic method for freeing individuals from personal problems, increasing human abilities, and speeding recovery from illness, injury, and mental disorder. V.

scope of services. the number, type, and intensity or complexity of *services* provided by a hospital or health program.

Scope of services is described or measured in a number of quite different ways so that the capacity and nature of various programs may be compared. A program's scope of services should reflect and be adequate to meet the *needs* of its *patient mix*. III.B.1., VII.D.

screen. 1. examine, usually methodically, in order to separate or sort into distinct groups, as well and sick; use of quick, simple *procedures* to separate apparently well people who have, or are *at risk* of having, a disease from those who do not. Multiple screening, or *multiphasic screening, is the combination of a battery of screening tests for various diseases applied to large groups of apparently well people. 2. initial, cursory *claims review* by insurance companies to identify claims which are obviously not covered or in some way are deficient.

See *green screen, phenylketonuria, preventive medicine, sensitivity*, and *specificity*. 1. VII.B.2.e., 2. IV.B.

screening clinic. an office, *department*, or other place where initial assessment or screening of patients seeking care is done to determine what services they need with what priority and, sometimes, where treatment of minor problems is provided; compare *triage*. III.B.1.

screening panel. in *malpractice*, a fact-finding group used in the early stages of a malpractice dispute. There are two types of screening panels: physician defense panels, which seek to develop the best possible defense for the physician who faces a real or potential malpractice claim; and joint physician and lawyer panels, which look at the facts of the case for both the defendant physician and the plaintiff and make recommendations on its merits. V.D.

scry. to use a crystal to obtain projected visual or *eidetic* imagery; to practice crystal gazing or divination; to employ a bright reflecting surface to facilitate visual hallucinations. A *scryer is a seer. I.A.2.d.

scut work. *house staff* slang, contemptible tasks, usually trivial in nature, paperwork, or work which could be done by anybody else. V., VIII.B.2.a.

seasonal affective disorder (SAD). a mental illness characterized by recurrent serious depression during winter, interspersed with periods of well-being during spring, summer, and fall.

The disorder is also associated with carbohydrate craving and weight gain, a 4 to 1 ratio of female to male incidence, and irritability and suspiciousness. It is treatable with large doses of light, as the grow lights that make plants grow in winter. II.B.2.

secondary. 1. second in time or development. 2. second in relation or *association;* subordinate; produced by a *cause* not considered *primary.* II.B.1.a.

secondary care. *medical care* and services provided by medical specialists, as by cardiologists or neurosurgeons, usually upon *referral* or *consultation.*

In the United States, there is much self-referral by patients for these services rather than referral by primary care providers. This contrasts with the path followed in Great Britain, where all patients first seek care from primary care providers and are referred for secondary or *tertiary care* as needed. V., VII.D.2.

secondary gain. any profit reaped by a patient, often unconsciously, from symptoms or illness, as relief from responsibility or increased personal attention, money, or disability benefits; contrast *primary gain* and *sick role.*

Secondary gain is often normal and proper. It is prominent in chronic illness and tends to perpetuate symptoms when greater than the costs of the illness. II.A.1.

secondary payer. see *primary payer.*

secondary prevention. see *preventive medicine.*

second-injury fund. in some states' *workmen's compensation programs,* a fund or *reserve* within the program used to pay full compensation to a *handicapped* or *disabled* worker who was hired despite his or her disability by an employer and subsequently received a second injury.

The employer is charged only for the benefits associated with the second injury, while the fund is charged the difference, i.e., the amount attributable to the original disability. Such funds are intended to make it possible for employers to hire the handicapped without risking eventual responsibility for the handicap. However, they are easily abused and hard to administer. VII.B.2.d.

second opinion. another recommendation or judgment concerning a problem on which a first recommendation has already been obtained.

Physicians have a traditional obligation to seek a second opinion, paid for by the patient, from a *consultant* whenever a patient desires one or they are themselves uncertain about diagnosis or treatment. *Third-party payers* sometimes suggest or require, and will then pay for, a second opinion when expensive *elective procedures* have been recommended in hopes of controlling costs by preventing *unnecessary surgery.* III.C., IV.B., V.A.

section 222. a section of the Social Security amendments of 1972, P.L. 92-603, which authorized the secretary of the Department of Health and Human Services to undertake, with respect to *Medicare,* studies, experiments, or demonstration projects on *prospective reimbursement* of ambulatory surgical centers (surgicenters), intermediate care facilities, and *homemaker services;* elimination or reduction of the three-day prior hospitalization requirement for admission to a skilled nursing facility; methods of reimbursing the services of *physician's assistants* and *nurse practitioners;* provision of day care services to older persons eligible under Medicare and Medicaid; and possible means of making the services of *clinical psychologists* more generally available under Medicare and Medicaid. IV.C.1., IV.C.2.

section 223. a section of the Social Security amendments of 1972, P.L. 92-603, which required the secretary of DHHS to establish limits on overall *direct* or *indirect costs* as *reasonable* under *Medicare* for comparable services in comparable facilities in an area. IV.C.1.

section 1122. a section of the Social Security Act that provides that payments will not be made under *Medicare* or *Medicaid* for *depreciation* on certain *capital* expenditures by *health facilities* found inconsistent with state or local *health plans* and is thus intended to help control unneeded capital development.

The National Health Planning and Resources Development Act of 1974 requires states participating in the section 1122 program to have the *state health planning and development agency* serve as the section 1122 agency for the required review. Section 1122 was an early but still active form of *capital expenditure review,* partly superseded by *certificate-of-need* programs. IV.C., VI.A.2.

selection bias. inadvertent selection of a nonrepresentative or nonrandom *sample* of subjects or observations, as by a 1936 *Literary Digest* poll which predicted Landon's victory over Roosevelt because telephone directories were used as the basis for selecting respondents.

See *bias* and *error.* VIII.D.

selective. in medical education, an *elective* selected from a limited list of available possibilities.

Many residency programs give participants some required rotations, some purely elective time, and some selective choice within specified limits. III.A.

self. the body, mind, and spirit, which together constitute the individual; the individual's characteristic *behavior.* I.A.2.

self-care (SC). *care* for one's self, usually without dependence on others except for education; compare *self-neglect.*

All people care for themselves, often well, some excessively, and always inadequately in some way. Getting them to correct the deficiencies can be very difficult; see *behavior therapy, compliance,* and *health education.* Self-care is often done in groups such as *Alcoholics Anonymous,* Parents Anonymous, *smokenders,* and *Weight Watchers.* The profit for others is in the education, see *alternative medicine,* and supplies, see *health food.* I.A.2.

self-help. synonym, *self-care.*

self-insure. the practice of an individual, group, employer, or organization assuming complete responsibility for *losses* which might be *insured* against, as malpractice losses or medical expenses and other losses due to illness; compare *go bare.*

With self-insurance, medical expenses are financed out of current income, personal savings, a fund developed for the purpose, and/or some other combination of personal or organizational assets rather than by insurance. IV.B., V.D.

self-neglect. in *adult protective services* law, inability of an adult, living alone, to provide or obtain for himself or herself the necessities and services required for personal health and welfare. I.A.2.

Semmelweis, Ignaz Philip. Hungarian physician, 1818–1865. While assistant at the Lying-in Hospital in Vienna, he recognized that puerperal or childbed fever was a communicable disease conveyed by the hands of the obstetrician. By insisting that their hands be washed, he succeeded in drastically reducing maternal mortality. For this Semmelweis, like *O.W. Holmes,* was scorned. V.C., VIII.A.1.

senescence.   aging, the process of growing old. *senile. characteristic of old *age,* afflicted with senile dementia. *senium. the last stage of life, old age; compare *child.*
    In environmental health, lakes nearing biologic extinction are senescent. In Roman law, the senium began at age 70 and relieved one of public obligations; compare modern mandatory retirement and availability of Social Security benefits. I.A.1.

senile dementia.   chronic progressive loss of mental powers in late life, characterized by failing memory, judgment, and other intellectual functions; synonym, senility; compare *imbecility* and *mental retardation.*
    Dementias caused by known diseases are often included. Some limit the term to those without known cause other than the normal decay of aging. I.A.1.

Senior Actualization and Growth Experience (SAGE).   a lovely nonprofit organization formed in 1974 to explore the myths and realities of the aging process.
    SAGE's premises hold that there is purpose to old age, people need special conditions for deep growth, well-being is enhanced by pleasurable experience, each person is unique and requires a unique therapeutic program, the old develop faster in some ways than the young, many of the ailments of age are reversible, old age may be a time of emancipation from inhibitions and habits of childhood, and old age may be a time of truth. SAGE has developed and published this philosophy of *holism* and successful aging with a variety of specific programs, skills, and exercises.
    Read Luce, Gay Gaer, *Your Second Life: Vitality and Growth in Middle and Latter Years from the Experiences of the SAGE Program* (New York: Dell Publishing Co., A Merloyd Lawrence Book, 1979. 465 pp.) I.A.1., III.B.2., VII.B.3.6.

senium.   see *senescence.*

sensitivity.   a measure of the ability of a diagnostic or screening *test* to correctly identify the positive or sick people; the proportion of *actual* positives correctly identified as positive.
    Sensitivity equals *true positives* divided by true positives plus *false negatives.* A test may be quite sensitive without being very *specific.*
    See *efficiency* and *predictive values.* VIII.D.

separation program number.   a number placed until 1974 upon servicepeoples' discharge papers by the armed forces which, unbeknown to the veterans, revealed confidential medical information to employers and others.
    There were codes for homosexuality, psychiatric disorders, bed-wetting, venereal disease, drug abuse, and obesity. The practice reflects the lack of *physician-patient privileges* in military law.
    Read Westin, Alan F., and Florence Isbell, *A Policy Analysis of Citizen Rights Issues in Health Data Systems,* National Bureau of Standards Spe-

cial Publication No. 469 (Washington: U.S. Government Printing Office, 1977). III.D.1.

septic tank. a watertight closed container, typically underground, that settles out solids from raw *sewage,* stores the sludge and the scum, and processes the sewage anaerobically and/or chemically.

Septic tanks are used in residential areas where there are no sewer systems. In portable applications they are used aboard boats, ships, and planes. Bacteria in the *waste* decompose the organic matter, while sludge settles to the bottom. *Effluent* flows through drains, ordinarily into the ground. Sludge is pumped out at regular intervals. I.C.4.

septic tank system. a series of seepage pits and/or leaching trenches for carrying off *effluent* from septic tanks in densely populated areas served by tanks rather than sewers. I.C.4.

sequela (pl. sequelae). a *complication* of a disease; an effect, result, or condition following and dependent on a disease or its treatment. II.A.2.

serious violation. in *occupational health,* a violation of the *general duty clause,* any *rule,* or an *occupational standard* imposed by the Occupational Safety and Health Act in which there is "a substantial probability that death or serious physical harm could result from a condition which exists, or from one or more practices, means, methods, operations, or processes...unless the employer did not, and could not with the exercise of reasonable diligence, know of the presence of the violation" [section 17(k)].

The Occupational Safety and Health Act provides special penalties for serious violations; an employer who receives a *citation* for one must be assessed a civil penalty not exceeding $1000 per violation. VII.B.2.d.

serum porcelain. a hypothetical chemical, porcelain is not found in the blood; the laboratory test to measure it; the sarcastic ultimate in expensive over-investigation of a patient, as, "She had a thousand dollar *work-up,* complete with serial serum porcelains." V.A., VIII.B.2.a.

serve. to care for, to work for.

service. 1. in economics, the performance or result of a labor having value to individuals or society without production of a tangible *good.* 2. in medicine, any unit of health care, whether or not tangible; the patients of a particular attending physician or health program; synonym, *department,* as the pediatric service.

Ordinarily plural, services in economics include legal, medical, and other forms of personal assistance; transportation; and entertainment. Service in medicine is synonymous with *procedure,* although the latter term is used for tangible services. It is sometimes synonymous with *encounter,* although, since there is little standardization or hierarchy of services, an encounter may both be a service and consist of multiple services.

A service is an action taken by the provider in order to improve or maintain the patient's and/or family's health and well-being.

Health services may be classified as follows:

1. diagnostic (investigative) services—these include a general assessment of any problem, annual health assessments, laboratory examinations performed both within and outside of the office setting, and others.

2. therapeutic services—these include pharmacological therapy, surgical therapy, physical therapy, psychotherapy, and others.

3. preventive services—these include immunizations, screening tests, education, pre- and postnatal checkups, well-baby care, family planning, and others.

Several items in the above classification may be classified in more than one section. A diagnostic service could be therapeutic or even preventive (*NAPCRG, 1978*).

See *ancillary service, channeling agency, charge, Current Procedural Terminology, debt service, operation,* and *unbundling.* VII.

service area.   synonym, medical trade area or, occasionally, catchment area.

service benefit.   a *benefit* in the form of a service rather than a cash payment, common in *Blue Cross/Blue Shield* plans.

Payment is made directly to the *provider* of *covered services* given to eligible people. Service benefits may be *full-service benefits, meaning that the plan fully reimburses the hospital, for example, for all services so that the patient has no *out-of-pocket* expenses. Full-service benefits may also be available when the program itself provides the service, as in a *prepaid group practice.* *Partial-service benefits cover only part of the expenses, the remainder being paid by the beneficiary through some form of *cost sharing.* See *indemnity benefit* and *vendor payment.* IV.B.1.

service-connected (SC) disability.   in the Veterans Administration health care program, a disease or *disability* incurred or aggravated in the line of duty in active military service. These disabilities are the primary concern of the program; compare *adjunct* or *non-service-connected disability.* III.D.1.

service patient.   a patient whose case is the responsibility of a health program or institution, as a hospital; contrast *private patient;* synonyms, *public, staff,* and *ward patients.*

Service patients are often cared for by an individual practitioner paid by the program, typically a member of a hospital's *house staff,* but the program, not the individual practitioner, is paid for the care. VII.A.1.

severity.   degree of seriousness, as severity of illness; probability of causing harm, pain, or death; compare *case-mix severity.*

*Severity of illness, how sick a patient is, is an important determinant of the cost of care and use of resources and is therefore measured by a variety of indices; see *acuity, Acute Physiology and Chronic Health Evaluation, Medical Illness Severity Grouping System, nursing intensity,* and *Patient Management Categories.* The *diagnosis related group*–based prospective payment system makes no allowance for severity of illness; every patient with the same diagnosis is reimbursed at the same rate no matter how sick, at least partly because reliable measures of severity with which to vary reimbursement that are independent of the diagnosis and costs of care are unavailable. II.A.2.

sewage.   the total of organic *waste* and wastewater generated by residential and commercial establishments.

Whether the wastes of domestic economy are considered sewage, garbage, or *solid waste* depends on how they are discharged. The unsanitary mess is called *sanitary sewage to distinguish it from water runoff, *storm sewage.

See *chlorination* and *septic tank.* I.C.4., I.C.5.

sewer.   any pipe or conduit used to collect and carry away domestic and commercial sewage, a *sanitary sewer,* storm water runoff, a *storm sewer,* or both from the generating source to treatment plants or receiving streams. Often storm water runoff and sewage are carried in the same system, a *combined sewer. I.C.4.

sewerage. 1. the collection and removal of sewage. 2. the entire system of conduits, sewers, and plants for sewage collection, treatment, and disposal. 3. effluent carried by sewers, whether sanitary sewage, industrial wastes, or storm water runoff. I.C.4.

Sex Information and Education Council of the United States (SIECUS). a multidisciplinary health agency concerned solely with human sexuality.

Founded in 1964 by Mary Calderone, U.S. physician, the organization has supported sex education by its programs of parent education, teacher training, consultation, conferences, and professional publications. Perhaps SIECUS's use of its vaguely obscene acronym as much as its concern for sexuality has made it a focus of conservative objections to modern sexuality. III.B.4., VII.B.2.b.

sexually transmitted disease (STD). a *contagious* disease ordinarily acquired during sexual intercourse or other intimate physical contact, current euphemistic synonym, *venereal disease.*

There are over 30 sexually transmitted diseases including gonorrhea, syphilis, chancroid, granuloma inguinale, lymphogranuloma venereum, some vaginitides, and acquired immune deficiency syndrome (AIDS). These diseases are the concern of special *reporting* requirements and control programs, as *reglementation.* II.B.1.a.

shadow gazer. slang, radiologist. VIII.B.2.a.

shaman. a priest-healer who uses *meditation,* magic, or traditional methods to cure the sick, divine the hidden, and control events that affect the welfare of people.

Many cultures have recognized healers, as *curanderos,* whom anthropologists generally call shamans, although the term originally referred to priests of a Ural-Altaic religion of northern Asia. III.A.

shared service. a medical or nonmedical *service* provided in a coordinated or otherwise explicitly agreed upon joint fashion by two or more otherwise independent hospitals or other health programs.

Sharing of medical services might include an agreement that one hospital will provide all open heart surgery needed in a community and no therapeutic radiology while another undertakes the reverse. Shared nonmedical services include joint laundry or dietary services for two or more nursing homes. Common laundry services purchased by two or more health programs from an independent retailer are not thought of as shared services unless the health programs own or otherwise control the retailer. VII.D.3.

shelter. a residential facility, as for delinquent or *abused* children or the homeless; irregularly distinguished from a *boarding home* by being publicly subsidized or providing organized programs of care for its residents; compare *halfway house* and *partial hospitalization.* III.B.1.

sheltered workshop. a program of structured, supervised employment for *mentally retarded* or otherwise *handicapped* people. II.B.2., III.B.1.

shiatsu. a *massage therapy,* developed in Japan in the eighteenth century, involving application of carefully gauged pressure at specific points, the *tsu bos, on bodily meridians. It combines Japanese massage with acupuncture.

Read Irwin, Yukiko, and James Wagenvoord, *Shiatzu: Japanese Finger Pressure for Energy.* (Philadelphia: J.B. Lippincott, 1976.) V.

ship's medicine chest.   the pharmaceuticals, surgical supplies and equipment, and other chemicals stored in the *sick berth* or bay of a ship.

Since 1790 federal law (46. U.S.C. 666) has required U.S. vessels to have a medicine chest. U.S. Public Health Service regulations detail its contents and use. Originally an actual chest to be removed from wrecked ships or taken ashore to be refilled by an *apothecary,* the "chest" is now a long list of the supplies with which sick bays must be furnished.

See *Deadhead Medico* and read the U.S. Public Health Service, *The Ship's Medicine Chest and Medical Aid at Sea* (HEW Publication No. (HSA) 78-2024. Washington: U.S. Government Printing Office, 1978). III.B.2.

shopper.   dental slang, a person who calls to price shop, or seek optimal insurance coverage; compare *doctor shopping,* which also happens to dentists.

The dentist's mildly hostile perception that such calls are wrong or unusual is interesting. Dentist collaboration with a shopper to fix charges to match insurance coverage may be illegal if charges to the shopper are inflated to avoid payment of *cost sharing.* V., VIII.B.2.

short.   dispense a quantity of a drug which is less than the quantity prescribed for the purpose of increasing profit by charging for the prescribed amount, compare *kiting;* a form of pharmaceutical *fraud.* III.B.3.

shroud waving.   British slang, the *administrative* practice of arguing that unless an area or health program is given additional resources, people will die unnecessarily. VIII.B.2.a.

sibling position.   the role one occupies as a child among one's siblings in the sibling subsystem.

Personality is in part determined by birth order. Family roles learned in families of origin, as by sibling position, operate, sometimes harmoniously, as the family constellations of families of procreation.

Read Toman, Walter, *Family Constellation* (New York, Springer: 1961). I.B.1.

sibling subsystem.   the group of children within a family.

Children learn peer relationships in the subsystem, including supporting, isolating, scapegoating, negotiating, cooperation, and competition. The boundaries of the sibling subsystem protect children from adults. I.B.1.

sick berth.   sick bay, the space on a ship which serves as both hospital and dispensary. Federal law (46 U.S.C. 660-1) and regulations require most U.S. merchant vessels to have a sick bay as well as a *ship's medicine chest.* III.B.1.

sick call (SC).   1. a time, place, or line where individuals report to a prison, ship, or other institutional medical officer or nurse for diagnosis and treatment. 2. a *visit* to a patient. VII.C.1., VII.C.5.b.

sick leave.   an absence from work, often paid, permitted because of illness; the days per year which an employer agrees to grant as leave because of illness. A *sick leave bank is a pool of sick leave to which some employers allow employees to contribute unused earned leave so that they may draw from the pool if their own illness requires more leave than they are entitled to. *Sick pay is pay during sick leave.

Sick leave, often granted only when a physician verifies the illness, is a major cost of illness and an important benefit of employment. It is typically earned in proportion to one's length of employment at a specified rate, often up to a maximum. It may be available for an employee's own illness, absence from work necessitated by caring for a sick family member, or obtaining health services.

See *blue flu*. VII.B.2.d.

sickness. synonym, *disease* and *illness;* common in *insurance.*

Sickness is irregularly defined. It implies perception of the self as sick, assumption of the *sick role,* and inability to function, none of which are necessarily the case with *disease*. II.

sickout. see *blue flu*.

sick role. the socially conventional *behavior* allowed and expected of one who is sick; compare *primary, secondary,* and *tertiary gain.*

Sick people are relieved of their usual responsibilities, are expected to rest, and are allowed to be unusually dependent and regressed. Failure either to take or to give up the role appropriately may be unhealthful. I.A.2.

sick tax. the part of a *charge* attributable to *bad debts;* not a tax at all, but slang for an accounting amount.

Hospitals and other programs often charge paying patients, and their insurers, the cost of caring for poor people, much as hospital pharmacy profits offset losses on pediatric services. IV.A., VI.C.1.

side effect. the cloud over the silver lining; an unintended, ordinarily undesired result or complication of treatment; compare *adverse drug reaction.*

They may also be unrecognized. Side effects are particularly associated with drugs and are the major complications to be balanced against benefits when establishing safety and dose for a drug.

Read Dukes, M.N.G. (ed.), *Meyler's Side Effects of Drugs: An Encyclopedia of Adverse Reactions and Interactions,* 10th ed. (New York: Elsevier Publishing Co., 1984. 966 pp.). III.B.3., V.B.

side-stream smoke. see *smoke*.

sign (Sx). an objective evidence or physical manifestation of a disease; contrast *symptom*. II.A.2.

significance level. the arbitrarily selected probability level for rejecting the *null hypothesis,* commonly .05 or .01. VIII.D.

significant difference. a difference between two statistical measures, calculated from two separate *samples,* which is of such magnitude that it probably did not occur by chance alone.

Usually the probability that the difference occurred by chance must be less than 1 in 20 ($p < .05$ or 5%) before the difference is accepted as significant. The smaller the probability, the more likely it is that the difference between the samples is real, i.e., that they came from different populations, although it may still not be important or correctly understood. VIII.D.

silent. of a disease which does not exhibit the usual *signs* and *symptoms;* characterized by a quiescent state; not clinically manifest, *subclinical*. II.

silicosis. *pneumoconiosis* caused by breathing silica or sand dust. II.B.2.

single-blind. see *double-blind study*.

single-handed practice. synonym, usually British, private practice.

skew. describes a family situation in which serious psychopathology of one marital partner is supported by the spouse, resulting in the distorted ideation being accepted in the family (folie a famille).

"There is considerable masking of conflict, creating an unreal atmosphere that does not help the child to trust his or her perception and judgment or learn social adaptive skills" (*Pinney and Slipp, 1982*).

skim. in health insurance or in health programs paid on a *prepayment* or *capitation* basis, enrolling only the healthiest people, as a way of controlling program *costs* since income is constant whether or not services are actually used; synonym, *creaming;* contrast *adverse selection.* III.B.1., IV.B.

skimp. deny or delay the provision of services, as cataract extraction, needed or demanded by *enrolled members* in a health program paid on a *prepayment* or *capitation* basis, as a way of controlling costs since income is constant whether or not services are actually used; contrast *adverse selection.* III.B.1.

skilled care. medical, nursing, and rehabilitative inpatient services at a *level of care* between hospital care and *intermediate care;* synonyms, skilled nursing care or services. VII.C.5.b.

skilled nursing facility (SNF). in Medicare and Medicaid, a facility, or distinct part of one, primarily engaged in providing skilled nursing care and related services for people requiring medical or nursing care, or *rehabilitation* services; formerly known as an *extended care facility.*

To be an SNF a facility must have a transfer agreement with one or more *participating* hospitals; formal policies for the services it provides; a physician, registered nurse, and medical staff responsible for execution of the policies; physician supervision of patients; physician availability for medical care in emergencies; medical records on all patients; 24-hour nursing service and at least one registered nurse employed full time; appropriate methods for dispensing drugs; a satisfactory *utilization review* plan; appropriate state and local licensure; an overall plan and budget; appropriate disclosure of ownership; an effective regular program of independent *medical review;* and evidence of compliance with applicable provisions of the *Life Safety Code.* III.B.1.

Skinner, Burrhus Frederic. American psychologist, 1904–. He is noted for his research and writings on operant conditioning. Many of the procedures of *behavior therapy* are based on laboratory research by Skinner and his students. III.C.

slicking. dental slang, unnecessary extracting of all remaining teeth to fabricate a denture. To "slick 'em" is to make the gums smooth. V., VIII.B.2.a.

sliding scale deductible. a *deductible* that is not set at a fixed amount but rather varies according to income.

A family is usually required to spend all, a *spenddown,* or a set percentage of their income above some base amount, as all or 25 percent of any income over $5000, as a deductible before medical care benefits are covered. There may be a maximum amount on the deductible. The sliding scale concept can also apply to *coinsurance* and *copayments.* IV.B.

Smith, Theobald. U.S. bacteriologist, 1859–1934. He separated bovine and human tubercle bacilli, contributed to the study of allergy, and showed the importance of insect *vectors* in the transmission of such diseases as cattle tick fever. VIII.A.1., VIII.C.

smog. properly, a combination of smoke and fog, see *particle;* commonly, any visible air *pollution.*

*Acid smog results from the combination in the atmosphere of a smoke aerosol retained in fog and of gaseous or liquid acid pollutants, originating primarily from stationary *emission* sources. *Photochemical smog results from the combination of gaseous photochemical oxidants and a liquid aerosol, originating from solar radiation action on pollutants from motor vehicle exhausts. I.C.1.

smoke. 1. the gaseous product of burning, made visible by suspension of solid and liquid *particles* in the gas. 2. emit, inhale, or make smoke. 3. as a medical concern, breathing, usually *habitually,* the smoke of burning plant material, especially marijuana or tobacco. 4. cure or preserve food by exposing it to smoke. 5. synonym, *fumigate.* *Main-stream smoke is cigarette smoke which has been exhaled. *Side-stream smoke is cigarette smoke which has never been inhaled. This is an important part of *passive smoking, breathing smoke from other people's cigarettes, a surprisingly serious problem. I.C.1., II.B.2.

smokenders. a common name for a group therapy program for smokers, usually combining education, *self-care* principles, and *behavior therapy;* compare *Weight Watchers.* V.C.

Snow, John. English physician and epidemiologist, 1813–1858. In 1854, Snow showed on the basis of brilliant *epidemiological* analysis that cholera is transmissible by water, from person to person, and by *contaminated* food. He inferred that the cause of the disease is a living organism. VIII.A.1., VIII.C.

SOAP. see *problem-oriented medical record.*

social benefit. antonym, *social cost.*

social cost. detrimental effect or *cost* imputable to an economic activity and borne not by the economic unit immediately involved but by other economic units not directly involved or by government or society as a whole; antonym, *social benefit;* compare *externality* and *internal cost.*

Social costs can be diffuse or concentrated, immediate or deferred, perceptible or not, monetary or nonmonetary. Environmental *pollution* is a social cost. *Herd immunity* is a social benefit of individual immunization. VII.D.1.

social good. see *good.*

social health maintenance organization (S/HMO). a project which integrates "health and social services under the direct financial management of a provider" (sec. 2355(b) of the Deficit Reduction Act of 1984).

This legislative authority continued demonstration funding by the Health Care Financing Administration of integrated provision of social services by a few *health maintenance organizations,* providing them 100 percent, rather than the 90 percent usually given HMOs, of the *average area per capita cost* for caring for Medicare beneficiaries to pay for the social services. Social services are not defined, although HCFA has implied that they include "chronic care benefits," which include home health care, *meals on wheels,* adult day care, transportation services, and nursing home custodial care. III.B.1.

social history. in an individual medical *history,* pertinent facts about the person's past and present social situation. There is no standard form or content.

Ordinarily only material of current relevance to the individual's health is recorded. However, a complete social history might cover salient parts of the family social history and the individual's places of residency, education, military experience, occupations, religion, habits, and usual recreation. II.A.1.

social insurance. a device for pooling *risks* by their transfer to an organization, usually governmental, that is required by law to provide *indemnity,* cash, or *service benefits* to or on behalf of covered persons upon the occurrence of specified *losses;* compare *social security* and *welfare.*

Social insurance is usually characterized by all the following conditions: Coverage is *compulsory* by law; eligibility for benefits is derived, in fact or in effect, from contributions made to the program by the claimant or a person upon whom the claimant is *dependent;* there is no requirement that the individual lack adequate financial *resources,* although eligibility may have to be established; methods for determining benefits are prescribed by law; benefits for an individual are not directly related to contributions made by or in respect of that individual but instead redistribute income so as to favor certain groups, as those with low former wages or a large number of dependents; there is a definite plan for financing the benefits designed to be adequate in terms of long-range considerations; the cost is borne primarily by contributions made by *covered* persons, their employers, or both; the plan is administered or at least supervised by the government; and the plan is not established by the government solely for its present or former employees. Examples in this country include Social Security, railroad retirement, and *workmen's* and *unemployment compensation.* In other countries, health insurance is often a government-sponsored social insurance program; see *national health insurance.* IV.B., IV.D.

socialized medicine. 1. medical care where the organization and provision of medical services is under direct governmental control and providers are employed by or contract for the provision of services directly with the government. 2. generally and irregularly any existing or proposed health *system* believed by the speaker to be subject to excessive governmental control. III.D., VIII.B.3.

social medicine. the study of the medical needs of society and of the influence of social factors and social organization on the promotion and protection of health and the cause and course of disease; compare *community medicine* and *public health.*

Social medicine is not an established or clinical *specialty.* It is practiced through efforts to create a *healthful* society; see *Health Research Group* and *Physicians for Social Responsibility.*

See *Rudolph Virchow.* III.C.

social problem. 1. a difficulty experienced by an individual arising from the nature of society or the individual's place in it, particularly one which contributes to illness in the individual, as inability to obtain needed medical care because of poverty from lack of work in a society with high unemployment. 2. a defect in a society, particularly one which is unhealthful, as subsidization of tobacco growing. 3. an individual who presents society with a *problem,* as a homeless waif. I.B.2.

social psychiatry. the field of *psychiatry* concerned with the cultural, ecological, and social factors that engender, precipitate, intensify, prolong, or otherwise complicate maladaptive patterns of behavior and its treatment; sometimes synonymous, *community psychiatry,* although the latter term should be limited to practical or clinical applications of social psychiatry. III.C.

social security. 1. the principle or practice of public provision for the economic security and social welfare of the individual and family, as through *social insurance* or *welfare.* 2. a U.S. government program for old age and survivors insurance, contributions to state unemployment insurance, and related purposes.

The program was established in 1935 by the *Social Security Act, which now includes authority for the *maternal and child health program,* (Title V), the Supplemental Security Income program (Title XVII), Medicare (Title XVIII), Medicaid (Title XIX), and social services grants to the states (Title XX). IV.D., VIII.B.3.

Social Security Administration (SSA). the administrative unit within the Department of Health and Human Services which manages the social security programs, other than Medicare and Medicaid, which are administered by the *Health Care Financing Administration.* III.B.1.

social service. synonym, *social work.*

social services designee. an individual identified in a *skilled nursing* or *intermediate care facility* to provide social services under the direction of a consulting social worker.

A designee should have at least two years of college education and, preferably, a bachelor of arts degree. State licensure is not required because the function of a social service designee is not an occupation but rather a role specified in regulations and assigned to an otherwise employed member of the facility staff. III.A.4.

social work. activity, service, or use of community resources and people's adaptive capacities to help individuals, families, and groups adjust to their social and environmental situations and deal with problems of social functioning affecting their health or well-being; synonym, social service. III.C.

social worker (SW). a *professionally* trained person who practices social work or provides social services.

Most social workers hold a master's degree in social work (MSW). The bachelor of arts in social work (BSW) is an entry-level professional degree. About a tenth of all social workers are in health care. Most of these work in health and government social service programs, although a few are engaged in independent private practice. Some states regulate social work, and a few require licensure for private practice. The National Association of Social Workers (NASW) requires that social workers in independent practice have at least an MSW and two years of professionally supervised practice in the methods to be employed in independent practice. III.A.4.

society. a *population* sharing common culture, institutions, and economic resources; compare *biome* and *community.* I.B.2.

socioeconomic status (SES). a measure of an individual's class or place in society, using education, income, occupation, or other attributes to locate the individual in one of up to six arbitrary hierarchical groups for research or demographic purposes. I.B.2.

sole community hospital (SCH). a hospital which (1) is more than 50 miles from any similar hospital, (2) is 25 to 50 miles from a similar hospital and isolated from it at least one month a year as by snow, or is the exclusive provider of services to at least 75 percent of its *service area* population, (3) is 15 to 25 miles from any similar hospital and is isolated from it at least one month a year, or (4) has been designated as an SCH under previous rules.

The Medicare *diagnosis related group* program makes special optional payment provisions for SCHs, most of which are rural, including providing that their rates are set permanently so that 75 percent of their payment is hospital-specific and only 25 percent is based on regional DRG rates.

Read "Sole Community Hospitals: Are They Different?" (NCHSR Publications Branch, 1-46 Park Building, Rockville, MD 20857). III.B.1, IV.C.1.

solid waste. useless, unwanted, or discarded material with insufficient liquid content to be free flowing; compare *sewage* and *waste*.

Various kinds of solid waste are named, generally by their origin, as *commercial waste from stores and other activities that do not actually make a product and *municipal waste, which is the domestic or residential and commercial waste generated within a community. I.C.4.

solo practice. *practice* of a health or other professional as a self-employed individual.

Solo practice is by definition *private practice* but not necessarily *general practice* or *fee-for-service* practice (solo practitioners may be paid by *capitation*, although fee-for-service payment is far more common). Solo practice is common among physicians, dentists, podiatrists, optometrists, and pharmacists and less common and sometimes illegal in other professions, as *denturism*, nursing, and social work. V.

somatic. bodily, corporeal; of or pertaining to the body or soma, rather than the psyche, sperm or ovum organs, or environment. I.A.1.

sound. free from injury or disease, robust, wholesome; correct, legal, reliable, valid. I.A.1.

sound. energy that by traveling in a medium elicits the sensation of hearing; mechanical radiating energy transmitted by longitudinal pressure waves in air or other media, the objective cause of hearing.

Sound is measured in *decibels*, is called *noise* when unwanted, and has many important physical, psychic, and social effects. Since sound is defined by hearing, a tree that falls in the forest where nothing can hear it makes no sound. I.C.2.

sound pressure level (SPL). a measure of *noise* in a given environment; the most used of a variety of distinct measures of sound, as sound energy, intensity, level, power, pressure, and spectrum.

The SPL is the value in *decibels* of 20 times the logarithm to the base 10 of the ratio of the pressure of a given sound to a reference pressure (commonly 20 micropascals, or 0.0002 microbar). (See Table p. 401.) I.C.2.

special care. synonym, *critical* or *intensive care*.

Special care has no special meaning and includes a great variety of special programs and units. Some generic technical definitions require specific physician or nurse staffing, equipment, and physical space in units recognized or reimbursed as providing special care; read *Federal Register,* 45: 21582–8, 1980. VII.C.5.a.

SOUND PRESSURE

Level, dB	Loudness	Noise Source
100–120	Deafening	Thunder, boiler factory, jet
80–100	Very loud	Noisy factory, cocktail party, loud hi-fi
60–80	Loud	Noisy office, average TV, loud conversation
40–60	Moderate	Noisy home, average conversation, kitchen noise, urban background noises
20–40	Faint	Quiet home, quiet conversation, rural background noise
0–20	Very faint	Whisper, rustle of leaves

specialist. one who practices or has special education in a specialty; a physician, dentist, or other health professional who limits his or her practice to a certain branch of medicine or dentistry.

Specialists usually have additional education and training related to their specialties, and most have *board certification* as specialists by the related specialty board. Increasingly hospitals, payment programs, and the profession itself define only physicians with board certification as specialists.

See *board eligible, general practice, secondary care,* and *relative value schedule.* III.A.1., III.C.

specialty. 1. a branch of medicine to which one devotes one's practice, whether full- or part-time and with or without special training and certification, usually to the partial or total exclusion of other specialties or *general practice.* 2. the group of persons, specialists, practicing the specialty. 3. the body of medical knowledge which such specialists use in their practice.

A specialty may be devoted to specific services or procedures, as radiology, surgery, and pathology; specific populations, as pediatrics and geriatrics; certain organs or body systems, as dermatology and orthopedics; or groups of diseases, as medical oncology and allergy and immunology. The recognized or established specialties are those with specialty boards. Geriatrics, for example, has no board but will have certificates of special competence from both family practice and internal medicine, i.e., be a subspecialty of both. Usage is irregular, usually referring to *subspecialties* as specialties; medical oncology is a subspecialty of internal medicine.

See *board eligible* and *certified, Graduate Medical Education National Advisory Committee to the Secretary, DHHS,* and *secondary care.* III.C.

specialty board. an organization that *certifies* physicians or dentists as specialists or subspecialists in one of various fields of medical and dental science.

The standards for certification may specify length and type of training and experience and include written and oral examination of applicants. The boards are not educational institutions, and the certificate of a board is not considered a degree. Specialties and their boards are recognized and approved by the American Board of Medical Specialties in conjunction with the American Medical Association Council on Medical Education. Some boards are called colleges. The certificate is called a *diploma, and one who holds it is a diplomate. III.A

specification standard. a *standard* specifying facilities or methods which must be used in doing a piece of work; the principal type of *occupational safety and health standard;* contrast *performance standard.*

Specification standards are easily enforced but inflexible because only one way of doing the job is allowed. Their inflexibility requires a *variance* procedure for any new or safer approach to the *hazard* or other problem with which the standard deals. VI.D., VII.D.2.

specificity. a measure of the ability of a diagnostic or screening *test* to correctly identify the negative or healthy people; the proportion of actual negatives correctly identified as negative.

Specificity equals *true negatives* divided by true negatives plus *false positives.* A test may be quite specific without being very *sensitive.* VIII.D.

specific learning disability (SLD). synonym, *learning disability.*

The addition of the word "specific" reflects the tendency to frequent, sloppy diagnosis of this rare, real problem. It did not prevent the U.S. Senate from passing legislation, refused by the House of Representatives, defining a specific learning disability as an "imperfect ability to read, write, listen, or do mathematical calculations." I.B.2.

specified disease insurance. insurance providing benefits, usually in large amounts with high maximums, for the expense of treating the specific disease or diseases named in the policy.

Such insurance is now rare except for cancer, although coverage of end-stage renal disease by Medicare may be thought of as an example. It used to be common for polio and spinal meningitis. IV.B.2.

speech and hearing (S&H, SH). *audiology* and *speech pathology* together. III.C.

speech therapist, pathologist. an individual trained in or practicing *speech therapy.*

The therapist may study and examine speech problems and conduct treatment programs to improve the communication of children or adults with difficulties arising from physiologic and neurologic disturbances, defective articulation, or foreign dialect. Licensure usually requires a master's degree. The American Speech and Hearing Association (ASHA) awards a certificate of clinical competence requiring academic training at the master's degree level, a year of experience, and passage of a national examination. Nearly half of the ASHA members are employed in elementary or secondary schools, and a large majority are engaged in clinical work, either diagnostic or therapeutic. Some speech pathologists are also trained as audiologists. III.A.4.

speech therapy. the study, examination, and treatment of defects and diseases of voice, speech, and spoken and written language; synonym, speech pathology. It is practiced by *audiologists, otolaryngologists,* and *speech pathologists.* V.

spell of illness. in Medicare, the *benefit period* during which Part A hospital insurance benefits are available.

A benefit period begins when an insured person enters a hospital and ends when that person has not been an inpatient in a hospital or *skilled nursing facility* for 60 consecutive days. During each benefit period, the insured individual is entitled to up to 90 days of hospital care, 100 days in a skilled nursing facility, and 100 home health visits. An additional *lifetime reserve* of 60 hospital days may be drawn upon when more than 90 days of hospital care is needed in a benefit period. There is no limit to the number of benefit periods an insured person may have. The spell of illness concept means the program may pay for more than 90 hospital days in a year, because with a new spell of illness the benefit becomes available again. When a spell continues for a long period, as several years, the program pays less than 90 days of care per year, because it does not pay in the second or third year if there has been no break in the spell of illness. Additionally, in Medicare, the deductible is tied to each spell of illness. Thus an individual hospitalized three times a year, each in a separate spell of illness, pays the deductible of the cost of an inpatient hospital day three times. IV.C.1.

spenddown. a method to establish eligibility for a medical care program by reducing gross income through incurring medical expenses until net income after medical expenses is low enough for program eligibility.

A spenddown is the same as a *sliding scale deductible* related to an individual's overall income. For example, if people are eligible for program benefits if their income is $200 per month or less, a person with a $300 monthly income would be covered after spending $100 *out of pocket* on medical care and one with an income of $350 would not be eligible until he or she incurred medical expenses of $150. The term originated in the Medicaid program. A *categorically related* individual whose income makes him or her ineligible for welfare but is insufficient to pay for medical care thus can become Medicaid eligible as medically needy by spending enough income on medical care. IV.C.2.

spillover benefit or cost. synonyms, social benefit, *spill-in, or *social cost,* *spill-out, respectively.

sponsored dependent. see *dependent.*

sponsored malpractice insurance. a medical *malpractice* insurance plan that includes an agreement by a professional society, as a state medical association, to sponsor a particular insurer's coverage and to cooperate with the insurer in administration of the coverage.

The cooperation may include participation in marketing, claims review, and review of rate making. Until 1975, this was a common form of coverage. It has since largely been replaced by professional society operated plans, *joint underwriting associations,* state insurance funds, and other arrangements. V.D.

sports medicine. the branch of medicine and surgery, typically of orthopedics, concerned with the health of athletes, the healthful conduct of athletic activity, and injuries and diseases associated with exercise and sports. III.C.

spurious association. irregularly, an artifactual, fortuitous, false secondary, or other noncausal *association* due to chance, *bias,* or failure to control for extraneous variables. VIII.C.

squeal rule.   slang, proposed requirement that federally assisted *family planning* programs notify the parents of teenagers who receive contraceptive prescriptions or information.

Efforts in 1982–1983 by the Reagan administration to impose such a rule on the family planning programs were rejected by the U.S. courts as inconsistent with congressional intent that teenagers be served *confidentially.* I.B.1., VII.B.3.b.

staff.   the personnel or corps of specially trained people concerned with the care of patients in a hospital or other health program.

Staffing a patient is group planning by a staff of a patient's care; an unfortunate use of the term as a verb is common among psychologists. See *house staff.* III.A., III.B.1., V.B.

staff patient.   synonym, *service patient;* antonym, *private patient.*

staff privilege.   the privilege given by a hospital or other inpatient health program to a physician or other professional to join the hospital's *medical* staff and hospitalize and/or treat patients; synonyms, admitting, clinical, hospital, and practice privilege.

A practitioner is granted privileges after meeting certain standards, being accepted by the medical staff and hospital board of trustees, and undertaking to carry out certain duties for the hospital, as teaching without pay or providing emergency or charitable services. Most U.S. hospitals are staffed by physicians who are *private practitioners* and obtain access to hospital facilities in this manner. A physician may have staff privileges at more than one hospital or may not have them at any hospital. Many hospitals limit privileges for certain services to *board certified* physicians. Full-time *hospital-based physicians* and physicians working in a system such as a prepaid group practice with its own hospital are not usually thought of as having staff privileges. Many hospitals have several different types or grades of privileges as active, associate, courtesy, or limited privileges. These have irregular meaning. III.B.1.

stage.   a phase or division of a disease characterized by particular symptoms or signs; a period or step in a process, activity, or development, as of anesthesia or an operation.

The courses of many cancers are divided into stages by the size and nature of the *tumor, nodes,* and *metastases. Work-up* to stage a cancer is necessary because the various stages often have quite different treatments and prognoses. II.A.2.

standard.   a thing, degree, or quality established by competent authority as the rule for judging the quantity or quality of a similar thing; something with the quality measured.

Conformity with standards may be a *condition of participation* or of *licensure, accreditation,* or payment for services or may be necessary to avoid penalties. In health care, standards may be defined in relation to the actual or predicted *outcomes* of care; the performance or credentials of professional personnel; and the physical plant, governance, and administration of programs. In the *peer review organization* program, standards are professionally developed ranges of acceptable variation from a *norm* or *criterion.* Thus, if the criteria for diagnosing a urinary tract infection were urinalysis and urine culture, then a standard might require urinalysis in all cases and culture only in previously treated cases.

See *American National Standards Institute, occupational safety and health standards, performance standard, specification standard,* and *variance.* VI.D., VII.D.2.

standard age groups.   "<1; 1–4; 5–14; 15–44; 45–64; >65. These groups may be further subdivided into smaller cohorts provided the standard division points are retained" (*NAPCRG, 1978*) I.A.1., VIII.C.

standard deviation (SD).   a mathematical measure of the dispersion or spread of scores about their *mean;* the square root of the average of the squares of the deviations of individual observations from the mean, conventionally represented by the Greek letter sigma.

The standard deviation measures the width of a *normal curve,* a small value being associated with observations which cluster around the mean and a large one deriving from widely scattered observations. About 65 percent of observed values fall within one standard deviation on either side of the mean, and 95 percent fall within two. VIII.D.

standard error.   the standard deviation divided by the square root of the number of items in a sample tested; the standard deviation of the sample mean.

The standard error measures the presumed distribution of measurement *errors.* For example, Wechsler IQ scores have a mean of 100, standard deviation of 15, and standard error of 3. This means that for any given test score, the probability that it is a true (*valid,* not erroneous) score can be estimated. The true value has a 65 percent probability of being in the range of the obtained score plus or minus 3, and a 95 percent probability of being the obtained score plus or minus 6. VIII.D.

standardized death rate.   in biometry, the number of deaths per 1000 which would have occurred in some standardized population, as the standard million, with a known age-specific death rate.

The rate may be standardized for race, sex, or other variables with known death rates. The *standard million is a population of 1 million divided in age groups in the same proportions as the age distribution in a designated population, as of England and Wales in 1901 or the United States in 1940. II.C.

standard methods.   common name for the American Public Health Association's *Standard Methods for the Examination of Water and Wastewater Including Bottom Sediments and Sludges.*

This bible for *sanitarians* is the source of instructions for such tests as *biologic* and *chemical oxygen demands* and a variety of other useful information. I.C.4.

standard metropolitan statistical area (SMSA).   a U.S. urban area specified by the Census Bureau with a central city with a population of over 50,000 people and including adjoining suburban areas. The bureau reports demographic and other census data in detail for SMSAs and their many divisions, *census tracts. II.C.

standing order (SO).   see *order.*

Stanford-Binet test.   see *intelligence quotient.*

stat.   at once, immediately; abbreviation of the Latin *statim.* V.

state comprehensive health planning agency (state CHP, 314(a) agency).   a state *health planning* agency formerly assisted under section 314(a) of the *Public Health Service Act.*

These agencies developed state *comprehensive health planning* programs with the assistance of a health planning council broadly representative of the state's *consumers* (who had a majority of the membership) and health organizations. The Comprehensive Health Planning and Public Health Service amendments of 1966, P.L. 89-749, began the program. It was superseded by the National Health Planning and Resources Development Act of 1974, P.L. 93-641, which authorized assistance for *State Health Planning and Development Agencies* as replacements for the 314(a) agencies. The agencies were quite variable in effectiveness and functions (some, but not all, having *certificate-of-need* power or administering the state *Hill-Burton* program).

See *areawide comprehensive health planning agency.* VI.A.2.

state cost commission. a state agency assigned health services *cost* and *charge* regulation or review responsibilities; synonym, state rate review commission.

Most commissions are solely or primarily concerned with hospitals. The duties of a commission may include assuring total hospital revenues are reasonably related to total services provided, rates bear a reasonable relationship to costs, and rates are calculated equitably to preclude discriminatory pricing among a hospital's various services and patients; see *sick tax.* VI.D.1.

state health planning and development agency (SHPDA). a state *health planning* agency assisted under section 1521 of the *Public Health Service Act.* Though Congress repealed the planning law in 1987, most states have retained SHPDAs.

The National Health Planning and Resources Development Act of 1974, P.L. 93-641, replaced existing *state comprehensive health planning agencies* with state health planning and development agencies and specified their structure, functions, and funding. SHPDAs prepare an annual preliminary state health plan for *health systems agencies* to use in their planning and a state medical facilities plan to guide the state *Hill-Burton* program which they administer. They also serve as the designated review agency for *section 1122* and administer a *certificate-of-need* program. VI.A.2.

statement of managers. see *conference.*

state rate review commission. synonym, *state cost commission.*

statewide health coordinating council (SHCC). a state council of *consumers,* who are in the majority, and *providers* that supervises the work of the *state health planning and development agency* and reviews and coordinates the plans and *budgets* of the state's *health systems agencies.*

static deductible. see *deductible.*

station. a place within a health facility or program where care is given; usually a *nurse's station,* occasionally an aide or medicine station. A *station hospital in the military is a fixed one at a military post or station; compare *mobile army surgical hospital.* III.B.1.

statistic. synonym, datum. *Statistics is the science of collecting, analyzing, and interpreting data. *Statistical inference is generalizing from observation of a specified *sample* to a whole *population;* making estimates concerning a population from information gathered from samples. VIII.D.

statute of limitation. a law specifying the time interval during which an injured party may sue for recovery of damages arising from an act.

The interval varies in different jursidictions.
See *discovery rule*. VIII.B.3.

statutory rape. sexual intercourse with a female under the age of *consent* in
the jurisdiction in which the event occurs, with or without her consent; synonym, second-degree rape.

Rape is often defined differently in modern statutory law than it is in
traditional common law, and these modern statutes are themselves variable in such as the above definition. VIII.B.3.

steer. direct a patient to a particular provider in violation of *freedom of choice,*
an unethical practice. VIII.B.3.

steerer. one who directs patients to a provider for a fee; synonym, *capper.*

Fee splitting is one result of steering. Being or using a steerer is expressly forbidden in some state medical practice acts. III.A., VIII.B.2.a.

stepfamily. synonym, blended or reconstituted family; see *family.*

stillbirth (SB). delivery of a fetus that died before or during delivery; refers
to either the delivery or the fetus; compare *fetal death* and *live birth.*

Usage is sometimes limited to fetuses of an age or weight potentially
or usually viable, as over 1000 grams.

See *death rate* and *perinatal mortality.* I.A.1.

stock insurance company. an insurance company owned by stockholders
and operated for the purpose of making a *profit;* contrast *mutual insurance
company.* In the former, the profits go to the owners; in the latter, to the
insured. IV.B.

storm sewer. a *sewer* that carries only rain or snow water runoff; contrast
sanitary sewer. I.C.4., I.C.5.

strain. see *stress.*

strategic family therapy. family therapy which solves problems by improving family patterns of behavior and functioning

Strategic and structural family therapy are two major variants of approaches to families which view the family as a *system* and are often combined in practice. Strategic approaches are theoretically rooted in theories
of how to change systems. Such therapy gives particular emphasis to fram-
ing solvable problems; use of tasks and directives, often paradoxical;
positive interpretation of symptoms, problems, and other homeostatic mechanisms; and achieving change outside the therapeutic session. This approach gives special attention to ethical and training issues, particularly
requiring direct observation of trainees at work. It has been used successfully with anorexia, psychosis, and depression in families.

Read Madanes, Cloe, *Strategic Family Therapy* (San Francisco: Jossey-
Bass Publishers, 1984). V.A.

stress. a physical, chemical, emotional, or other force applied to an organism, system, or thing which requires it to adjust to maintain homeostasis
or avoid injury; the exertion of such force; the state of being subject to such
force. A *stressor is such a force. *Strain is the state of being subject to
stress, or the resulting adjustment, although the terms are often used interchangeably.

Stressed people fatigue and age more rapidly than others and are more
likely to make mistakes, suffer injury, and develop disease. Some of these
diseases, as ulcers and alcoholism, are produced directly by the stress and
how it is handled. In others, stress increases *susceptibility* without being
an apparent cause. While stress is a normal part of life and is found ev-

erywhere, it is particularly important in *occupational health,* where stressors are many and often unnatural and may be severe but should be controllable. Important sources of occupational stress are *noise* and the pressure of piecework.

See *relaxation response.* I.A., I.C.

stressful life event. any event, good or bad, in personal or family life which puts substantial stress on the people involved, as birth, marriage, death, moving, or changing jobs; compare *life change event.*

People who undertake and suffer such events are so predictably more likely than those who do not to experience unexpected illness or dysfunction that the events may be assigned graded values and used to give odds on developing illness in the coming year; see *health hazard appraisal.*

Read Holems, T.H., and R.H. Rahe, "The Social Readjustment Rating Scale" (*J Psychosom Res,* 11: 213–18, 1967). I.A.2.

stroke. informal synonym, cerebrovascular accident; damage to part of the brain from interruption of its blood supply, whether because an artery breaks and bleeds into brain tissue, *cerebral hemorrhage, or is blocked by locally forming clot, *cerebral thrombosis, or by lodging of a clot formed elsewhere and carried to the brain in the blood stream, *cerebral embolism.

Strokes kill tissue and may produce loss of sensation, paralysis, seizures, coma, and death. They are a major cause of morbidity and mortality in the United States and therefore, along with *cancer* and *heart disease,* have been the subject of *categorical* health programs, as the *Regional Medical Program.* II.B.2.

stroke clinic. euphemism, the golf course, as in, "I'm sorry, the doctor can't see you Wednesday afternoon, he'll be in stroke clinic." VIII.B.2.a.

strontium 90 (^{90}Sr). a *radioactive isotope* of strontium, a malleable, ductile metal with atomic number 38.

Strontium has little significant medical use. ^{90}Sr is a product of uranium fission and a major component of *fallout.* It has a half-life of 28 years, enters the diet through grain and milk, and becomes concentrated in bone. I.A.1., I.A.3.

structural family therapy. family therapy which solves problems by improving family structure and boundaries.

Structural approaches are rooted in family theory and images of appropriate family structure and functioning for each family's development stage, tasks, and socioeconomic circumstances. Unbalancing dysfunctional systems and intensifying symptoms are seen as inevitable concomitants of change and thus are often induced. Desired change is enacted within the therapeutic session. This approach has been effective with children with school and behavioral problems. Neither strategic, structural, nor other family therapy has been subject to much long-term follow-up, *random controlled trial,* or even analysis of large series of cases.

See Minuchin, Salvador, and H. Charles Fishman, *Family Therapy Techniques* (Cambridge, MA: Harvard University Press, 1981). V.

structural integration. a deep *massage* technique, developed by Ida P. Rolf (U.S. biochemist), which is designed to help a person realign the body by altering the length and tone of myofascial tissues; compare *Alexander technique.*

Practitioners of rolfing, as the technique is commonly known, believe that misalignment resulting from inaccurate learning about posture and from emotional and physical trauma may have a detrimental effect on one's health, energy, self-image, perceptions, and muscular efficiency. Rolfers use ten one-hour sessions to achieve a correct vertical posture in their subjects.

structural measure. see *input measure.*

study. a considered endeavor toward some object, usually acquiring knowledge of a particular subject.

There are many formal types of study, see *case control, cohort, crossover, double-blind, longitudinal,* and *random controlled.* VIII.D.

Study on Surgical Services for the United States (SOSSUS). a major federally funded study of the supply, distribution, and workloads of U.S. surgeons, *Surgery in the United States,* done by the American College of Surgeons and the American Surgical Association and published by them in 1975.

When some people still thought there was a physician shortage, it concluded most U.S. surgeons' workloads were light and made recommendations, never followed, for limiting the number of surgeons. III.A.1.

study population. "all patients included in a study during the period of a project" (*NAPCRG, 1978*).

See *rate.* VIII.D.

subclinical. of a disease with manifestations so slight as to go unnoticed or not to be demonstrable; compare *clinical* and *preclinical.* II.

subject. in research, an individual who is studied physiologically or psychologically in an experiment.

Using subjects as their own *controls* compares them with themselves before and after treatment or after different treatments. This has the advantage of decreasing error variance and the likelihood of showing significant differences with relatively small groups and the disadvantage of risking *practice effects* that occur with repeated measurements. VIII.D.

subjective, objective, assessment, and plan (SOAP) notes. see *problem-oriented medical record.*

subluxation of the spine. an incomplete or partial dislocation of two adjacent vertebrae.

Normally the vertebral bodies are squarely situated atop one another, but such things as trauma and arthritis may shift one vertebral body with respect to its neighbor. When the shift does not abolish contact between normally adjacent surfaces but does alter their position with respect to each other, the abnormally positioned vertebra is subluxed or partially dislocated. Services of *chiropractors* are covered under Medicare only when subluxation is demonstrated on x-ray. II.B.2., IV.C.1.

subrogation. succession or acquisition by an insurance company, after payment of a *loss,* to or of the insured's rights against any other party responsible for the loss, as against a person *negligently* causing the loss or another insurer covering the same loss.

Health insurance does not ordinarily subrogate the insured as auto and property insurance often do. If it did, companies could sue when negligence caused covered expenses or recover from other insurers. This might limit expenses and avoid some *duplication of benefits* but would be time-consuming and expensive.

subscriber. casual synonym, *member* or *beneficiary;* strictly, only individual family heads or employees who have elected to contract for, participate in, or subscribe to insurance or a health maintenance organization plan for themselves and their eligible *dependents;* compare *guarantor.* IV.B.

subsequent injury fund. synonym, *second-injury fund.*

subspecialty. a part of a *specialty.*
   Subspecialization is often achieved with an extra year or more of training as a *resident* or *fellow.* The recognized subspecialties in U.S. medicine are those in which a *certificate of special competence is awarded by the appropriate *specialty board,* as those of *internal medicine,* or those which have wholly separate residencies from the parent specialty's, as those of *preventive medicine.* There are many unofficial subspecialties, as diabetology. III.C.

substance abuse. any illegal or hazardous use of a chemical, typically a drug; compare *designer drug.* Often used as a synonym for *drug dependence,* sometimes includes legal, nonmedical, or recreational uses, even when not hazardous. II.B.2., VIII.B.3.

substitution. the filling of a *prescription* by a pharmacist with a drug product *therapeutically* and *chemically equivalent* to, but not, the one prescribed.
   Some states have *antisubstitution* laws which prohibit the pharmacist from filling a prescription with any product other than the specific product of the manufacturer whose *brand name* is used on the prescription.
   See *generic name* and *maximum allowable cost.* III.B.3.

subsystems. one part of a system, particularly a family system normally differentiated into a variety of smaller units that serve certain functions. Family subsystems include dyads such as the parental subsystem and those formed by generation, by sex, by interest, or by function. Individuals may belong to a number of subsystems, but in each subsystem different levels of power exist for each individual. I.B.1.

suburb. an outlying, typically residential area of a city or town, often including adjacent but separate smaller towns and villages within commuting distance; compare *rural* and *urban.* I.B.2.

suffer. to submit to, be forced to endure, labor under, undergo, experience; to sustain loss or damage; to be subject to *disability* or *handicap.*
   Suffering usually, but not necessarily, involves some experience of physical or emotional pain. Similarly, people with pain may not suffer from it.

sufficient cause. see *cause.*

summary. see *discharge summary.*

superbill. jargon, a combined *encounter* form and statement of *charges* which may be used by either a provider or patient to *file* for insurance *benefits.*
   To serve these purposes the bill must properly identify the patient, provider, insurance policy, *diagnoses* treated, services or *procedures* performed, and charges for the encounter. Often computer-generated, the appearance of superbills in physicians' offices has been accompanied by increased demand for cash at the time of service and decreased acceptance of *assignment* and other forms of assistance to the patient in filing insurance. VII.D.1.

SuperPro. an organization which contracts with the federal Department of Health and Human Services to review the operation of *peer review orga-*

nizations, particularly their work on admission rates and diagnosis related group validations. VI.D.2.

Supplemental Feeding Program for Women, Infants, and Children (WIC). a federally funded and guided program administered by state and local health departments that provides food supplements, as powdered milk, and other services to poor pregnant women and children who have, or are at high risk for, illness, anemia, or pregnancy at an early age. VII.A.1.

supplemental health insurance. health insurance that covers medical expenses not covered by separate insurance already held by the insured. For example, insurance companies sell policies to people covered by Medicare that cover *cost-sharing* expenses required by Medicare, services not covered, or both. Where cost sharing is intended to control *utilization,* the availability of supplemental health insurance for cost-sharing expenses limits its effectiveness. IV.B.2.

supplemental health service. an *optional service* which *health maintenance organizations* may provide in addition to *basic health services.*

The supplemental services may be anything; the law includes a long laundry list of possibilities, as dental and additional mental health services, which would be good but are too costly to be required or competitive. III.B.1.

Supplemental Security Income (SSI) program. a program of income support for low-income aged, blind, and *disabled* persons, authorized by title XVI of the Social Security Act.

SSI replaced state *welfare* programs for the aged, blind, and disabled in 1972. It is a federally administered program. States may supplement the basic benefit amount. Receipt of a federal SSI benefit or a state supplement under the program often establishes Medicaid eligibility. I.A.2.c.

Supplementary Medical Insurance Program (Part B, SMI). the voluntary portion of Medicare in which all persons entitled to the *hospital insurance program* (Part A) may enroll.

The program is financed on a current basis from monthly premiums paid by people insured by the program and a matching amount from federal *general revenues.* About 95 percent of eligible people are enrolled. During any calendar year, the program pays, with certain exceptions, 80 percent of the *reasonable charge* for covered services after the insured pays an initial deductible. Covered services include physician services, home health care, medical and other health services, outpatient hospital services, and laboratory, pathology, and radiology services. Any individual over 65 may enroll in Part B. Individuals not eligible for Part A who elect to buy into Part A must also buy into Part B. State welfare agencies may buy Part B coverage for elderly and disabled public assistance recipients and pay the premiums on their behalf. The program contracts with *carriers* to process *claims* under the program. Part B refers to part B of title XVIII of the Social Security Act, the legislative authority for the program. IV.C.1.

supplementation. partial payment for a portion of the cost of nursing home care by a patient or the patient's family.

Supplementation was a common requirement in state Medicaid programs before it was stopped by a directive of the Senate Finance Committee in its report on the 1967 Social Security amendments. Supplementation should be distinguished from the practice of requiring an individual to contribute his or her excess income to offset state payment for care. Generally, under Medicaid, a nursing home must agree to accept reimbursement from the state as the full amount of its payment for service. As an example of the present Medicaid approach, a state may pay $500 a month for nursing home care for which a home charges $600. If an individual has $125 in personal income, he or she is allowed to retain $25 for personal incidental expenses and pays $100 to help meet the $500 rate for his or her care. The state pays the other $400, and the home must settle for $500. With supplementation, a state pays $500 but the nursing home does not accept it as full payment, requiring supplementation of the state rate by the individual or the individual's family. The amount a home collects in supplement is not under state control. Supplementation, albeit subject to abuse, was used where the state rate was admittedly insufficient to pay the cost of the care. III.B.1., IV.C.2.

supplier.   1. any program or individual that furnishes supplies or services. 2. in Medicare, a physician, nonhospital laboratory, ambulance company, or other *provider* paid by *carriers* on the basis of *reasonable charges;* contrast *institutional provider.* III., IV.C.1.

supplies.   items or a quantity, usually readily available for use and disposable, as bandages, tongue depressors, or drugs; distinguish fixed and durable *capital goods,* i.e., those whose use lasts over a year. III.B.2.

supply.   in economics, the quantity of *goods* or *services* offered for sale at various prices, with *income* and other factors held constant.
   Increases in price usually induce increases in supply. Increases in *demand* (but not necessarily in *need*) normally induce increases in price. VIII.B.1.

supply-push inflation.   see *inflation.*

support group, support system.   the people, resources, and organizations that help an individual exist and endure. Some usage limits the meaning to people outside the immediate family, although usually one's family is one's major support.
   Old people particularly may have inadequate support from dwindling family, friends, and social connections as well as inadequate financial and other resources. This may cause them to present *problems,* even medical ones, which will get better only if the person's support group or system is improved. I.B.2.

surgeon (S).   a physician specializing by practice or education in surgery or any of its specialties.
   See *itinerant surgeon* and *A. Pare.* III.A.1.

surgeon general (SG).   the chief medical officer of an armed force or public health service unit.
   The *Surgeon General of the United States is the chief medical officer of the *Commissioned Corps* of the U.S. Public Health Service. In recent decades this is neither the highest ranking nor most important health office in the U.S. government. III.A.1.

surgery (S).   1. the science and specialty devoted to trauma and diseases requiring operative treatment or *manipulation.* 2. any of the *operations,* procedures, and treatments developed and applied in surgery. 3. in Great Britain, a practitioner's *office* or place of consultation and treatment.
   There are 10 surgical specialties—*colon and rectal surgery, general surgery, neurologic surgery, obstetrics-gynecology, ophthalmology, orthopedic*

surgery, otolaryngology, plastic surgery, thoracic surgery, and *urology*—and one surgical subspecialty, pediatric surgery.

See *ambulatory, cosmetic, elective, major, minor,* and *unnecessary* surgery and *psychosurgery.* III.C.

surgicenter. a registered trademark and now a synonym for an ambulatory surgical center; a facility that serves outpatients requiring surgical treatment exceeding the capability of a physician's office but not requiring hospitalization as an inpatient. Such centers are not necessarily part of a hospital. The surgery is known as ambulatory surgery, day surgery, or in-and-out surgery. III.B.1., VII.C.4.

surplus. in insurance, the excess of a company's assets, including any *capital,* over *liabilities.*

Surpluses may be used for future dividends, for expansion of business, or to meet possible unfavorable future developments. They are developed and increased intentionally by including an amount in *premiums* in excess of the pure premium needed to meet anticipated liabilities, the *risk charge.* Surpluses are sometimes earmarked in part as *contingency reserves* and in part as unassigned surplus. IV.B.

surveillance system. a monitoring system to determine environmental quality.

Surveillance systems monitor progress toward attainment of environmental standards and identify potential *episodes* of high *pollutant* concentrations in time to take preventive action. I.C.

survivor benefit. synonym, *death benefit.*

susceptibility. capability or probability of developing a disease, given the opportunity; lacking *immunity.*

Susceptibility may be inherited or acquired. Increased susceptibility, sometimes called *hypersusceptibility, is found with *accident proneness,* in *allergies,* and in people *at risk* for something. I.A.

susceptibility bias. see *bias*

Sutton's law. (Willie "the Actor" Sutton, U.S. bank robber, 1901–1980) go where the money is.

Mr. Sutton told the judge he robbed banks because "that's where the money is." In diagnosis of disease one may properly, even legally, be guided by this principle. As they say, "If you hear hoofbeats, don't look for zebras; common disease is common; rare disease, rare." Test for the best bet first. VIII.B.3.

swap maternity. a provision in group health insurance providing immediate *maternity benefits* to a newly covered woman but terminating coverage of pregnancies in progress upon termination of a woman's employment.

See *flat* and *switch maternity.* IV.A.

swine flu. influenza of the specific antigenic type that caused the pandemic of 1918 in humans and is normally endemic in swine.

Swine flu is famous because it appeared briefly in early 1976 in soldiers at Fort Dix, N.J. Since it was unusually virulent in 1918, and because a worldwide epidemic of a new type of influenza was due at the time, a special program, the *swine flu program, was undertaken in the United States in 1976 to immunize Americans against it. II.B.2.

swing bed. a *bed* which may be used interchangeably by a *health facility* for providing different *levels of care,* i.e., as either an acute hospital or skilled nursing bed, and will be reimbursed for whichever use by Medicare, Medicaid, or similar financing programs.

Medicare and Medicaid historically required that facilities with more than one kind of bed have them in distinct parts of the facility, thus requiring that they always be used for the same purpose, but now allow some rural facilities to swing beds. Swing beds would have to meet *standards* set for both hospital and skilled nursing beds. Whether use of the bed is reimbursed at hospital or skilled nursing rates would depend on the level of care required by the patient using the bed. Financing programs generally have not allowed facilities to swing beds among different levels of care as needed. Allowing beds to swing makes it easier for facilities to achieve the economics of maintaining full *occupancy* and for communities to meet shifting needs for different kinds of beds. I.B.1.

switch maternity. a provision in group health insurance providing *maternity benefits* to female employees only when their husbands are covered in the plan as their *dependents.*

This has the effect of denying maternity benefits to single women and married couples who choose separate plans because it is free to the employee but costly to add a dependent.

See *flat* and *swap maternity.* IV.A.

Sydenham, Thomas. English physician, 1624–1689. He developed the useful but incorrect atmospheric-miasmatic theory of disease and gave it an important place in public health thought well into the nineteenth century; known as the English Hippocrates. VII.B.2.e., VIII.A.1.

sylvatic. pertaining to or occurring in the woods or wild animals, as sylvatic plague, which is widely distributed in American wild rodents and their fleas but rarely affects humans. II.

symmetrical association. see *association.*

symptom (Sx). a manifestation or phenomenon of a physical or mental disease or disorder of which the host is subjectively aware, as pain or weakness; contrast an objective *sign,* as a characteristic x-ray change. *symptomatic. of or pertaining to symptoms.

Asymptomatic disease, without symptoms, is hardly *illness* since it produces no awareness of dysfunction or trouble. *Symptomatic treatment responds to symptoms rather than their cause. Characteristic or *pathognomonic* symptoms of a particular disease are called symptomatic, as anginal chest pain is symptomatic of ischemic heart disease. II.A.1.

syndrome. a set or constellation of concurrent symptoms and/or signs which together characterize or identify a specific condition, disease, or disorder. Used particularly of congenital conditions and those with poorly understood causes. II.

synecology. see *ecology.*

synergy. combined or cooperative action or operation, as of drugs, *health hazards,* or muscles and nerves, such that the total action or effect is greater than the sum of the actions taken independently, as carbon monoxide and heat *stress* are more *toxic* together than the sum of their separate actions.

Synergy is common in biology and an important problem in determining doses, *threshold limit values,* and such for individual agents whose true values and dangers may require synergists to be fully expressed. I.A.1.

syniatrist. obsolete, synonym, physician assistant or nurse clinician.

system. a complex unity of diverse parts serving a common plan or purpose; such a unity as a functional whole; related things, organs, or organisms joined by nature or art in regular interaction and interdependence; synonyms, classification, method, network, order, and scheme; compare *economy.*

In systems analysis the *environment* of a system includes whatever it does not control but with which it does interact. What it does control is considered part of the system. What has no effect on it is not even part of the environment.

See *health care delivery system.* I.C.

systematic error. *bias* or false result due to factors other than chance, as faulty measuring instruments; contrast *sampling error.* VIII.D.

Systematized Nomenclature of Dermatology (SNODERM). a microglossary or extract from SNOMED prepared by the American Academy of Dermatology. II.B.1.

Systematized Nomenclature of Medicine (SNOMED). a complete list or catalogue of approved terms and codes for describing and recording pathologic and clinical observations and attributes of *encounters* and patients; the first edition was known as the *Systematized Nomenclature of Pathology (SNOP).

SNOMED is a five-digit hierarchical approach which serves as a classification system as well as a *nomenclature.* It has seven axes (topography or anatomic location, morphology or structure, *etiology,* function, disease, procedure, and occupation) and will add additional axes as they are developed and found useful. Developed by the College of American Pathologists and many collaborating organizations and individuals, it is more coherent, complete, and flexible than major existing systems, as *ICD* and *CPT.*

Read *Systematized Nomenclature of Medicine (SNOMED),* 2d ed. (Skokie, IL: College of American Pathologists, 1979) and Cote, Roger A., and Stanley Robboy, "Progress in Medical Information Management: Systematized Nomenclature of Medicine (SNOMED)," *JAMA,* 243(8): 756–62, 2/22/80). II.B.1., VIII.

Système International d'Unites (SI units). see *International System of Units.*

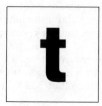

tachyphylaxis. decreasing response to stimulation with repeated exposure, as with desensitization to toxic substances or allergens by previous inoculation of subtoxic doses or with loss of responsiveness to a drug. III.B.3., V.B.

T'ai Chi Ch'uan. an ancient Chinese system of exercise, including some elements of *meditation* and self-defense.

There are several variants, and some overlap with other Chinese practices, see the *Tao of Loving*. As with many probably valid *alternative medical* practices, motivation is crucial to success, since it may take years of practice to acquire the skills involved. These may then help slow aging, ease tension, strengthen muscles, exercise joints, and control breathing. T'ai Chi Ch'uan is used by the *Senior Actualization and Growth Experience* program.

Read Liang, T.T., *Tai Chi Ch'uan for Health and Self-Defense* (New York: Random House, 1977). V.

tail. in malpractice, a provision of a *claims made policy* covering claims made during specified years after the original policy period is over which arise out of injuries occurring during the policy period.

The tail ordinarily must be bought while the original policy is in force. It has the effect of converting claims made to *claims incurred* coverage. V.D.

Take Off Pounds Sensibly (TOPS). a group treatment program for obesity, comparable to *Weight Watchers*. I.A.2.a., V.B.

talk down. treat a panic reaction to use of a *psychotropic*, a *bad trip or high, or another hallucinatory, agitated, or abnormal mental state with calm, firm, reassuring conversation intended to hold the patient's attention and maintain the patient's contact with reality.

This approach is often more effective than medication or restraints, as

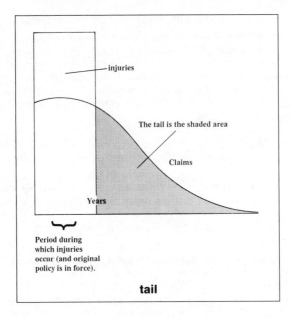

injuries

The tail is the shaded area

Claims

Years

Period during
which injuries
occur (and original
policy is in force).

tail

it would be for many other acute and chronic conditions (if there were enough talkers). V.B.

talking book. a recording of a book read out loud.

In the United States talking books are available free to anyone legally *blind,* incapable of reading standard print, physically incapable of holding a book or turning pages, or certified by a physician as having an organic dysfunction severe enough to prevent normal reading. The service provides playback equipment, catalogues, and recordings postage free through regional libraries and state commissions for the blind to about 1 million of 8 million potential users. III.B.2.

Tao of Loving. part of ancient Chinese medicine which teaches men to control their ejaculations; an aspect of Taoism, an ancient Chinese religion which seeks unity with the Tao, or universal source.

The Tao contributes to personal well-being, harmony, and love between couples and acts as a method of contraception. Popular recently in the United States for obvious reasons.

Read Chang, Jolan, *The Tao of Loving and Sex* (New York: E.P. Dutton, 1977). V.

Target Health Hazard Program. an *Occupational Safety and Health Administration* program which concentrated its early *health hazard abatement* efforts on five major or *target health hazards: asbestos,* cotton dust, see *brown lung,* silica, lead, and carbon monoxide.

These hazards were chosen for their seriousness, the fact that they can be effectively measured and monitored, and the large number of workers *exposed* to them. Despite the enormous importance of these and other health hazards, the basic *safety* bias of the OSHA effort is exemplified by the fact that only a small percentage of inspections are concerned with health hazards. The THH program is now defunct. VII.B.2.d.

Target Industry Program (TIP).   an *Occupational Safety and Health Administration* program which focused enforcement efforts on five specific target industries with especially high injury rates: marine cargo handling or longshoring, roof and sheet metal work, meat and meat products, miscellaneous transportation equipment (primarily mobile home manufacturing), and lumber and wood products.

These industries have *industrial accident rates* about twice the average for manufacturing. In the early 1970s about 40 percent of OSHA inspections were of target industries. This program is now defunct. VII.B.2.d.

tax.   1. a charge or burden, usually pecuniary, laid upon a person or property for public purposes; a forced contribution of wealth to meet the needs of a government. 2. to assess or determine by law or judicially such a charge or contribution.

See *excise, payroll, progressive, proportional,* and *regressive taxes,* and *marginal tax rate.* IV.C

tax credit.   a reduction of liability for federal or other income tax.

Several *national health insurance* proposals allow businesses and/or individuals to reduce their taxes dollar for dollar for specified medical expenses. Using a tax credit rather than a tax deduction gives people and business an equal benefit for each dollar spent on health care. A tax credit favors lower- over higher-income people. A tax deduction increases in value with the *marginal tax rate.* IV.C.

tax deduction.   a reduction in the *income* base on which federal or other income tax is calculated.

Health insurance expenditures are deductible by businesses as a business expense. This means there is a reduction of tax liability of about $1 times the tax rate for each $1 a business spends on health insurance. Individuals may take a *medical deduction* on personal income tax of half the cost of health insurance premiums up to $150 plus all medical expenses and premiums that exceed 3 percent of income. Nationally, each deduction amounts to several billion dollars a year. Since the *marginal tax rate* increases with income, the value of a tax deduction for income spent on medical care increases as income increases. Thus the subsidy is greater for the higher-income person or more profitable corporation. IV.C.

tax expenditure.   revenue lost to government because of a legal tax reduction or tax forgiveness, including tax credits and deductions.

The term emphasizes that such revenues forgone for specific purposes, as subsidizing private purchase of health insurance through federal income tax deductions, are budgetarily equivalent to actual federal expenditures. IV.C.

tax expenditure budget.   in the federal *budget,* an enumeration of revenue losses resulting from tax expenditures. Section 301 of the Congressional Budget and Impoundment Control Act of 1974 requires that estimated levels of tax expenditures be presented by major *functions* in the *congressional* and *presidential budgets.* IV.C.

teaching hospital.   a hospital which provides *undergraduate* or *graduate medical education,* usually with one or more medical, dental, or osteopathic *residency* programs and *affiliation* with a medical school.

Hospitals which educate nurses and other health workers without training physicians are not generally thought of as teaching hospitals, nor are those that have only programs of continuing education for practicing professionals.

See *affiliated hospital* and *house staff.* III.B.1.

teaching physician.   a physician responsible for training and supervising medical students and *residents.*

Teaching physicians are often but not necessarily salaried by the institutions for which they teach. Reimbursement of these physicians has been a subject of considerable controversy. *Medicare* reimburses hospitals through the *hospital insurance program* (Medicare Part A) for costs incurred in compensating physicians for teaching and supervisory activities and in paying the salaries of residents in approved teaching programs. In addition, *reasonable charges* are paid under the *supplementary medical insurance program* (Medicare Part B) for teaching physicians' services to patients. The double payment occurring when Part A pays a resident for performing a service while Part B pays the teaching physician for supervising it was limited by the federal Health Care Financing Administration, DHHS, by allowing Part B payment only when the teaching physician directly and personally participates in the patient's care.

See *private patient.* III.A.1.

technical component.   see *professional component.*

technician (T).   synonym, *technologist;* compare *paraprofessional.*

In *occupational health,* a technician is defined by the *National Institute of Occupational Safety and Health* as a high school graduate trained through short courses and related in-service programs in occupational health and/or safety, typically as an *industrial hygienist* or *inspector.* III.A.4.

technique.   the way in which technical details are treated; method or manner; synonym, *procedure.* V.B.

technologist (T).   one who has learned the practical details, special methods, and use of the *technology* of a subject, as a *medical technologist.*

Technician and technologist are used irregularly, often interchangeably, and are thus best treated as synonyms, with the latter preferred. They may be distinguished by saying technologists learn, usually at a college level, a technology, while technicians are trained, typically in high school, to practice a technique. Technologists do x-rays, laboratory procedures, and such under the direction of and for *professionals* who remain responsible for the quality and for interpreting the meaning of the results. III.A.4.

technology.   1. the application of knowledge to practical purposes; applied science. 2. the means, methods, or language of achieving such purposes.

Technology is *curing* not *caring,* the things used and the technical and scientific knowledge behind them.

See *technologist* and *health care technology.* III.C.

technology assessment.   the *study* of *technology* and specific technologies, including their *use, safety, efficacy,* and *cost-effectiveness,* and of the social and ethical implications of their use.

Conscious efforts to assess medical and surgical *procedures* are a necessary part of their social control. The development of methods of assessment and control has become necessary only in recent years as *health care technology* has become astonishingly powerful and expensive. III.C., VI.D.2.

telephone order (TO).   see *order.*

tension.   inner unrest, striving, imbalance; a feeling of psychologic *stress* manifested by increased muscular tone and other physical indicators of emotion; synonym, *stress.*

teratogen.   substance or agent inducing a *congenital anomaly,* birth defect, or *malformation* in an embryo, as a virus, chemical, or radiation; compare *carcinogen* and *mutagen.* *teratogenesis. embryonic maldevelopment. I.C.

tertiary care.   medical care and services provided by highly specialized providers, as in dialysis or transplant programs.
Such services frequently require highly sophisticated technological and support facilities. The distinction between *secondary* and tertiary care is one of degree, arbitrary and irregular, and not very useful. There is a useful separation of the continuous responsibility for a whole person's needs taken by a *primary* provider, as a family physician, and the episodic role of the specialist seen on *referral* or in *consultation;* even this distinction is blurred by chronic tertiary care, as ongoing dialysis. VII.D.2.

tertiary prevention.   see *preventive medicine.*

test.   1. a trial or examination. 2. a procedure to identify a constituent, detect changes of function, or establish the true nature of a condition.
Tests are evaluated by their *efficiency* and *predictive values, sensitivity,* and *specificity.* For many *laboratory* tests the *normal range* is defined as between two *standard deviations* below and above the *mean.* This means 5 percent of normal people have *false-positive* abnormalities.
See *Ames test.* III.B.2.

test of significance.   a measure of statistical *significance;* a comparison of the observed and predicted probabilities of an event.
If the probabilities are substantially different, the assumptions used in calculating the predicted probability, see *null hypothesis,* are likely to be wrong. VIII.D.

therapeutic.   curative, pertaining to therapy. *therapeutics. the branch of medical science concerned with therapy and the *treatment* of the sick and diseased. V.B.

therapeutic abortion.   see *abortion.*

therapeutic community.   a social organization of patients and personnel in a structured mental hospital setting or milieu, hence also *therapeutic milieu, intended to help patients function within the range of social norms, overcome their dependency needs, and assume responsibility for their own and each other's rehabilitation. The term originated in Great Britain.
See *token economy.* V.B., VII.C.5.b.

therapeutic contract.   in *family therapy,* an agreement by a "family and therapist, at the start of therapy,... on the nature of the problem and on the goals for treatment.
"This contract may or may not have a clearly defined objective, but it must be initially agreed upon, even though at a future time it can be changed" *(Pinney and Slipp, 1982).*
All therapy is at least an unspoken contract. In regular medical practice the patient contracts to pay the physician to tell him or her what to do

about a symptom. Family physicians may further contract to exchange specified desired behaviors with patients. V.B.

therapeutic equivalents. *drug* products from different sources with indistinguishable effects in the treatment of a disease or condition.

Such products are usually but not necessarily *chemical equivalents* or *bioequivalent.* Therapeutic equivalents are sometimes limited to those which are chemical equivalents. Drugs with the same treatment effect which are not chemically equivalent are called *clinical equivalents. This is a useful but inconsistent distinction. III.B.3.

therapeutic index, ratio. the ratio of a toxic dose or one causing unacceptable side effects of a substance to its therapeutic dose.

The index is a measure of a drug's *safety* and *efficacy.* III.B.3.

therapeutic privilege. a physician's common law right to withhold from a patient information about the patient's condition or the risks of treatment if, in the physician's judgment, full disclosure might have a detrimental effect on the physical or psychologic well-being of the patient.

The therapeutic privilege is well recognized in law and serves as a defense for failure to obtain *informed consent* for treatment, although guidelines for its appropriate use have never been specified and obtaining consent from a *competent* close relative is wise.

See *physician-patient privilege.* V.B., VIII.B.3.

therapeutic radiology. see *radiology.*

therapeutic test. a trial of therapy for a specific disease as an aid in the diagnosis of an undiagnosed condition. V.A.

therapy (Rx, Tx). 1. the means of caring for the *sick* and curing their ills. 2. aid for the mentally ill, dysfunctional families, or community problems. Often used in combination, as chemotherapy or psychotherapy; compare *regimen.*

See *art, massage, music, occupational, physical, play, recreation,* and *speech therapy,* among others. V.B.

thermography. a technique for measuring variation in the heat emitted by various parts of the body and recording it as a photographic image for diagnostic purposes, as screening for breast cancer; compare *xeroradiography.* III.B.2., III.C.

third-party payer. an organization, public or private, that pays or *insures* health or medical expenses on behalf of *beneficiaries* or recipients, as Blue Cross, commercial insurance companies, *Medicare,* and *Medicaid.* *Third-party reimbursement is payment by such organizations and comes in many forms and with many rules.

The beneficiary generally pays a *premium* for coverage in all private and some public programs. The organization then pays bills on the patient's behalf. The payments are called third-party payments because of the separation between the individual receiving the service, the first party; the individual or institution providing it, the second party; and the organization paying for it, the third party.

See *indemnity* and *service benefit.* IV.B.

threshold. the minimum *exposure* to or amount of a stimulus, toxic substance, drug, or other agent needed to produce a recognizable effect or response. A *threshold dose is the minimum amount of a drug needed to obtain a therapeutic effect.

The threshold is the point on the exposure-response curve where a response can be first measured. Thresholds may be different for the same substance in different individuals since they are a result of individual *susceptibility*, the circumstances of the *exposure*, and the substance itself. They may also be different for acute and chronic effects of the substance. They may be determined by limitations in our ability to measure small doses and responses rather than by actual failure of the exposed organism to respond. Whether substances, particularly *carcinogens*, have a safe *threshold exposure, below which no response is actually present, or have zero thresholds is a matter of scientific and legal debate, as the argument over changing the *Delaney Amendment,* which treats carcinogens in foods as having zero thresholds. I.C.

threshold limit value (TLV).   in *occupational health,* a guideline for general worker *exposure* to a chemical or physical *hazard;* synonym, permissible concentration. They specify maximum allowable *exposure* in terms of an eight-hour, time-weighted average, as an average for eight hours of less than two fibers per cubic centimeter of *occupational air* for *asbestos.* *Ceiling limits or values control exposure to fast-acting substances by specifying a maximum concentration (the ceiling) as their TLV which must not be exceeded for more than 15 minutes in a work cycle; these substances are marked with a C in TLV tables.

The TLVs have been developed by the American Conference of Governmental Industrial Hygienists and in many cases used by the Occupational Safety and Health Administration as *health standards.* They do not denote a precise demarcation between *safe* and unsafe exposures and are not meant to protect all workers no matter how *susceptible,* although a safety factor is used so that the TLV should be below the level at which any toxic effects occur. Some are based on animal rather than human data.

See *excursion factor* and *synergy.* I.C.

throwaway literature.   clinical reading matter, particularly magazines, which is provided free to the reader and neither indexed in *Index Medicus* nor *reviewed.*

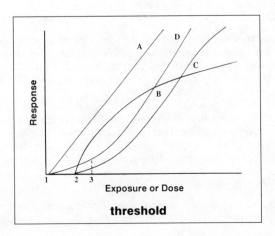

threshold

The costs of throwaways are borne by advertisers, and authors are often paid for their contributions, typically review articles on new drugs or particular diseases.

See *medical literature*. III.C.

tissue bank. see *blood bank*.

tissue committee. a committee, usually of a hospital *medical staff*, which does *tissue review*.

The name derives from the use of pathologic findings from tissue removed at surgery as one element in the review. III.B.1.

tissue remedies. in *homeopathy*, the 12 remedies which, according to homeopathic biochemical theory, form the mineral bases of the body; compare *concordant* and *inimic remedies*. V.

tissue review. an evaluation of surgery performed in a hospital based on the extent of agreement among the preoperative, postoperative, and pathological diagnoses; the appropriateness of the *procedures* done; and other considerations.

The pathological or tissue diagnosis helps determine if the procedures were necessary. Hospitals with tissue committees have been shown to have lower rates of *unnecessary surgery* than do those without. Tissue review is a form of *utilization review*. VI.C.2.

Title XVIII. the part of the Social Security Act which contains the principal legislative authority for the *Medicare* program, and therefore a common name for the program. IV.C.2.

Title XIX. the part of the Social Security Act which contains the principal legislative authority for the *Medicaid* program, and therefore a common name for the program. IV.C.1.

token economy. use of plastic coins or other tokens in a *therapeutic community* or such institutional setting as rewards for patient good behavior, work, or other desired activity. Patients use the tokens in turn to purchase personal items and privileges.

Such *behavior therapy* simulates the real world and avoids the need to use punishment for failure to behave or work. V.B., VII.C.5.b.

tolerance. 1. relative ability of an organism to endure, without physiologic or psychologic modification or *trauma*, the effects of an unfavorable environmental factor or toxic or polluting substance or agent, particularly when acquired by continued use of or exposure to the substance. 2. the amount of a chemical considered safe in a food to be eaten by a person or animal. 3. the allowable deviation from a standard, as the range of variation permitted the content of a drug in one of its dosage forms.

A **tolerance limit* is the maximum level, intensity, accumulation, or duration of a factor, substance, or agent that can be endured by an organism before physiologic or psychologic modifications occur. I.A.1., I.A.2.a., I.C., III.B.3.

tomato effect. failure to use effective treatment for a disease because it does not "make sense" in light of accepted theories of disease mechanisms and drug action, for example, the failure to use aspirin in treating rheumatoid arthritis despite proven efficacy during the first half of this century, when rheumatoid arthritis was thought to be a chronic infection, because aspirin does not control infection. Named after the long-standing refusal of

North Americans to eat tomatoes because, since they are of the nightshade family, they were obviously poisonous; compare *placebo effect.*

Read Goodwin, James S., and Jean M. Goodwin, "The Tomato Effect: Rejection of Highly Efficacious Therapies" (*JAMA*, 251(18): 2387–90, 5/11/84). V.B., VIII.D.

topsy.   slang, *autopsy* (lay, southern). II.B.1., VIII.B.2.a.

to the house (TTH).   slang, to discharge a patient home; often in acronym form, as "let's send her TTH." VIII.B.2.a.

toxic.   of, relating to, or caused by a *toxin* or *poison;* affected by a toxin or poison, as a toxic patient. *toxicant. a substance that acts as a poison, especially an insect control preparation that kills rather than repels. *toxicity. the quality, state, or degree of being poisonous or harmful to life.
See *median lethal concentration.* II.B.1.a.

toxicology.   the science and study of poisonous substances; their nature, detection, effects, and treatment; and the clinical, legal, occupational, and other problems they cause. III.C.

toxic substance.   a *poison;* any agent which is *carcinogenic, mutagenic,* or *teratogenic;* produces discomfort, disease, or injury; adversely affects health; or endangers life; compare *toxin.*
Toxic substances include toxic chemicals, *pollutants,* and *wastes.* Some substances are toxic only at *exposures* exceeding some *threshold,* and many have different dose-response curves for acute and chronic effects. I.C.

Toxic Substances Control Act (TSCA).   the principal federal legislative authority for regulating the development, sale, use, and disposal of *toxic substances.* III.C.

Toxic Substances List.   a list of known toxic substances prepared and maintained by *National Institute of Occupational Safety and Health.*
It is required by the Occupational Safety and Health Act. I.C.

toxic waste.   usually a synonym for hazardous waste but irregular, see *waste.*

toxin.   properly, a substance produced by a living organism and poisonous to other organisms; commonly, any *poison;* compare *toxic substance.*
Toxins can be produced by fungi (mycotoxins), plants (phytotoxins), animals (zootoxins), and bacteria (bacterial toxins). Bacterial toxins are either excreted normally (exotoxins) or retained inside the bacteria and released only after their disintegration (endotoxins). Something which neutralizes a toxin is an *antitoxin. I.A.1.

tracer.   a condition or disease, usually common, chosen for appraisal to assess the *quality* of medical care in a program because the quality of care given for the tracer is believed to be representative of the quality of care given generally or to all diseases. VI.D.2.

trade name.   synonym, *brand name.*

trainable.   see *mental retardation.*

training center.   for *allied health professions,* a junior college, college, or university with at least one curriculum in allied health and at least 20 students, a *teaching hospital affiliation,* and *accreditation* (section 795 of the Public Health Service Act). III.A.4.

tranquilizer. a drug or agent used in humans or animals to produce sedation, reduce anxiety, or correct mental disturbance.

So many and varied drugs are called tranquilizers that the term has little specific meaning. Use of *major tranquilizers to mean antipsychotic and antidepressant agents and of *minor tranquilizers to mean anxiolytics, as the benzodiazepines and simple hypnotics, is also irregular, mixes apples and oranges, and is to be discouraged. III.B.3.

transactional analysis. the study of and therapy for human interactions or transactions.

Read Berne, Eric, *Games People Play: The Psychology of Human Relationships* (New York: Ballantine Books, 1973).

transcendental meditation (TM). a program of *meditation.*

The name is trademarked, and the classes are franchised for profit. The meditational skill successful students acquire is real and useful. V.

transinstitutionalization. ugly synonym, *deinstitutionalization,* which is bad enough already.

transitional year. a year of *residency,* replacing the old rotating *internship,* with rotations in more than one specialty and intended to allow future training in more than one possible discipline; compare *flexible residency.*

This allows graduating medical students who have not decided what to do next to make the transition to the real world easily. III.A.

trauma. 1. an injury caused by a mechanical or physical agent. 2. a severe psychic injury. A *trauma center is a program or facility specializing in treating trauma, usually the worst trauma from a whole *catchment* area. See *tolerance.* II.B.1.a.

treatment (Rx, Tx). 1. application of measures for combating disease; *therapy;* the action or manner of caring for the sick or dysfunctional. 2. anything used in therapy. 3. application of a chemical agent or physical process to a substance or object to make it fit for use or disposal; compare *regimen* and *remedy.*

Treatment is both *caring* for the sick person and *curing* the illness, although actual practice is irregular, with the former often being omitted. 1. V.B.3., I.C.4.

triage. to sort or screen people seeking medical care to determine which service is initially required and with what priority. Triage originally described the sorting of battle casualties into groups that could wait for care, would benefit from immediate care, and were beyond care.

A patient coming to a facility for care may be seen first by a triage nurse to ascertain whether he or she has a medical or surgical problem or requires a nonphysician service, as social work consultation. Places for this purpose are known as *triage, *screening, or *walk-in clinics. Such rapid assessment units may merely refer patients to the most appropriate treatment service or may also give treatment for minor problems. V.A.

trial. act of trying or testing; synonym, *study.*

triangle. the fundamental relationship in families (along with many other parts of nature, including all mechanical engineering), consisting of an established pattern of behavior among three individuals.

Both the structure and function of families with several members can be mapped by describing their triangles. Many dysfunctional dyads can be understood only as one side of a triangle. Change in one triangle must change them all. I.B.1.

triple blind. see *double-blind study.*

troll. *house officer* slang, a patient who never dies, no matter how reasonable doing so might be; compare *gomer.*
    Usually old, debilitated, and incompetent, such patients have none of the malevolence of the gnomes under the bridge. VIII.B.2.a.

trolley car policy. facetiously, an insurance policy so hard to collect benefits from that it is as though it covered only injuries resulting from being hit by a trolley car, typically used of *mail-order insurance.* IV.B.2., VIII.B.2.a.

trophic. relating to or functioning in nutrition; nutritional.
    See *ecological pyramid* and *food chain.* I.A.2.a.

tropical medicine (Trop Med). the branch of medical science concerned with problems of health and disease found commonly or exclusively in tropical regions. III.C.

true negative (TN). a correct or valid negative or *normal* reaction to a *test;* contrast *false negative.* VIII.D.

true positive (TP). a correct or valid positive or *abnormal* reaction to a *test;* contrast *false positive.* VIII.D.

trust fund. a fund created and used by the federal government for a specific purpose or program according to the terms of a trust agreement or statute, as the Social Security and unemployment trust funds.
    Trust funds are administered by the government in a *fiduciary* capacity for those benefited and are not available for the general purposes of the government. Trust fund receipts whose use is not anticipated in the immediate future are invested in interest-bearing government securities and earn interest for the trust fund. The *Medicare* program is financed by two trust funds, the Federal Hospital Insurance Fund for Part A and the Federal Supplementary Medical Insurance Trust Fund for Part B.
    See *congressional* and *Presidential budgets, funded,* and *social insurance.* IV.C.

Tuke, William. U.S. Quaker, 1732–1822. He founded the Retreat at York in 1794, a humane asylum for the mentally ill, and with *Pinel* and others led the movement to treat the insane as humans. III.C., VIII.A.1.

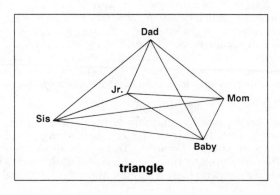

triangle

tumor. see *cancer*.

tumors, nodes, metastases (TNM). a common system for *staging* a *cancer* which scores three important determinants of the cancer's *prognosis:* the size or nature of the tumor itself, the extent of lymph node or gland involvement, and the presence and nature of any *metastases*. II.B.2.

turkey. a deprecating *house staff* term for an inpatient who is not believed to need hospital admission. Such patients are not usually *malingerers*. VII.C.5.a., VIII.B.2.a.

type I error. synonym, alpha error; see *sampling error*.

type II error. synonym, beta error; see *sampling error*.

type A behavior, personality. behavior which, or an individual who, is impatient, aggressive, ambitious, restless, and time-pressured, even when relaxing. *Type B is anything that is not type A. Type A people have more heart attacks, hypertension, and other *stress*-related illnesses than the general population.

Read Friedman, Meyer, and Ray Rosenman, "Type A Behavior Pattern: Its Association with Coronary Heart Disease" (*Ann Circ Res,* 3: 300–12, 1971) and *Type A Behavior and Your Heart* (New York: Alfred A. Knopf, 1974).

unallocated benefit provision.   see *allocated benefit provision.*

unbundling.   separating a group of related but distinguishable *services* normally *charged* as a single service into multiple services and charges; synonym, *fractionation.*

For example, a charge of $75 for a history and physical which includes tonometry and a Pap smear can be unbundled into charges of $40 for a history and physical, $15 for tonometry, and $20 for the Pap. There is no regular use or meaning for a bundle of services. VII.D.1.

unclear medicine.   slang, *nuclear medicine.* VIII.B.2.a.

uncompensated care.   *charity* care and care of patients who presumably could pay but do not, i.e., produce *bad debts.*

What counts is the value of uncompensated care, i.e., bad debts plus the cost of charity care. The difference between costs and charges for *cost-based* payers and the losses arising from discounts negotiated by some powerful payers, as the *Blue Cross discount,* are not usually included in estimates of uncompensated care. Such care is provided disproportionately by *teaching hospitals* and urban public hospitals as compared to *proprietary* and nonteaching *voluntary* ones. III.B.1., IV.A.

undergraduate medical education.   medical education given before receipt of the M.D. or equivalent degree, usually four years of study in medical, osteopathic, dental, or podiatric school leading to a degree.

This use contrasts with that in general education, where the term refers to college education leading to a bachelor's degree. III.C.

underwrite.   in insurance, to assume a *risk;* to become answerable for a designated *loss* on consideration of receiving a premium; to select, classify, evaluate, and assume risks according to their *insurability.*

Underwriting seeks to assure that the group insured has the same probability of loss and probable amount of loss, within reasonable limits, as the

428

universe on which the premium rates were based. Since rates are based on an expectation of loss, the underwriting process classifies risks with about the same expectation of loss into homogeneous groups or classes. IV.B.

underwriting profit.   the part of the earnings of an insurance company that comes from the function of underwriting.

The profit is found by deducting incurred *losses* and expenses from earned *premium,* after excluding earnings from investments (other than interest earnings required by law or regulation to be assumed to have been earned for purposes of determining *reserves* held). Investment earnings include income from securities or from sale of securities at a profit. IV.B.

undifferentiated family ego mass.   "describes a family's lack of separateness, consisting of a fused cluster of egos of individual family members as if they all had a common ego boundary. The ego fusion is the most intense in the least mature families, but fusion is present to some degree in all families" (*Pinney and Slipp, 1982*); compare *enmeshment.* I.B.1.

unemployment insurance.   *social insurance,* provided by state laws adopted pursuant to the federal Social Security Act and funded by *payroll taxes,* which pays calculated cash *benefits* for defined periods to people who qualify, typically by virtue of accumulated amounts of covered employment, and are involuntarily unemployed.

People receiving unemployment insurance do not usually continue to receive group health insurance coverage obtained through their most recent place of employment or any other health insurance. The federal government has therefore debated ways of providing them with health insurance, without result, since at least 1974. IV.C.

uniform cost accounting.   the use of a common set of accounting definitions, procedures, terms, and methods for accumulation and communication of quantitative data concerning their activities by separate enterprises. VI.C.1.

Uniform Hospital Discharge Data Set (UHDDS).   a defined set of data which give a minimum description of a hospital episode or *admission.*

Collection of a UHDDS is required upon discharge for all hospital stays reimbursed under *Medicare* and *Medicaid.* The UHDDS includes data on the age, sex, race, and residence of the patient; *length of stay;* diagnosis; responsible physicians; *procedures* performed; disposition of the patient; and sources of payment. The *peer review organization* program uses a slightly larger data set called the *Peer Review Organization Hospital Discharge Data Set (PHDDS). The *Uniform Hospital Discharge Abstract (UDHA) used to collect the UHDDS is one example of a *discharge abstract.* VII.C.5.

uniform individual policy provisions.   a set of provisions regarding the nature and content of individual health insurance policies, developed as a recommended model by the National Association of Insurance Commissioners, adopted with minor variations by almost all jurisdictions, and permitted in all. IV.B.

union.   a confederation or league of independent individuals, as nations or persons, for a common end or purpose. A *labor union is an organization of workers, usually with a common occupational interest and sometimes a common employer, whose purpose is obtaining, as by collective bargaining, its members' interests, as in wages and working conditions.

Unions have made notable contributions to occupational health and health insurance. In the United States, unlike other parts of the world, health personnel unions lack influence, unless one includes *professional associations*. III.A.

unit-dose system. dispensing of drugs in a hospital or other inpatient program in individual doses prepared and separately packaged in the institution's pharmacy rather than at the patient's nurse's station; packaging all medications for one patient at one time. In the traditional system, nurses measured liquids and took individual doses of tablets from stock bottles. IV.B.3.

United Nations International Children's Emergency Fund (UNICEF). an organization, created by and dependent on the General Assembly of the United Nations, which deals with *rehabilitation* of children in war-ravaged countries, *maternal and child health* and welfare, and development of technical and health programs, particularly for children. III.D.2.

United States Adopted Names Council (USAN). a private group responsible for assigning *established names* to *drugs;* made up of representatives of the American Medical Association, American Pharmaceutical Association, Food and Drug Administration, and the public. III.B.3.

United States Pharmacopeia (USP). a *compendium* of *standards* for *drugs*.
The USP is revised and published every five years by the United States Pharmacopeial Convention under the direction of a national committee of physicians, pharmacists, and academicians. It includes assays and tests for determination of strength, quality, and purity. A **USP drug,* as aspirin, USP, is one *compounded* according to and meeting the pharmacopeia's standards. III.B.3

United States Public Health Service (USPHS). the agency of the U.S. government responsible for most federal public health, biomedical research, health services, and health resources development programs.
Originating in 1798 as the Marine Hospital Service, the PHS has become the part of the Department of Health and Human Services headed by the assistant secretary for health.
See *Commissioned Corps*. III.D.1.

University Group Diabetes Program (UGDP). a multicenter, *random controlled trial* of several different therapies for non-insulin-dependent diabetes mellitus.
The study is known first for finding that the popular and profitable oral hypoglycemics are more dangerous and no more effective than dietary and insulin therapy and second for the extensive argument over this finding. The argument produced important lessons for study design and bias control and legal precedents on confidentiality of trial data and use of final results.
Read the University Group Diabetes Program, "A Study of the Effects of Hypoglycemic Agents on Vascular Complications in Patients with Adult-Onset Diabetes" (*Diabetes,* 19(suppl 2): 747–830, 1970) and correspondence by T.C. Chalmers and D.B. Martin (*N Engl J Med,* 315(19): 1233–4, 1985). VIII.D.

unnecessary surgery. surgery that is inappropriate for the condition or patient being treated or is done by a surgeon who is not qualified to do the operation.
These criteria were attributed to George Crile (U.S. surgeon) in *American Medical News,* 19(7): 2/16/76.

See *acute remunerative appendectomy, hip pocket hysterectomy,* and *second opinion.* V.B.

unnumbered hospital. in the U.S. Army, a fixed hospital ordinarily designed for permanent operation in the continental United States or any of its possessions. Unnumbered hospitals have names, as Letterman Army Hospital or U.S. Army Hospital, Fort Belvoir. III.B.1., III.D.1.

unofficial. of or pertaining to a drug or remedy that is not included in the *United States Pharmacopeia* or *National Formulary;* compare *official.* III.B.3

unscheduled benefit. in insurance, a *benefit* that pays the actual charge for the given service without a limit specified in the policy, albeit still usually not more than the *usual* and *customary charge;* compare *fixed* and *scheduled benefit.* IV.B.2.

unwarrantable failure. occurs when a coal mine operator *negligently,* recklessly, or intentionally does not comply with a mandatory health and safety standard.

Two such failures in 90 days, when they present more than a speculative possibility of causing disabling injury or death, are grounds for immediate closure of a mine under section 104 of the Federal Mine Safety and Health Act of 1977. VII.B.

upgrade. slang, charge for services more extensive than actually given, as billing for an extended office visit when only an intermediate visit's worth of time was spent. VII.D.1., VIII.B.2.

urban. of, relating to, or characteristic of a city or densely populated area; contrast *rural* and *suburb.* I.B.2.

urgent care center. see *episodic care center.*

urgicenter. corruption of *urgent care center.*

urologist. a physician specializing by practice or education in urology. III.A.1.

urology. the science and surgical specialty devoted to the study and care of the urinary tract, including the kidneys, ureters, bladder, urethra, and male genitalia.

Urology has an ancient existence because of kidney stones, see the *Hippocratic Oath,* for extraction of which specialized equipment has evolved. Urology shares the kidneys with *nephrology* and yields the female genitalia to *gynecology.* III.C.

use. employment, *utilization,* or ordinary purpose. VII.D.

use permit system. an alternative to the use of *occupational safety and health standards* for regulating *health hazards,* particularly *carcinogens* with possible zero *thresholds.*

The use permit system was considered by the *Occupational Safety and Health Administration* in the early 1970s but was not adopted because of questions about its legality and administrative feasibility. It would have required employers proposing any use of specified *toxic substances* to obtain prior to such use a permit from OSHA describing the proposed use and its risks to workers. VII.B.2.d.

use screen. a *norm* or *standard* for use of a diagnosis, diagnostic procedure, or therapy used by a utilization review committee, third-party payer, or other interested party to identify for full investigation possible wrong patterns of practice or charges.

Use screens are often computer-applied and identify providers whose services may be inappropriate to their diagnoses or overpriced or who make particular diagnoses with unusual frequency. VII.D.

usual charge. see *customary charge.*

usual, customary, and reasonable plan (UCR). a health insurance plan that pays a physician's full *charge* if it does not exceed the physician's usual charge; does not exceed the amount customarily charged for the same service by other physicians in the area, often defined as the ninetieth or ninety-fifth percentile of all charges in the community; and is otherwise *reasonable.* In this context, usual and customary charges are similar but not identical to *customary* and *prevailing charges,* respectively, as used by *Medicare.* Many private health insurance plans use the UCR approach. IV.B.

utilization. usually an affected five-syllable synonym for *use,* so common in health care as to be an acceptable long variant.

There were once useful distinctions; employing "utilize" for uncommon uses, as using a chair for sitting but utilizing it as a weapon, or for good, optimal, or purposeful uses. "Use" is measured by rates per unit population at risk for a given period, as number of admissions to hospital per 1000 persons over age 65 per year or number of visits per person per year for family planning services. VI.D.2., VIII.D.

utilization review (UR). *evaluation* of the *necessity, appropriateness,* and *efficiency* of the use of medical *services* and *facilities.*

In a hospital this includes review of the appropriateness of *admissions,* services ordered and provided, *length of stay,* and discharge practices, both on a concurrent and a retrospective basis. Utilization review may be done by a utilization review committee, *peer review organization,* or other group, or public agency.

See *medical* and *tissue review.* VI.D.2.

utilization review committee. a staff committee of an institution or a group outside the institution responsible for conducting *utilization review* activities for that institution. *Medicare* and *Medicaid* require, as a *condition of participation,* that hospitals have an operating utilization review committee. VI.D.2.

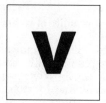

vaccine. a preparation administered to induce *immunity* in the recipient to something antigenically represented by the preparation.

A vaccine may be a suspension of living or dead organisms or parts of organisms or pollens. Vaccines induce production of antibodies which serve as protection against infection with the naturally occurring bacterium or virus. The federal Food, Drug, and Cosmetic Act regulates vaccines as *biologics*.

See *E. Jenner*. III.B.3., VII.B.3.b.

validity. the degree to which data or results of a *study* are correct or true, occur in the real world; the extent to which a situation as observed reflects the true situation; compare *external validity* and *reliability*. VIII.B.

variable. any characteristic in a *study* which may change or assume different values.

A *dependent variable is one which is measured after manipulation of an independent variable and whose variation is assumed to be a function of the variation in the independent variable, see *control*. An *independent variable is one which is under the experimenter's control and whose effects are being studied.

See *intervening variable* and *quantitative variable*. VIII.B.

variable cost. in accounting, a *cost*, as of raw materials, that changes proportionately with a change in productivity or activity; contrast *fixed cost*. VI.C.1.

variance. a permission or license to do an act contrary to the usual rule, especially to build or operate in violation of an applicable *standard* or code.

Variances from *occupational safety and health standards* are available by petition for experimental purposes, for national defense, temporarily to employers who cannot comply for such reasons as unavailability of equipment or personnel, and permanently to employers who show that their safety measures are as safe as those required by a standard. VI.D., VII.D.2.

vector. intermediate *carrier* agent, as an insect or rodent, that transmits *pathogens* from one *host* to another; compare *fomite*. *Vector control includes any activity which kills or otherwise limits vectors, as spraying pesticides to eliminate insects.

See *G.M. Lancisi, W. Reed, R. Ross, T. Smith,* and *sylvatic.* VIII.C.

vegan. see *vegetarianism*.

vegetarianism. the theory or practice of living solely upon vegetables, fruits, grains, or nuts.

Vegetarian diets include *lactovegetarian (plant foods with dairy products), *lactovovegetarian (plants, milk, and eggs), and pure vegetarian (without dairy products or eggs). *Vegans are pure vegetarians who also share a particular philosophy and lifestyle. There is a lot of variation in vegetarian diets, associated beliefs, and motivation. Such a diet may be *nutritionally* complete, guard against *obesity,* and lower cholesterol.

See *macrobiotic,* and read American Academy of Pediatrics, "Nutritional Aspects of Vegetarianism, Health Foods, and Fad Diets" (*Pediatrics,* 59(3): 460–4, 3/77).

vegeto-therapy. practically obsolete, a therapy developed by *Wilhelm Reich* (German psychoanalyst, 1897–1957) which seeks to restore harmonious functioning of the vegetative energies of the body by improving muscle balance, breathing, and attitudes. Reich subsequently supplemented the vegetative energies with *orgone*.

Vegeto-therapy was an early form of biofunctional therapy—therapy built on the principle that a sound body helps make a sound mind, to whatever extent they are not the same thing. V.B.

vendor. synonym, *provider;* an institution, agency, organization, or individual who provides health or medical *services.* III.

vendor payment. in a public assistance program, a payment made directly to a *vendor* of service, compared with a cash income payment or payment for a service made to an assistance recipient.

Vendors, or providers of services, are reimbursed directly by the program for services they provide to eligible recipients. Vendor payments are analogous to *service benefits* provided by health insurance and prepayment plans. IV.B.1., IV.C.

venereal disease (VD). contagious disease ordinarily acquired during sexual intercourse or other intimate physical contact; currently known as *sexually transmitted disease.* II.B.1.a.

verbal order (VO). see *order*.

vertical categorization. see *categorization*.

Vesalius, Andreas, of Brussels. European anatomist and physician, 1514–1564. A wonderful man. His *De Humani Corporis Fabrica* was published in 1543, revolutionizing anatomy by its repudiation of *Galen* and use of actual observation of human material. The book remains a masterpiece of the printer's art; its illustrations, done by Vesalius and others including Titian, illustrated the first edition of this dictionary (*Discursive, 1976*). VIII.A.1.

Veterans Administration (VA). the agency of the U.S. government responsible for benefit programs, including the Veterans Administration Health

Program, for those who served in the government's uniformed services; see *Commissioned Corps*. III.D.1.

veterinarian (DVM, MV, VM, VS). a person educated in, licensed in, and/or practicing veterinary medicine; synonyms, *veterinary* and veterinary surgeon. III.A.5.

veterinary. of or pertaining to the practice of medicine with animals, particularly domestic animals; synonym, *veterinarian*. III.A.5.

veterinary medicine. the branch of medical practice which treats diseases and injuries of animals.

Animals, as human food, sources of labor, and *vectors* of human disease, with their largely human biology, require care that is essentially part of medicine. Therefore, veterinary medicine is included in federal health personnel programs and organized and credentialed in ways similar to the rest of medicine. III.C.

Virchow, Rudolph. German pathologist, 1821–1902. He developed the concept of cellular pathology and was also an eminent anthropologist and politician. Early in his career Virchow developed a theory of social *epidemiology*, compare *social medicine*, which he used to improve community *public health* in Berlin. II.B.1., III.C., VIII.A.1., VIII.C.

virucide. see *pesticide*.

virulence. *malignancy*, noxiousness; the *pathogenicity* or disease-producing power of an organism. *virulent. having virulence, unusually great virulence.

See *herd effect* and *palliate*. II.A.2.

Visa Qualifying Examination (VQE). an exam administered to *foreign medical graduates* seeking entry into the United States for *graduate medical education*. Passage is required prior to the granting of the necessary visa and is equivalent to passing parts I and II of the *National Board Examination*. III.A.1.

visit. an *encounter* between a patient and a health professional requiring the patient to travel from his or her home to the professional's usual place of practice, an *office visit, or vice versa, a *house call or home visit by the professional.

See *gang visit*. VII.C.5.

visiting nurse (VN). a nurse who provides care to people in their homes.

Most visiting nurses are registered nurses and work as *public health nurses* or for *voluntary agencies*. A *private duty nurse* working in someone's home would not usually be thought of as a visiting nurse. III.A.2.

visiting nurse association, visiting nurse service (VNA, VNS). a *voluntary health agency* which provides *nursing services* in the home using nurses and other personnel, as home health aides trained to give bedside personal care; compare *home health agency*.

These agencies had their origin in the visiting or district nursing provided to the sick poor in their homes by voluntary agencies, as the New York City Mission, in the 1870s. The first visiting nurse associations were established in Buffalo, Boston, and Philadelphia in 1886–1887. VII.C.1.

vital statistics. data concerning *births* (natality), *deaths* (*mortality*), marriages, *health*, and *disease* (*morbidity*); the study of such data.

Vital statistics for the United States are published annually by the *National Center for Health Statistics* of the Health Resources and Services Administration, DHHS. It is a branch of biostatistics, compare *demography*. See *J.S. Billings, W. Petty,* and *J.G. Grawnt.* II.C.

vitamin.   an organic compound present in variable, minute quantities in *natural* foodstuffs and required for the normal qrowth and maintenance of life of an animal, as a person, that is unable itself to synthesize the compound.

Vitamins are fully effective in very small amounts and do not furnish energy but are *essential* to the organism's functioning. They are divided into two major groups: water soluble, the B vitamins; and fat soluble, all others.

See *J. Goldberger* and *J. Lindy.* I.A.2.a.

vitamin therapy.   treatment with vitamins, see *megavitamin therapy;* synonym, orthomolecular therapy or treatment.

vocational rehabilitation (voc rehab, VR).   habilitation and rehabilitation for people unable to find work because of *handicaps, disability,* or lack of job skills; an organized, usually state-operated, vocational rehabilitation program. VII.B.3.b.

voluntary health agency.   a nonprofit nongovernmental organization, governed by lay or professional individuals, organized on a national, state, or local basis whose primary purpose is health-related.

Voluntary health agencies are usually *charities* primarily supported by contributions from the public. Most engage in a program of service, education, and research related to a particular disease, disability, or group of diseases and disabilities, as the American Heart Association, American Cancer Society, and National Tuberculosis Association, and their state and local affiliates. The term can apply to nonprofit hospitals, *visiting nurse associations,* and other local service organizations which may be supported by both contributions and charges for services provided.

See *L.F. Flick.* III.B.4.

volunteer bias.   the *bias,* or deviation from findings in a whole population, attributable to using, as a *sample* for a study, individuals who volunteer, since they are not generally representative of the total population.

Self-selected patients who seek treatment in response to newspaper publicity, for example, are likely to do significantly better than randomly selected patients. VIII.D.

voucher system.   government funding for services, as education or health care, in which eligible beneficiaries are given some form of paper with which to buy the services themselves in the marketplace; an idea whose time has never come, food stamps for health care.

Various proposals along these lines for funding *national health insurance* have never been enacted. IV.C.

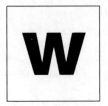

waiting period. an interval which must pass before an individual becomes eligible either for insurance coverage or for a given benefit after overall coverage has commenced; compare *exclusion*.

This does not generally refer to the time needed to process an application for insurance but is a period defined in the policy before benefits become payable, as one that will not pay *maternity benefits* until the policy has been in force for nine months, or in *group insurance* offered as a benefit of employment when coverage does not start until one has been employed for 30 days. There is a two-year waiting period before disabled persons can be covered under *Medicare,* i.e., the disabled must draw Social Security benefits for two years before their medical benefits begin. IV.B., IV.C.

waiver of premiums. a provision in an insurance policy which exempts the *insured* from paying *premiums* when the insured is disabled during the life of the contract. IV.B.

Wald, Lillian. U.S. nurse, 1867–1940. She established *public health nursing* in the United States and founded the Henry Street Settlement in New York, a famous early social work agency. III.A.2., VIII.A.1.

walkaround right. the requirement, in section 8(e) of the *Occupational Safety and Health Act* that representatives of both an employer and his or her employees be given an opportunity to accompany and assist an inspector during any inspection of their workplace.

Where no authorized employee representative, as one chosen by a union, is available, the inspector is required to consult with a reasonable number of employees concerning the *healthfulness* and *safety* of the workplace. VII.B.2.d.

walk-in. a patient who seeks care without an appointment.
See *episodic care center.* VII.A.1.

war. armed, open, hostile conflict between political units or states; a state of hostility, conflict, opposition, or antagonism between mental, physical, social, or other forces.

War and starvation are principal sources of *death, injury,* and *malnutrition.* War is particularly perverse for killing the *fittest* first (only humans could be counterevolutionary) and its apparent preventability.

See *nuclear winter.* I.B.

ward. a large *service* or *department* in a health facility, often for patients with the same disease or similar problems, as a burn ward or isolation ward. III.B.1.

ward. a person subject to guardianship or custody, as a ward of a court. VIII.B.3.

ward patient. synonym, *service patient;* antonym, *private patient.*

warranty. in malpractice, an action against a physician on the basis of a warranty rather than the usual action based on *negligence.*

A warranty arises when the physician promises or seems to promise that a procedure to be used is *safe* or will be *effective.* An advantage of bringing an action on warranty grounds rather than negligence is that the *statute of limitations* is usually longer. V.D.

waste. solid, liquid, or gaseous material or substance remaining from human activities, particularly from production, processing, and consumption of goods.

Because of the large and continuous production and frequent toxicity of wastes, their disposal into the *environment* is the major cause of *pollution.* There are many types of waste, often named for their origin, as *agricultural waste from agriculture. *Bulky waste includes any item whose large size precludes easy handling. *Hazardous or special waste requires special handling to avoid risk to health or damage to property. *Incombustible waste cannot be burned at normal solid waste incinerator temperatures (800–1000°F), as glass and metal. The most effective, but generally costly, method of eliminating wastes is to recover and recycle them by various treatments and processes as reusable by-products.

See *food waste, radioactive waste, sewage,* and *solid waste.* I.C.4.

wastewater. water carrying waste from homes, businesses, and industries; water mixed with dissolved or suspended *solid waste.* I.C.5.

water quality. biologic, chemical, and physical characteristics of water that are *healthful* and aesthetically pleasing in use.

Water may be treated at the water supply intake, *water treatment, and after use, *liquid waste treatment, to control toxic or infectious agents, objectionable taste or odor, turbidity, coloration, hardness, alkalinity, salinity, dissolved oxygen, foaming agents, or temperature.

See *drinking water* and *fresh water.* I.C.5.

water quality criterion. a maximum acceptable level of a pollutant that affects the suitability of water for a given use, particularly one of the four commonly classified uses: public water supply, recreation, propagation of fish and other aquatic life, and agricultural and industrial use. I.C.5.

water treatment. see *water quality.*

Weight Watchers. a group treatment program for obesity, comparable to *smokenders* and *Take Off Pounds Sensibly.*

Members are given a good diet to follow and recipes consistent with it. They meet weekly in local chapters or groups to weigh and encourage each other. I.A.2.a., V.B.

welfare. 1. state of faring; condition of *health,* happiness, prosperity; negatively, freedom from evil or calamity of an individual, group, or institution, as in the welfare of the troops. 2. organized public or private efforts for social betterment of a specified class or group. 3. aid or relief in the form of money or necessities for the indigent, aged, handicapped, or otherwise *disabled.*

In the United States, the term is irregularly used. Usage is often limited to programs for the poor, typically federally assisted, state-administered *income* support programs for certain of the *poor,* specifically *Aid to Families with Dependent Children.* In this context the term has a largely unwarranted connotation of *abuse,* tax support for the promiscuous and lazy. As defined, welfare programs include many employer, union, and other private health and welfare plans and some health insurance programs (many feel *Medicaid* is a welfare program, if only because it is *categorically related*). Conventionally, *social insurance* programs are not thought of as welfare. 1. II., 2. I.B.2., 3. I.A.2.c.

Wernicke rounds. (K. Wernicke, German neurologist, 1848–1905) slang, a gathering at which alcohol is consumed, as a regular Friday afternoon celebration by *house staff* of the end of the week. Wernicke was the first to characterize the pathologic effects of alcohol on the brain. VIII.B.2.a.

wetfingered. describes a dentist who actually practices; compare dryfingered, one who does not. V., VIII.B.2.a.

wet nurse. a woman who furnishes breast feeding to an infant not her own. III.A.4.

wholistic. synonym, *holistic.*

Will Rogers phenomenon. the taxonomic and statistical consequences of *stage migration, the moving of cancer patients from one clinical stage to another caused by changes in diagnostic techniques, not by any real change in their disease.

Will Rogers (American humorist) observed that "When the Okies left Oklahoma and moved to California, they raised the average intelligence in both states." When improved diagnostic techniques discover tumors earlier, *zero-time shift* occurs. When lymph node spread and metastases are discovered earlier, cancers are assigned to more severe stages, as in *TNM* staging systems. This improves survival in both groups, removing sicker people from earlier stages and assigning healthier ones to the worse stages, although the total survival for the whole *cohort* is unchanged.

Read Feinstein, Alvan R., et al., "The Will Rogers Phenomenon: Stage Migration and New Diagnostic Techniques as a Source of Misleading Statistics for Survival in Cancer" (*N Engl J Med,* 312(25): 1604–8, 1/20/85). VIII.D.

witch doctor. a professional worker of magic in a primitive society, occupying a tribal position similar to that of a *shaman,* who seeks to cure illness, detect witches, and counteract malevolent magical influences by use of charms, herbal remedies, and incantations. III.A.

withdrawal. taking away or removing anything, as coitus interruptus or discontinuance of a drug.

The *withdrawal syndrome is the complex of physical and psychologic disturbances observed in addicts upon withdrawal of an addicting agent. The severity of the syndrome varies with the agent and the duration and magnitude of the addiction. II.B.2., III.B.3.

withdrawal syndrome. see *addiction* and *withdrawal.*

women's auxiliary. see *auxiliary.*

wonder drug. lay term, a *drug* with therapeutic properties or safety substantially better than or different from earlier drugs; any new drug introduced by lots of advertising; a drug whose importance brings its introduction to public attention; the first drug in any substantially new therapeutic area, as smallpox vaccine, penicillin, chlorpromazine, propranolol, and the first clinically useful monoclonal antibody; synonym, miracle drug.

Originally common in press reports of new antibiotics, it is heard less frequently now that drugs with real *efficacy* are fairly common. III.B.3.

work. synonym, *occupation.*

work capacity. see *occupation.*

workmen's compensation act. a state statute making employers liable without fault for injury, illness, disability, and death of their employees occurring as a result of employment.

These acts, enacted in all states early in the century, fix awards for injuries; dispense with proof of *negligence* and most legal actions, including the employee's right to common law recovery; and usually go beyond simple determination of compensation to create programs of insurance. The acts are quite variable among states. Some allow either employers or employees to elect not to participate in the compensation system, although not doing so typically forfeits otherwise available rights and defenses, as *contributory negligence.* VII.B.2.d.

workmen's compensation insurance. state operated or supervised *social insurance,* provided by workmen's compensation acts, against statutory damages arising from injury to employees while in the employ of an insured employer.

The insurance is purchased by the employer, who is responsible for the injuries and damages. Its purchase is usually required by law. The insurance provides cash benefits to workers and their dependents for loss of wages and, ordinarily, all medical services necessary for treatment and restoration to health and productive work arising out of injury, illness, or disability occurring as a result of employment. VII.B.2.d.

workmen's compensation program. a state-operated program, under authority of the state's workmen's compensation act, which provides or supervises the state's workmen's compensation insurance and *vocational rehabilitation* services and works to assure safe and healthful workplaces.

See *scheduled benefits* and *second-injury fund.* VII.B.2.d.

work history. see *occupation.*

working capital. properly, current *assets* minus current *liabilities,* sometimes called *net working capital; commonly, synonym, *current assets.*

See *capital.* VI.C.1.

work test. a trial of something by use; a measure or trial of someone's ability to work or work capacity; distinguish *means test.*

See *occupation.* I.A.2.c.

work-up. an investigation of a problem or of a patient and his or her problems, typically including a *complete history* and *physical examination* and laboratory and other diagnostic procedures appropriate to the problems presented; to do such a work-up. V.A.

World Health Organization (WHO). a specialized agency of the United Nations generally concerned with *health* and *health care.*

The WHO assists governments upon request in the health field, promotes research and cooperation among scientific and professional groups, and studies administrative and social techniques in preventive medicine. It has authority to make sanitary and quarantine regulations, regulate morbidity and mortality *nomenclature,* and set standards for purity and potency of drugs and biologics. III.D.2.

World Organization of National Colleges, Academies, and Academic Associations of General Practitioners/Family Physicians (WONCA). the international organization of family physicians.

WONCA sponsors *ICHPPC, FAMLI,* and other primary documents in family medicine. III.D.2.

wrongful life. a legal action filed on behalf of an infant born with a genetic or other congenital birth defect seeking damages for physician failure to inform and advise parents adequately about foreseeable fetal risks, thus precluding parental choice to avoid conception or birth and leading to the child's birth.

This controversial birth-related legal claim is the child's action and is distinguished from *wrongful pregnancy, the parents' cause of action for negligent performance of a sterilization resulting in an unplanned, but healthy birth; *dissatisfied life, a child's cause of action for birth with an impairment of status, usually illegitimacy; and *wrongful birth, the parental action, corresponding to wrongful life, based on the loss and expenses from birth of a defective child. Wrongful pregnancy and birth have gained general judicial acceptance; wrongful and dissatisfied life have not.

Read Schmidt, Susan M., "Wrongful Life" (*JAMA,* 250(16): 2209–10, 2/28/83). VIII.B.3.

xenodochium. synonym, *hospital;* a Latin term used in medieval and common English law for a place that offers refuge to dispossessed people, the sick, and the *infirm.* III.B.1., VIII.B.3.

xenograft. (Greek, *xenos,* foreigner) a graft of tissue transplanted between animals of different species, as with a baboon's heart in a human child; synonyms, heterograft, heterologous graft, and heteroplastic graft; compare *allograft.* I.A.1.

xeroradiography. radiography that records a roentgen image with a dry process, *xerography, which uses the powdered surface of an electrically charged selenium plate to record the image. III.C.

x-ray. 1. electromagnetic *radiation* having wavelengths in the range of 0.1 to 100 angstroms, usually produced by bombarding a metal target with fast electrons in an evacuated tube. 2. a photograph taken with x-rays.

X-rays penetrate substances to varying degrees or distances, ionize tissues, affect photographic plates, and cause some substances to fluoresce. See *radiology* and *W. C. Roentgen.* I.C.3., III.C

x-ray technologist. a *technologist* trained in *radiology.* III.A.4

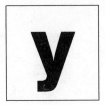

yellow beret. slang, a member of the *Commissioned Corps* of the U.S. Public Health Service, particularly one like the author who served a two-year Selective Service obligation in the corps during the war in Vietnam, when the Green Berets were widely known. III.D.1., VIII.B.2.a.

yellow rain. an alleged *biologic weapon* containing fungal F2 (trichothecene) mycotoxin.

Yellow rain was alleged by the U.S. State Department to have been used by the Soviets and Soviet allies in Afghanistan and southeast Asia during the late 1970s. A panel of American scientists, while not denying the possibility of *chemical warfare,* found persuasive evidence that yellow spots on leaf samples from Thailand and Laos were pollen-filled drops of bee excrement released while the bees were in flight during an annual purging by the wild southeast Asian honeybee, *Apis dorsata.* I.B.

yoga. 1. an orthodox system of Hindu philosophy, theistic and characterized by the teaching of raja yoga as a practical method of self-liberation. 2. a system of *exercises* and *meditations* for attaining bodily and mental control. 3. health and well-being; union of the self with the universal being.

The meditations relieve *stress* and tension, hence yoga's renewed popularity as a *healthful* practice. V.

Zen macrobiotics. see *macrobiotics.*

zero population growth (ZPG). 1. balance of birth, death, and migration rates in a *population* such that the whole population is stable, neither growing nor shrinking. 2. an organization dedicated to achieving zero population growth in the human world population.

If the world does not soon achieve zero population growth by *family planning,* then population control by war and starvation may be inevitable. 1. II.C., 2. III.B.1.

zero threshold. see *threshold.*

zero threshold phenomenon. any situation in which there is no *dose* or *exposure* level, or *threshold,* which must be attained before there is an effect, as a gene mutation, and below which no effect occurs. I.C.

zero-time shift. the change in date of diagnosis of a disease which occurs when a screening test or other appropriate new diagnostic procedure leads to detection of the disease before symptoms appear or otherwise earlier than was previously the case; synonym, lead-time bias; compare *Will Rogers phenomenon.*

This phenomenon may extend the statistical length of a patient's survival without necessarily prolonging the patient's life.

Read Feinleib, M., and M. Zelen, "Some Pitfalls in the Evaluation of Screening Programs" (*Arch Environ Health,* 19: 412–5, 1969). VIII.D.

zones. climates; regions; layers; belts; girdles. I.C.1., VIII.B.3.

zone therapy. synonym, *Ingham Reflex Method of Compression Massage.*

zoonosis. a disease of animals, particularly lower animals, transmissible to vertebrate animals, especially humans; plural, zoonoses. II., VIII.C.

zygosity. the genetic state of a *zygote, a fertilized ovum or other organism produced by union of two gametes.

Zygosity usually refers to the identity, *homozygosity, or nonidentity, *heterozygosity, of one or more gene pairs. *Dizygotic or fraternal twins grow from two different fertilized ova. They have the genetic relationship as any two siblings. *Monozygotic, or identical, twins are the product of a single fertilized ovum. I.A.1.

Annotated Bibliography

☐

The following references include major glossaries and dictionaries of health, health care, and related fields for the reader who wishes to extend this dictionary's scope and coverage in any area in which it is found deficient.

The bibliography is annotated and also includes references to works concerning and using the language of health care and lexicography. When available, addresses for obtaining obscure references have been included.

The bibliography does not include references pertaining to a particular term. A reference enlarging on a specific term will be found in its definition. Sources simply justifying definitions are available from the author.

Conspectus locations at which a reference is cited by subject are noted. References on any given subject may be found by locating that subject in the Conspectus where references are listed by subject.

Abel, Ernest L. (compiler). *Dictionary of Alcohol Use and Abuse: Slang, Terms, and Terminology*. Westport, CT: Greenwood, 1985. 191 pp. $29.95. II.B.2.

Adams, Margaret. *Bailliere's Midwives Dictionary*. 7th ed. New York: Bailliere Tindall, 1983. 368 pp. $6.75, softcover. III.C.

Age Words: A Glossary on Health and Aging. Bethesda: National Institute on Aging, 1986. 65 pp. I.A.1

Alderson, Michael. *An Introduction to Epidemiology*. New York: Macmillan Press Ltd., 1976. VIII.C.

A Manual of Style. 12th ed., revised by the editorial staff. Chicago: The University of Chicago Press, 1976. 546 pp. First edition, 1906.
  The reference style and usage manual for this work. VIII.B.

American Board of Medical Specialties. *Directory of Medical Specialists.* 19th ed. 3 vols. Chicago: Marguis Who's Who, Inc., 1979.
  Information concerning the approved medical specialties and each of their certified specialists. III.A.

American Medical Records Association. *Glossary of Hospital Terms.* 2nd ed. Chicago: American Medical Records Association (875 N. Michigan Ave. - Suite 1850), 1983. 111 pp.
  A careful, formal work with fairly official status. III.B.1.

American Psychiatric Association (APA). *Diagnostic and Statistical Manual of Mental Disorders, DSM-III.* 3rd ed. Washington, DC: American Psychiatric Association, 1978.
  Completely revised psychiatric nomenclature. III.B.2.

Anderson, Scarvia B. et al. *Encyclopedia of Evaluation: Concepts and Techniques for Evaluating Education and Training Programs.* San Francisco: Jossey-Bass, Inc., Publishers, 1975. 515 pp.
  Short essays with references. Well done. VI.D.

Apple, Rima D. (compiler). *Illustrated Catalogue of the Slide Archive of Historical Medical Photographs at Stony Brook.* Center for Photographic Images of Medicine and Health Care. Westport, CT: Greenwood Press Inc., 1984. 442 pp. 3171 illus. $55. VIII.A.

Ashford, Nicholas A. *Crisis in the Workplace: Occupational Disease and Injury. A Report to the Ford Foundation.* Cambridge, MA: The MIT Press, 1976. 589 pp.
  Source of much of the occupational health material in the second edition. VII.B.2.

Attwood, H.D. "Xhumation: A Dissertation upon the Lung of the Late Dr. Samuel Johnson, the Great Lexicographer." *The Lancet,* II (8469/70): 1411–3,*12/85.
  He had emphysema at autopsy, along with an "exceedingly large" heart, an aortic valve "beginning to ossify," a gallstone "about the size of a pigeon's head," ascites, an early peritonitis, and a right varicocele. VIII.B.

Ayers, Donald M. *Bioscientific Terminology: Words from Latin and Greek Stems.* Tucson, AZ: University of Arizona Press, 1972.
  More a treatise than a dictionary on the use of these languages in scientific terminology. Organized in a logical sequence of lessons for students' use. VIII.B.

Bander, Edward J., and Jeffrey J. Wallach. *Medical Legal Dictionary.* Dobbs Ferry, NY: Oceana, 1970.
  Selective list of 400 terms geared toward the legal and medical professions. Stresses practical definitions. Useful material in the appendix includes lists of reference sources and the text of the Uniform Anatomical Gift Act. VIII.B.3.

Beighton, Peter, and Greta Beighton. *The Man behind the Syndrome.* New York: Springer-Verlag, 1986. 250 pp. Illustrated. $36.
  Biographies of the physicians after whom syndromes are known with portraits, histories, and references. II.B.2., VIII.A.1.

Bender, Arnold E. *Dictionary of Nutrition and Food Technology.* 4th ed. New York: Chemical Publishing, 1976. First edition, 1960.
    Authoritative definitions that apply to food study. Includes appropriate terms from medicine, chemistry, home economics, etc. I.A.2.a.

Bennington, James L. (ed.). *Saunders Dictionary and Encyclopedia of Laboratory Medicine and Technology.* Philadelphia: W.B. Saunders, 1984. 1674 pp. $47.95. III.B.1.

Bierce, Ambrose. *The Devil's Dictionary.* New York: Dover Publications, 1958. 145 pp. First edition, 1911. VIII.B.2.b.

Bishop, Claude T. *How to Edit a Scientific Journal.* Professional Editing and Publishing Services. Philadelphia: ISI Press, 1984. 138 pp. $21.95, hardcover; $14.95, softcover. VIII.B.

Bittel, Lester R., and Jackson E. Ramsey (eds.). *Handbook for Professional Managers.* New York: McGraw-Hill Book Company, 1985. 1000 pp. $59.95.
    A magnificent new version of the *Encyclopedia of Professional Management* with 235 signed major articles. Includes references and an index. VI.

Black, Henry Campbell. *Black's Law Dictionary.* St. Paul, MN: West Publishing Co., 1968.
    The primary law reference for this dictionary and an excellent work. The legal system of definition by citation takes some getting used to on the part of the nonlawyer. VIII.B.3.

Blades, C.A. et al. *The International Bibliography of Health Economics: A comprehensive annotated guide to English language sources since 1914.* New York: Macmillan, 1986. 1092 pp. $180. VIII.B.1.

Blakiston's Gould Medical Dictionary. 4th ed. New York: McGraw-Hill Book Company, 1979. 1632 pp. $26.95.
    The primary medical reference for this dictionary, since it was in a current edition, is well done, and is the primary reference for the G. C. Merriam Company's medical lexicographer, R. Pease. III.C.

Bloomfield, Robert L., and E. Ted Chandler. *Mnemonics, Rhetoric and Poetics for Medics: Knowledge Worth Spewing Not Requiring Emetics.* Winston-Salem (NC 27106): Harbinger Press (Box 17201), 1982. 222 pp.

Bloomfield, Robert L., and Carolyn F. Pedley. *Mnemonics, Rhetoric and Poetics for Medics: With a Preface for Those Who Think This Pathetic.* Vol II. Winston-Salem: Harbinger Medical Press, 1984. 167 pp. Illustrated. $10.
    Erudite, occasionally contrived, collections of mnemonics and such. V.A., VIII.B.

Borgenicht, Louis. "American Medicine: An Annotated Bibliography." *N Engl J Med,* 304(18): 1112–6, 4/30/81.
    A discussion of literature about medicine for lay people, particularly of the 1970s. VIII.A.

Boucher, Carl O. (ed.). *Current Clinical Dental Terminology: A Glossary of Accepted Terms in all Disciplines of Dentistry.* 2nd ed. St. Louis, MO: C.V. Mosby, 1974.
    Includes over 10,000 clinical dental terms; definitions supplied by over 40 contributors are concise and cross-referenced. Includes appendices of chemical names and miscellaneous information. III.C.

Bowker, R.R. (preparer). *Medical and Health Care Books and Serials in Print 1986: An Index to Literature in the Health Sciences,* vol 1, *Books—Subjects,*

Authors Index, vol 2, *Books—Titles; Serials—Subjects, Titles; Publishers.* New York: R.R. Bowker Co., 1986. 2039 pp. $110. III.C.

Brace, Edward R. *A Popular Guide to Medical Language.* New York: Van Nostrand Reinhold, 1983. 279 pp. $19.50. V.C., VIII.B.

Brace, Paul. *Glossary of the Environment.* New York: Praeger Special Studies in International Economics and Development, Praeger Publishers, 1977. 117 pp.
    An excellent vocabulary and the source of much of this work's environmental material. I.C.

Bricklin, Mark. *The Practical Encyclopedia of Natural Healing.* Emmaus, PA: Rodale Press, 1976.
    A volume of folk medicine and nondrug therapies. V.

Brieland, Donald, and John Lemmon. *Social Work and the Law.* St. Paul, MN: West Publishing Co., 1977.
    An overview of social work related subjects with definitions. III.C.

Bynum, W.F., E.J. Browne, and Roy Porter (eds.). *Dictionary of the History of Science.* Princeton, NJ: Princeton University Press, 1981. 494 pp. $40. Reprinted in paper, 1985, $12.95.
    Traces the evolution of 134 medical concepts among over 700 entries. Illustrated. VIII.A.2.

Campbell, Robert T. *Psychiatric Dictionary.* 5th ed. New York: Oxford University Press, 1981. $35. III.C.

Cape, Barbara F. (ed.). *Bailliere's Nurses Dictionary.* 18th ed. Baltimore, MD: Williams & Wilkins, 1974. III.C.

Chabner, Davi-Ellen. *The Language of Medicine.* 3rd ed. Philadelphia: W.B. Saunders Company, 1985. $24.95, softcover. 687 pp. Illus. VIII.B.

Chaplin, James P. *Dictionary of Psychology.* Rev. ed. New York: Dell Pub. Co., 1975. 576 pp. $2.95. III.C.

Chen, Ching Chih. *Health Sciences Information Sources.* Cambridge, MA: (02142): The MIT Press, 1981. 767 pp.
    A guide for health science librarians and text for students of the biomedical literature. Good lists of bibliographies, dictionaries, statistical sources, organizations, periodicals, and data bases. VIII.D.

Collocott, T.C. (ed.). *Chambers Dictionary of Science and Terminology.* New York: Barnes & Noble, 1972. Expanded edition of *Chambers Technical Dictionary.*
    One of the best one-stop technical dictionaries available. Over 40,000 terms. III.C.

Corsini, Raymond J. et al. (eds.). *Concise Encyclopedia of Psychology.* New York: John Wiley, 1987. 1242 pp. $74.95. III.C.

Critchley, Macdonald (ed.). *Butterworths Medical Dictionary.* 2nd ed. London: Butterworths, 1978.
    A comprehensive standard British medical dictionary, with 8000 new entries in the second edition, clear format, and thorough definitions. It ignores American conventions. III.C.

Crowley, Ellen T., and Helen E. Sheppard (eds.). *Acronyms, Initialisms, & Abbreviations Dictionary.* 9th ed. Detroit: Gale Research Company, 1984. 2048 pp.

Curran, William J. "Titles in the Medicolegal Field: A Proposal for Reform." *American Journal of Law and Medicine,* 1(1): 1–11, 1975.
    Medicolegal studies have been unable to develop consistent and lexicographically defensible descriptive titles for the field itself. This offers an analysis of the historical roots of the terminology which has been applied in the field, an examination of current confused usage, and a proposal for reform. VIII.B.3.

Davis, Neil M. (ed.). *Medical Abbreviations: 2300 Conveniences at the Expense of Communications and Safety.* 2nd ed. Huntingdon Valley, PA: Neil M. Davis Associates, 1985. 61 pp. $3.25, softcover.

Darnay, Brigitte T., and John Nimchuk (eds.). *Subject Directory of Special Library and Information Centers,* vol. 3: *Health Sciences Libraries.* Detroit: Gale Research Co., 1985. 270 pp. $145. III.C.

Deblock, J.I. *Elsevier's Dictionary of Public Health.* New York: American Elsevier Publication Company, 1976. VII.B.2.e.

Delk, James H. *A Comprehensive Dictionary of Audiology.* Sioux City, IA: Hearing Aid Journal, 1973.
    Includes 5500 entries which provide definitions, pronunciations, and abbreviations. Illustrates hearing equipment. Provides word equivalent list. V.

Delong, Marilyn Fuller. *Medical Acronyms & Abbreviations.* Oradell, NJ: Medical Economics Books, 1985. 312 pp. $10.95.

DeLorenzo, Barbara. *The Pharmaceutical Word Book.* Philadelphia: W.B. Saunders Company, 1985. 158 pp. $14.95. III.B.3., III.C.

Department of Labor. *Dictionary of Occupational Titles.* Washington: U.S. Government Printing Office, 1977. 1371 pp. $13.
    Contains titles, alphabetically and by industry, with a glossary of defined technical terms. VII.B.2.

Deutsch, Albert (ed.). *Encyclopedia of Mental Health.* 6 vols. New York: Watts, 1963.
    Includes bibliography, index, and a list of mental health agencies. II.B.2.

Dirckx, John H. *The Language of Medicine: Its Evolution, Structure, and Dynamics.* 2nd ed. New York: Praeger, 1983. 193 pp. $22.95. First edition, 1976.
    A fond exploration of the informal language of medicine. VIII.D.

A Discursive Dictionary of Health Care. Subcommittee on Health and the Environment of the Committee on Interstate and Foreign Commerce, U.S. House of Representatives. Washington, DC: U.S. Government Printing Office, 1976. 182 pp. Originally, $2.40, softcover.
    The first edition of this dictionary. Hastily prepared by the author in about six months. Inconsistent in scope, coverage, and style.

Downes, John, and Jordon Elliott Goodman. *Dictionary of Finance and Investment Terms.* Woodbury, NY: Barron's Educational Series, Inc., 1985. 495 pp. $6.95.
    Brief but formal, includes U.S. slang. VI.

Dox, Ida, Biagio J. Melloni, and Gilbert M. Eisner. *Melloni's Illustrated Medical Dictionary.* 2nd ed. Baltimore, MD: Williams and Wilkins, 1985. 533 pp. $22.50. First edition, 1979.

Consists of 2500 illustrations prepared by the distinguished medical illustrators Ida Dox and Biagio Melloni, with definitions. Useful for allied health personnel. III.A.4., III.C.

Drever, James, rev. by Harvey Wallerstien. *A Dictionary of Psychology*. Rev. ed. Baltimore: Penguin Books, Inc., 1964.
British. Dated. III.C.

Duncan, A.S., G.R. Dunstan, and R.B. Welbourn. *Dictionary of Medical Ethics*. Rev. ed. New York: The Crossroad Publishing Company, 1981. 459 pp. $24.50.
Very British and very discursive. A valuable dictionary which includes detailed, undogmatic explanations. V.

Duncan, Helen A. *Duncan's Dictionary for Nurses*. New York: Springer Publishing, 1971.
Defines 11,000 terms from nursing, medicine, and related disciplines. Definitions are clear and include pronunciations. Etymology and chemical formulas are omitted. Small line drawings. For professional nurses, paramedical personnel, and students. III.C.

Duncan, Ronald, and Miranda Weston-Smith. *The Encyclopedia of Medical Ignorance: Exploring the Frontiers of Medical Knowledge*. New York: Pergamon Press, 1984. 253 pp. $17.95.
About two dozen essays on what we do not know about various major medical topics from genetics to medical care itself. III.C.

Durrenberger, Robert W. *Dictionary of the Environmental Sciences*. Palo Alto, CA: National Press Books, 1973.
Includes approximately 4000 terms related to the environmental sciences, with concise definitions, and illustrations. Appendices include geologic time, and equivalents and conversion tables. I.C.

Eidelberg, Ludwig (ed). *Encyclopedia of Psychoanalysis*. New York: Macmillan, 1968.
Highly specialized encyclopedia. Includes bibliographies, definitions, interpretations. III.C.

Elling, Ray H. *Cross-National Study of Health Systems: Concepts, Methods, and Data Sources*. Vol. 2 in the Health Affairs Information Guide Series. Detroit: Gale Research Co., 1980. 293 pp.
Annotated listing of major works, data sources, bibliographies, and journals. VIII.D.

Encyclopedia of Sociology. Guillford, CT: Dushkin, 1974.
Comprehensive encyclopedia with references. Alphabetical articles cover major areas of sociology. I.B.2.

Energy Terminology. 2nd ed. New York: Pergamon, 1986. 539 pp. $112.50, hardcover; $45, softcover. I.C.

Erlen, Jonathon. *The History of the Health Care Sciences and Health Care, 1700–1980: A Selected Annotated Bibliography*. (Vol. 10 in the *Bibliographies of the History of Science and Technology*, Robert Multhauf and Ellen Wells, eds., *Garland Reference Library of the Humanities*, vol. 398) New York: Garland Publishing, Inc., 1984. 1028 pp. $100. VIII.A.

Estes, Ralph. *Dictionary of Accounting*. Cambridge, MA: The MIT Press, 1981. 161 pp. $4.95.
The much appreciated reference dictionary for accounting for this effort. VI.C.1.

Estrin, Norman F. (ed.). *CTFA Cosmetic Ingredient Dictionary*. Washington, DC: The Cosmetic, Toiletry, and Fragrance Association, 1973.

Compiles pertinent data on substances frequently used in the cosmetic industry. Attempts to standardize cosmetic ingredient nomenclature. Monograph format lists adopted names, synonyms, CAS registry numbers, structural formulas, and reference sources. III.B.

Etter, Lewis E. *Glossary of Words and Phrases Used in Radiology, Nuclear Medicine, and Ultrasound*. 2nd ed. Springfield, IL: Charles C. Thomas, 1970.

Over 5500 words and definitions including abbreviations, cross-references, and footnotes. Prepared for medical secretaries, x-ray technicians, and medical students. III.C.

Evans, Anthony (compiler). *Glossary of Molecular Biology*. New York: Halsted Press, 1975.

About 350 entries related to molecular biology. Cross-references and bibliography of 139 citations. Useful for molecular biologists as well as individuals with backgrounds in biology and chemistry. I.A.1.

Eysenck, Hans J., and W.A.R. Meili (eds.). *Encyclopedia of Psychology*. 3 vols. London: Search Press, 1972.

Articles vary in length, depending on subject, but are well-referenced. Authors from 22 different countries. III.C.

Farber, Lawrence (ed.). *Medical Economics Encyclopedia of Practice and Financial Management*. Oradell, NJ: Medical Economics, 1984. 1253 pp. $69.95. VI.

Fergusson, Rosalind. *The Penguin Dictionary of Proverbs*. New York: Penguin Books, 1983. 331 pp. $5.95.

Subjects include cleanliness, death, health, and remedies. VIII.B.

Food and Nutrition Terminology: Definitions of Selected Terms and Expressions in Current Use. FAO Terminology Bulletins, no. 28. Rome: Food and Agriculture Organization, 1974.

The definitions, in English and intended to facilitate the work of the U.N. system, are not official or definitive. Prepared by the FAO and WHO in collaboration with the International Union of Nutritional Sciences. I.A.2.a.

Food: Multilingual Thesaurus. 4 vols. New York: K.G. Saur, 1978.

An English, German, French, and Italian index to a controlled vocabulary on food. I.A.2.a.

Frenay, Agnes Clare, and Rose Maureen Mahoney. *Understanding Medical Terminology*. 7th ed. St. Louis, MO: Catholic Hospital Association, 1984. 618 pp.; 85 illustrations. $19.50, softcover. First edition, 1958.

An easy-language dictionary devoted to biologic disorders and medicine. Contains illustrations, charts, a bibliography, and an index. Written for the public and students of pharmacy, nursing, medical technology, physical therapy, and hospital administration. III.A.4. and 6., VII.B.2.b.

Friel, John P. (ed.). *Dorland's Illustrated Medical Dictionary*. 26th ed. Philadelphia: W.B. Saunders Company, 1985. 1485 pp. $39.95. First edition, 1900.

A standard medical dictionary for 80 years with over 120,000 entries contributed by 80 authorities. Contains illustrations and plates; now available on computer tape. A high-quality, recommended dictionary. III.C.

Garb, Solomon, Eleanor Krakauer, and Carson Justice. *Abbreviations and Acronyms in Medicine and Nursing*. New York: Springer Publishing, 1976.
A compilation of medical abbreviations and acronyms. Includes 400 terms, with brief explanations, and Greek and Roman abbreviations.

Gibson, Mary Jo Storey, and Charlotte Nusberg (eds.). *International Glossary of Social Gerontology*. New York: Van Nostrand Reinhold Co., 1985. 96 pp. $28.95. III.C.

Glossary of Terms: Used in the "Health for All" Series, Nos. 1–8. Geneva: World Health Organization, 1984. II.C.

Glossary on Air Pollution. WHO Regional Publications, European Series No. 9. Copenhagen: World Health Organization, Regional Office for Europe, 1980. 114 pp. Sw. fr. 12. Correspondence should be directed to the Director, Promotion of Environmental Health, WHO Regional Office for Europe, Scherfigsvej 8, 2100 Copenhagen 0, Denmark. I.C.1.

Goldberg, Marcia et al. *A Worker's Guide to Winning at the Occupational Safety and Health Review Commission*. 2nd ed. Washington (2000 P St., N.W., DC 20036): Health Research Group, 1981. $5.
Has basic glossary. Otherwise helpful. VII.B.2.d.

Goldenson, Robert M. (ed.). *Encyclopedia of Human Behavior: Psychology, Psychiatry, and Mental Health*. 2 vols. Garden City, NY: Doubleday, 1970.
Includes terms, theories, biographies, and treatment techniques. I.A.2., III.C.

Gould, Julius, and William L. Kolb (eds.). *Dictionary of the Social Sciences*. Compiled under the auspices of the United Nations Educational, Scientific, and Cultural Organization. New York: The Free Press, 1964. 761 pp.
Somewhat dated but encyclopedic, with references and high quality. I.B.2.

Gove, Philip Babcock, and the Merriam-Webster Editorial Staff. *Webster's Third New International Dictionary of the English Language Unabridged*. Springfield, MA: G & C Merriam Company, Publishers, 1976. 2662 pp.
The reference English language dictionary for this work, and a deservedly famous work. VIII.B.

Graf, Rudolph F., and George J. Whalen. *The Reston Encyclopedia of Biomedical Engineering Terms*. Reston, VA: Reston Publishing Co., 1977.
Biomedical and engineering terms briefly defined with cross-references. Many interdisciplinary terms are included. Not overly technical. III.B.2.

Grant, Roger, and Claire Grant (eds.). *Grant & Hackh's Chemical Dictionary*. 5th ed. New York: McGraw-Hill Book Company, 1987. 641 pp. $74. I.A.1.

Greenwald, Douglas. *The McGraw-Hill Dictionary of Modern Economics: A Handbook of Terms and Organization*. New York: McGraw-Hill Book Company, 1965. VIII.B.1.

Griffiths, Mary C., Carolyn A. Fleeger, and Lloyd C. Miller (eds.). *USAN and the USP Dictionary of Drug Names*. 1986 ed. Rockville, MD: U.S. Pharmacopeial Convention, 1985. 678 pp. $54.95. III.B.3.

Grzimek, Bernhard. *Grzimek's Animal Life Encyclopedia*. 13 vols. New York: Van Nostrand Reinhold, 1972–1975.
The set is arranged by animal groups, with the material in each volume arranged by animal orders and families. Includes a systematic classification index and multilingual glossary. I.A.1.

Hamilton, Betty, and Barbara Guidos. *MASA: Medical Acronyms, Symbols and Abbreviations*. New York (23 Cornelia St.): Neal-Schuman Publishers, 1984. 186 pp. $39.95.

Handbook for Foreign Medical Graduates. Philadelphia: Educational Commission for Foreign Medical Graduates, 1976. Glossary, pp. 68–73. III.B.1.

Hampel, Clifford A., and Gessner G. Hawley. *Glossary of Chemical Terms*. 2nd ed. Jersey City, NJ: Unz & Co., 1982. 320 pp. $28.75.
    Over 2000 terms in the several subdivisions of chemistry and the chemical industry with an expanded treatment of toxic materials and waste control. I.C.

Haubrich, William S. *Medical Meanings: A Glossary of Word Origins*. San Diego: Harcourt Brace Jovanovich Publishers, 1984. 285 pp. $9.95, softcover.
    Ordinary, informal clinical etymology. VIII.A.2., VIII.B.

Hawley, Gessner. *The Condensed Chemical Dictionary*. 10th ed. Jersey City, NJ: Unz & Co., 1981. 1472 pp. $49.50.
    Covers alternative energy sources, derivation of chemical terms, TLVs for workroom environments, FDA regulations, hazard and handling information, and technical descriptions of chemicals raw materials, and processes I.C.

Health Information Resources in the Federal Government. Washington, DC: U.S. Department of Health and Human Services, 1984. 128 pp. III.D.1.

Health Insurance Institute. *Source Book of Health Insurance Data*. 1986–87. New York: Health Insurance Institute, 1987.
    Updated annually, contains a good brief glossary of health insurance. IV.B.

Heyel, Carl (ed.). *The Encyclopedia of Management*. 2nd ed. New York: Van Nostrand Reinhold Company, 1973. 1161 pp.
    Signed articles with references and other supporting material on subjects from accounting to zero deficits. Has a brief conspectus. VI.

Hinsie, Leland E., and Robert J. Campbell. *Psychiatric Dictionary*. 4th ed. New York: Oxford University Press, 1970. 816 pp.
    A standard psychiatric dictionary. Includes over 1400 words with pronunciations, illustrations, and references. Maintains a multidisciplinary approach to psychiatry. III.C.

Hill, Austin Bradford. *A Short Textbook of Medical Statistics*. London: Hodder and Stoughton, 1977. Glossary, pp. 297–301. VIII.D.

Hochberg, Burt. "The Making of a Dictionary from Aardvark to Zyzzogeton." *Games*, 14–19, 8/85.
    Nice brief description of making dictionaries. VIII.B.

Hodgkin, K. "Diagnostic Vocabulary for Primary Care." *Journal of Family Practice*, 8(1): 129–144, 1979. V.A.

Hogarth, James. *Glossary of Health Care Terminology*. Public Health in Europe Series, No. 4. Copenhagen: Regional Office for Europe, World Health Organization, 1975.
    A collection of published WHO definitions. Therefore does not define terms which have not been defined elsewhere. III.

Hooper, Robert. *Lexicon Medicum: or Medical Dictionary*. 6th ed. London: A. & R. Health and Co., 1977. III.C.

Hughes, Harold K. *Dictionary of Abbreviations in Medicine and the Health Sciences.* Lexington, MA: Lexington Books, 1977.
More than 12,000 entries with some definitions. Contains a handy guide to construction and use of acronyms. A valuable tool for health and allied professionals.

Hulke, Malcolm. *The Encyclopedia of Alternative Medicine and Self-Help.* New York: Schocken Books, 1979.
A lovely book with fair perspective and references. V.

Hukill, Peter B. "The Spoken Language of Medicine: Argot, Slang, Cant." *American Speech,* 36: 145–8, 1961. VIII.B.

Hyman, Albert S., Leonard A. Larson, and Donald E. Herrmann (eds.). *Encyclopedia of Sport Sciences and Medicine.* New York: Macmillan, 1971.
International work on a wide range of subjects, as intellect, disease, environment, and rehabilitation. Contributions from over 500 authors. Well-written, indexed. III.C.

The International Encyclopedia of Pharmacology and Therapeutics. New York: Pergamon, 1973.
A multivolume reference encyclopedia with articles by authorities. For researchers in medicine and pharmacology. III.B.3., III.C., V.B.

International Labour Office. *Encyclopedia of Occupational Health and Safety.* 2 vols. 2nd ed. New York: McGraw-Hill Book Company, 1971. 1621 pp.
Enormous, semiofficial, slightly dated, well-referenced, fairly clinical and technical. Includes helpful appendices and bibliographies, and a comprehensive analytic index. VIII.B.2.d.

International Labour Office. *Occupational Health and Safety.* 2 vols. Washington, DC: International Labour Office, 1972.
Contains 900 articles which deal with the health and safety of people at work. International contributions cover occupations, industrial processes, chemical hazards, and statistics. VII.B.2.d.

Jacob, Alphons, and Herbert L. Jackson. *Dictionary of Radiologic Terminology.* St. Louis, MO: Warren H. Green, 1979.
A comprehensive, complete dictionary which defines terms used in all specialized branches of radiology. Among those covered are pediatric, diagnostic, therapeutic, and anatomic radiology. III.C.

Joint Commission on Accreditation of Hospitals. *Accreditation Manual for Hospitals.* 1980 edition. Chicago (Ill. 60611): JCAH (875 N. Michigan Ave.), 1979. 225 pp. Glossary pp. 211–5. III.B.1.

Jerrard, H.G., and D.B. McNeill. *A Dictionary of Scientific Units.* 5th ed. New York: Chapman and Hall (Methuen), 1986. 222 pp. $39.95, hardcover; $19.95, softcover. VIII.D.

Kasner, Kay, and Dennis H. Tindall. *Bailliere's Nurses' Dictionary.* 20th ed. Philadelphia: W.B. Saunders, 1984. $9.95, hardcover; $5.95, softcover. III.C.

Kaufman, Martin et al. (eds.). *Dictionary of American Medical Bibliography.* 1027 pp. in 2 vols. Westport, CT: Greenwood Press Inc., 1983. $55/vol, $95/set.
Over 1200 sketches of people who died before 1977 including nonphysicians, blacks, women, and alternative practitioners. Each biography contains family background, education, career, bibliography, and references. VIII.A.1.

Kelly, Emerson C. *Encyclopedia of Medical Sources*. Baltimore, MD: Williams & Wilkins, 1948.
Covers major medical discoveries alphabetically with original references for the discoveries. VIII.A.2.

Kelly, Howard Atwood, and Walter L. Barrage. *Dictionary of American Medical Biography*. Longwood Press, 1978. VIII.A.1.

Kerr, Avice. *Medical Hieroglyphs: Abbreviations and Symbols*. Chicago, IL: Clissold, 1970.
Over 8400 abbreviations and symbols extracted from medical records.

Kiger, Anne Fox (compiler). *Hospital Administration Terminology*. 2nd ed. Chicago: American Hospital Publishing Inc., 1986. 61 pp. $18.75 (AHA members, $15). III.B.1.

King, Robert C., and William D. Stansfield. *A Dictionary of Genetics*. 3rd ed. New York: Oxford University Press, 1985. 480 pp. $29.95, hardcover; $17.95, softcover. I.A.1.

Klein, Barry T. (ed.). *Reference Encyclopedia of American Psychology and Psychiatry*. Rye, NY: Todd Publications, 1975.
A compilation of associations, research centers, periodicals, audiovisual aids, and hospitals for psychologists and psychiatrists; a directory-encyclopedia for college, medical, and public libraries. III.C.

Koch, Michael S. *Biomedical Thesaurus and Guide to Classification*. New York: CCM Information, 1972.
A compilation of medical terms from the National Library of Medicine, the Library of Congress, and MeSH. The thesaurus includes 5000 headings and cross-references emphasizing clinical terms, and works as a guide in classification schemes. III.C.

Kohler, Eric L. *A Dictionary for Accountants*. 5th ed. Englewood Cliffs, NJ: Prentice-Hall, Inc., 1975. 498 pp.
A discursive dictionary of accounting. VI.C.1.

Kolin, Philip C. "The Language of Nursing." *American Speech: A Quarterly of Linguistic Usage*, 48(1–2), 1973.
A great collection in narrative of the argot, slang, and cant of nursing. III.C.

Kotz, Samuel, Normal L. Johnson, and Campbell P. Read (eds.). *Encyclopedia of Statistical Sciences*. Vol. 6, *Multivariate Analysis to Plackett and Burman Designs*. New York: Wiley-Interscience, 1985. 758 pp. $85. VIII.D.

Krauss, Stephen. *Encyclopaedic Handbook of Medical Psychology*. London: Butterworths, 1976.
Over 200 articles written by psychiatrists, neurologists, and psychologists. III.C.

Kruzas, Anthony T. et al. (eds.). *Medical and Health Information Directory*. 3rd ed. 3 vols. Detroit: Gale Research Co., Book Tower, 1985.
Vol. 1: *Organizations, Agencies, and Institutions*.
Vol. 2: *Libraries, Publications, Audiovisuals, and Data Base Services*.
Vol. 3: *Health Services*. III.

Lagua, Rosalinda T., Virginia S. Claudio, and Victoria F. Thiele. *Nutrition and Diet Therapy; Reference Dictionary*. 2nd ed. St. Louis, MO: C.V. Mosby, 1974.
Covers 3500 terms in biochemistry, nutrition, dietetics, physiology, and related topics with some terms of historic value. Appendices cover the clas-

sification of carbohydrates, lipids, and proteins, and describe minerals, vitamins, and enzymes. Written for the student and public. I.A.2.a.

Landau, Sidney I. *Dictionaries: The Art and Craft of Lexicography*. New York: The Scribner Press, Charles Scribner's Sons, 1984.
Required reading for the author and his colleagues on how to write a dictionary; an excellent work. VIII.B.2.

Landau, Sidney I. et al. *International Dictionary of Medicine and Biology*. New York: John Wiley, 1986. 3200 pp. $395.
Nearly a decade in preparation, this dictionary contains 151,000 terms and 159,000 definitions in 70 subjects with useful descriptive and usage information. III.C.

Lapedes, Daniel N. (ed.). *McGraw-Hill Encyclopedia of Food, Agriculture, and Nutrition*. New York: McGraw-Hill, 1977.
Presents an overview of the world food problem. Contains 400 signed articles. Includes tables of food composition. A handy, authoritative reference for general libraries. I.A.2.a.

Last, John M. et al. *A Dictionary of Epidemiology*. New York: Oxford University Press, 1983. 114 pp. $21.95, hardcover; $10.95, softcover. Illus. VIII.C.

Leigh, Denis, C.M.B. Pare, and John Marks (eds.). *A Concise Encyclopedia of Psychiatry*. Baltimore, MD: University Park Press, 1977.
Includes biographical as well as conceptual information, charts, and diagrams. III.C.

Levine, Milton L., and Jean H. Seligmann. *The Parents' Encyclopedia of Infancy, Childhood, and Adolescence*. Philadelphia, PA: Harper & Row, 1978.
Pediatricians cover some 1000 topics. Appendices provide useful directory information: poison control centers, community mental health programs, and genetic counseling agencies. Extensive beginner's bibliography. No index, adequate cross-references. VII.B.2.b.

Lingeman, Richard R. *Drugs from A to Z: A Dictionary*. 2nd ed. New York: McGraw-Hill, 1974.
Reference tool which lists drug terms, including slang, defined from both a pharmacological and sociological point of view. Entries include synonyms, cross-references, and quotations from authors. Four appendices of legal classifications of drugs. III.B.3.

Lipton, Morris A., Alberto Di Mascio, and Keith F. Killam (eds.). *Psychopharmacology: A Generation of Progress*. New York: Raven Press, 1978.
An extensive encyclopedia of basic and clinical psychopharmacology. Covers ethics and the strategy of administering psychotropic drugs; describes common withdrawal syndromes. A thorough reference for those who use psychotropic drugs. III.C., V.B.

Logan, C. *Medical Abbreviations, 1987*. New York: Harper & Row, 1987. $22.50.

Lourie, John. *Medical Eponyms: Who Was Coude?* London: Pitman Publishing Ltd., 1982. 220 pp. $12.75 paper. Available in the U.S. from Urban & Schwarzenberg, Medical Publishers, 7 East Redwood Street, Baltimore, MD 21202
A dictionary of the origins of eponymous names. II.B.2., VIII.B.

Maddox, George L. et al. *The Encyclopedia of Aging*. New York: Springer Publishing, 1987. 890 pp. $96. I.A.1.

Magalini, Sergio. *Dictionary of Medical Syndromes.* Philadelphia, PA: J.B. Lippincott, 1971.

    An alphabetical listing of over 1800 defined medical syndromes with eponyms. Provides references for the etiology, pathology, symptoms, therapy, and prognosis of each syndrome. Includes bibliography and index. II.B.2.

Manhold, John H., and Michael P. Balbo (eds.). *Illustrated Dental Terminology: With Spanish, French, and German Correlations.* Philadelphia: J.B. Lippincott, 1985. 370 pp. $15.75. III.C.

Manning, Robert T. "A Glossary of Statistical Words and Expressions Commonly Used in Scientific Writing." *Continuing Education,* 81–93, 7/81. VIII.D.

Manuila, Alexandre (ed.). *Progress in Medical Terminology.* Basel: S. Karger, 1981.

    Extensively used by *Landau, 1984.* VIII.B.2.

McAnish, T. F. (ed.). *Physics in Medicine and Biology Encyclopedia: Medical Physics, Bioengineering, and Biophysics.* 2 vols. New York: Pergamon Press Inc., 1986. 980 pp. $245. III.C.

McDavid, Raven I., and Audrey R. Duckert (eds.). "Lexicography in English." *York Academy of Sciences,* 211: 1–342, 6/8/73.

    A lexicographer's delight. Perhaps there are so few good books on lexicograhy because the lexicographers are forever busy with their files. Such harmless drudgery is not very theoretical. VIII.B.

McGraw-Hill Dictionary of the Life Sciences. New York: McGraw-Hill, 1976.

    A practical guide to the biologic sciences with 20,000 definitions covering 49 fields of science. Good cross-referencing and over 800 illustrations. Serves both the specialist and general public. I.A.1.

McGrew, Roderick E. *Encyclopedia of Medical History.* New York: McGraw-Hill International Book Co., 1985. 400 pp. $34.95. VIII.A.

    103 essays on selected medical topics, no definitional entries or biographical sketches.

Merriam-Webster Editorial Staff. *Webster's New Collegiate Dictionary.* Rev. 8th ed. Springfield, MA: G & C Merriam, 1973.

    A standard English dictionary used as the reference dictionary for this work when vacationing. VIII.

Metz, Robert. "Principles of Medicine." *Journal of the Tennessee Medical Association,* 70(4): 261–3, 4/77.

    Sixty-seven facetious and ironic principles of medicine, like but not including *ox's laws.* VIII.B.2.b., VIII.B.3.

Michael, Max et al. *Biomedical Bestiary: An Epidemiologic Guide to Flaws and Fallacies in the Medical Literature.* Boston: Little, Brown, 1984. 161 pp. $12.95.

    A clever guide to the classic pitfalls of clinical epidemiology and research. VIII.C.

Miller, Benjamin F., and Claire B. Keane. *Encyclopedia and Dictionary of Medicine, Nursing, and Allied Health.* 3rd ed. Philadelphia: W. B. Saunders Company, 1983. 1270 pp. $24.95. First edition, 1972.

    Contains photographs, line drawings, and anatomic plates. Useful for the nurse, paramedic, or lay person. III.A.4., III.C.

Miller, William C., and Geoffrey P. West. *Black's Veterinary Dictionary*. London: Black, 1972.
    Encyclopedic dictionary of veterinary care, similar to *Black's Medical Dictionary* in format. Includes causes, symptoms, and treatment of disease. Illustrated. III.C.

Millodot, Michel. *Dictionary of Optometry*. Boston: Butterworths, 1986. 187 pp. $19.95, softcover. III.C.

Mishler, Elliot G. *The Discourse of Medicine: Dialectics of Medical Interviews*. (Language and Learning for Human Service Professions, Cynthia Wallet and Judith Green, eds.) Norwood, NJ 07648: Ablex Publishing Corp. (355 Chestnut St.), 1984. 211 pp. $29.50, hardcover; $18.95, softcover. VIII.B.

Modern Drug Encyclopedia and Therapeutic Index. 17th ed. New York: Yorke Medical Books, 1985. Annual.
    Monographs on drugs, listed alphabetically by nonproprietary names or drug groups, giving description, indications, contraindications, dosage, and administration. Also has availability information, which includes trademark, packaging, dose forms, and manufacturer. III.B.3., V.B.

Moerman, Daniel E. *American Medical Ethnobotany: A Reference Dictionary*. New York: Garland Publishing, 1977.
    Over 3500 entries arranged according to standardized contemporary botanical nomenclature. Lists plants with medical properties with a full bibliographical citation for each entry. V.B.

Moffat, Donald W. *Economics Dictionary*. New York (NY 10017): American Elsevier Publishing Company, Inc. (52 Vanderbilt Avenue), 1976. 301 pp.
    Regularly and gratefully used in preparing this dictionary. VIII.B.1.

Morgan, Peter. *An Insider's Guide for Medical Authors and Editors*. (Professional Editing and Publishing Series) Philadelphia: ISI Press, 1986. 111 pp. $23.95, hardcover; $14.95, softcover. VIII.D.

Morris, Dwight A., and Lynne Darby Morris. *Health Care Administration: A Guide to Information Sources*. Vol. 1 in the Health Affairs Information Guide Series. Detroit: Gale Research Co., 1978. 264 pp.
    An annotated bibliography of references, statistical sources, periodicals, and so forth. VI.C., VIII.D.

Morton, Leslie T. *A Medical Bibliography (Garrison and Morton): An Annotated Check-list of Texts Illustrating the History of Medicine*. 4th ed. Lexington, MA: Lexington Books, 1983. 1000 pp. $52.
    Known as *Garrison and Morton*, this work lists the important contributions in each major medical subject (books and journals) in chronological order, usually with an annotation describing the work reported in the publication. The fourth edition has 7830 entries. VIII.A.

Morton, L.T., and S. Godbolt (eds.). *Information Sources in the Medical Sciences*. (*Butterworths Guides to Information Sources*, D.J. Foskett and M.W. Hill, eds.) 3rd ed. Woburn, MA: Butterworths, 1984. 534 pp. $89.95. III.C.

Nicolosi, Lucille, Elizabeth Harryman, and Janet Kreschek. *Terminology of Communication Disorders: Speech, Language, and Hearing*. Baltimore, MD: Williams & Wilkins, 1978.
    Comprehensive vocabulary of audiology, otolaryngology, neurology, and psychology. Over 10,000 definitions cover language, voice, rhythm, struc-

ture, and hearing. Intended for speech, language, and hearing professionals. V.

Nohring, Jurgen (compiler). *Dictionary of Medicine: English-German.* New York: Elsevier Scientific Publishing Co. Inc., 1984. 708 pp. $113.50. III.C.

North American Primary Care Research Group (NAPCRG). "Glossary for Primary Care: Report of the Committee on Standard Terminology." *The Journal of Family Practice,* 7(1): 129–34, 1978. V.

> Incompetent, dated glossary by a competent body. Cited as *NAPCRG, 1977.* V.

O'Brien, Robert, and Sidney Cohen. *The Encyclopedia of Drug Abuse.* New York: Facts on File, 1984. 454 pp. $40. II.B.2.

Occupational Safety and Health Information Centre. *CIS Thesaurus.* Washington, DC: International Labour Office, 1976.

> French-English dictionary of more than 10,000 terms relating to occupational safety and health. Includes systematic and alphabetic sections. Also published under the title *Thesaurus CIS.* VII.B.2.d.

Office of Human Development Services, Administration for Children, Youth, and Families, Children's Bureau, U.S. National Center on Child Abuse and Neglect. *Interdisciplinary Glossary on Child Abuse and Neglect: Legal, Medical,* and *Social Work Terms.* DHEW Pub. No. (OHDS) 78-30137. Washington, DC: U.S. Government Printing Office, 1978. I.B.1., II.B.2.

Omega 1987 Complete Handbook of Scientific and Technical Books. Annual ed. Stamford, CT: Omega Press, 1987. Free, to qualified people. III.C.

Oran, Daniel. *Law Dictionary for Non-Lawyers.* St. Paul, MN: West Publishing Co., 1978. 333 pp.

> Useful work with some helpful appendices on sources and legalities but not as good as Black or Ballentine. VIII.B.3.

Osler, Robert W., and John S. Bickley (eds.). *Glossary of Insurance Terms.* Santa Monica, CA: Insurance Press, Inc., 1972. IV.B.

Parker, Sybil P. et al. *McGraw-Hill Encyclopedia of Science and Technology.* 6th ed. 20 vols. New York: McGraw-Hill, 1987. 12,700 pp. $1600.

> "One of the world's leading works on all aspects of science for the lay reader." I.

Patrick, P.K. (compiler). *Glossary on Solid Waste.* Copenhagen: World Health Organization Regional Office for Europe, 1980. 92 pp. I.C.4.

Pearce, David W. (ed.). *The Dictionary of Modern Economics.* Rev. ed. Cambridge: The MIT Press, 1983. 481 pp. $12.50, softcover. First, clothbound edition, 1981.

> Extensive and well cross-referenced. VIII.B.1.

Peterson, Martin S., and Arnold H. Johnson. *Encyclopedia of Food Science.* Westport, CT: Avi Publishing, 1978. I.A.2.a.

Pinney, Edward L., and Samuel Slipp. *Glossary of Group and Family Therapy.* New York: Brunner/March, 1982. 149 pp. $15.

> Two separate vocabularies with many brief biographical definitions of people. Relied on by this author for much family therapy material. I.B.1., III.C.

Pomeranz, Virginia E., and Dodi Schultz. *The Mothers' and Fathers' Medical Encyclopedia*. Boston: Little, Brown, 1977. Revised and expanded version of the *Mother's Medical Encyclopedia*.

Over 2000 entries with many illustrations, useful appendices, and room for charting medical histories. An excellent home reference. Includes a particularly helpful section on poisonous household substances with appropriate antidotes. VII.B.2.b.

Purdom, P. Walton. *Environmental Health*. 2nd ed. New York: Academic Press, 1980. 714 pp.

Reich, Warren T. *Encyclopedia of Bioethics*. 4 vols. New York: The Free Press, 1978. 1933 pp.

A massive work by multiple contributors with extensive references. V.

Research Documentation Section, U.S. National Institutes of Health. *Medical and Health Related Sciences Thesaurus*. Public Health Service Pub. No. 1031. 2nd ed. Washington, DC: U.S. Government Printing Office, 1969.

Entries compiled as an indexing authority list for a research grants index. Contains 9200 terms with cross-references. VIII.B., VIII.D.

Rhodes, Philip. *An Outline History of Medicine*. Woburn, MA: Butterworths, 1985. 219 pp. $29.95. VIII.A.

Rieger, R. et al. *Glossary of Genetics and Cytogenetics*. New York: Springer-Verlag, 1976. I.A.1.

Rigal, Waldo A. *The Inverted Medical Dictionary: A Method of Finding Medical Terms Quickly*. Westport, CT: Technomic Publishing, 1976.

Almost 13,000 medical terms with each definition reduced to a brief key phrase. Arranged alphabetically by descriptive subject. Reference tool for medical writers. VIII.B.

Rinzler, Carol Ann. *The Dictionary of Medical Folklore*. New York: Crowell, 1979.

A collection of some 500 medical old wives' tales. I.B.2., V.

Roody, Peter, Robert E. Forman, and Howard B. Schweitzer. *Medical Abbreviations and Acronyms*. New York: McGraw-Hill, 1976. 255 pp.

Abbreviations and acronyms used in medicine, dentistry, audiology, psychology, etc. Indexes 14,000 terms. Cross-referenced. Heavy emphasis on American terminology. Lacks a section listing full terms followed by the corresponding shortened form.

Roper, Fred W., and Jo Anne Boorkman. *Introduction to Reference Sources in the Health Sciences*. 2nd ed. Chicago: Medical Library Association, 1984. 302 pp. $27. VIII.D.

Roper, Nancy. *Livingstone's Dictionary for Nurses*. 14th ed. Edinburgh: Churchill Livingstone, 1973.

Over 5000 definitions. Appendices of common prefixes and suffixes and their meanings, procedures for urine and blood tests, and common toxic substances. III.C.

Rosen, George. *A History of Public Health*. MD Monographs on Medical History, number one. New York: MD Publications, Inc., 1958.

The source of many of the descriptions of people included in this work and itself a lovely effort. VII.B.2.e., VIII.A.

Rothenberg, Robert E. *The New American Medical Dictionary and Health Manual*. 3rd ed. New York: New American Library, Signet Books, 1975.

An American lay medical dictionary. VII.B.2.b.

Ruiz Torres, Francesco. *Diccionaro de Terminos Medicos.* 4th ed. Philadelphia: W.B. Saunders, 1982. 612 pp. $39.95. VIII.B.

Ruiz Torres, Francesco. *Vocabulario De Medicina.* Philadelphia: W.B. Saunders, 1982. 102 pp. $9.95, softcover. VIII.B.

Rycroft, Charles. *A Critical Dictionary of Psychoanalysis.* Totowa, NJ: Littlefield, Adams, 1973.
Over 600 terms, cross-referenced. Emphasizes conceptual and theoretical use. Includes medical, Jungian, anthropological, and biologic terms. III.C.

Safire, William. *Safire's Political Dictionary.* 3rd ed. of *The New Language of Politics.* New York: Random House, 1978. 845 pp. First edition, 1968.
A discursive work similar to this one, only better. VI.A., VIII.B.3.

Sampson, P. *Glossary of Bacteriological Terms.* London: Butterworths, 1975.
A glossary of over 1000 medical bacteriology terms with definitions, cross-references, drawings, and an extensive bibliography. I.A.1.

Sarnoff, Paul. *The New York Times Encyclopedic Dictionary of the Environment.* New York: Equinox Books, 1971.
Complete, discursive, polemical, and dated. I.C.

Saunders Health Care Directory. Philadelphia: W.B. Saunders, A Norback Book, 1984. 960 pp. $85. III.

Schertel, Albrecht. *Abbreviations in Medicine.* 2nd ed. Basel: S. Karger, 1977.

Schmidt, J.E. *(Schmidt's) Attorney's Dictionary of Medicine and Word Finder.* 17th ed. 3 vols. New York (NY 10017): Mathew Bender (235 E 45th St.), 1982. First edition, 1962.
Subscription updating available. 61,000 entries. VIII.B.3.

Schmidt, Jacob E. *Index of Paramedical Vocabulary: An Index-Indicator Enabling the User Not Versed in Greek and Latin to Locate the Terminology of Any Given Subject in a Paramedical, Medical, or Biological Dictionary.* Springfield, IL: Charles C. Thomas, 1974.
To be used as a key to alphabetical medical dictionaries. Cross-references English to Latin prefixes. Helpful to lawyers, managers, paramedics, and others seeking to acquaint themselves with medical vocabulary. III.A.4., VIII.B.

Schmidt, Jacob E. *Structural Units of Medical and Biological Terms.* Springfield, IL: Charles C. Thomas, 1969.
A guide to dissection of the medical vocabulary. Each of the 1000 main entries includes definition, origin, combining stem, and examples of compound words. VIII.B.

Sewell, Winifred (series ed.). *Health Affairs Information Guide Series.* Published by the Gale Research Company, Book Tower, Detroit, MI 48226. Eighteen volumes are contemplated of which three are available; see *Morris, 1978, Elling, 1980,* and *Weise, 1979.* VIII.D.

Sichel, Beatrice, and Werner Sichel. *Economics Journals and Serials: An Analytical Guide.* New York: Greenwood Press, Inc., 1986. 285 pp. $45. VIII.B.1.

Sienklnecht, Charles W. "A Primer in the Rheumatic Diseases for East Tennessee." *American Journal of Medicine,* 78: 182–4, 2/85.
Southern mountain lay language for disease; corruption, pones, and such. VIII.B.2.a.

Simon, Fritz B., Helm Stierlin, and Lyman C. Wynne. *The Language of Family Therapy: A Systemic Vocabulary and Sourcebook.* A Family Process Press book distributed by Norton Professional Books. New York: W.W. Norton, 1985. 408 pp. $30.
Well-done exploration of many concepts; essays with references. V.

Singer, Richard B., and Louis Levinson (eds.). *Medical Risks: Patterns of Mortality and Survival.* Lexington, MA: Lexington Books, D.C. Heath and Company, 1976. $27.50.
A reference volume sponsored by the Association of Life Insurance Medical Directors of America and the Society of Actuaries. An enormous compendium of tables of comparative mortality and survival data. III.C., IV.B., VIII.C.

Singleton, P., and D. Sainsbury. *Dictionary of Microbiology.* New York: John Wiley, 1978.
Definitions of terms, techniques, and concepts in microbiology with descriptions of over 1000 taxa. I.A.1.

Sippl, Charles J., and Roger J. Sippl. *Computer Dictionary.* 3rd ed. Indianapolis (IN 46268): Howard W. Sams & Co., Inc., 1980. 624 pp. $16.95, softcover. First edition, 1974.
Brief formal definitions (and many of them). III.B.2.

Sittig, Marshall. *Pharmaceutical Manufacturing Encyclopedia.* Park Ridge, NJ: Noyes Data, 1979.
Describes drug manufacturing processes. Arranged alphabetically by generic name. III.B.3.

Skinner, Henry Alan. *The Origin of Medical Terms.* 2nd ed. New York: Hafner Publishing Company, 1970. 437 pp.
Many minibiographies and a great deal of history combined with commentaries on the origin of terms. VIII.A.2., VIII.B.1.

Slee, Virgil N. *Health Care Terms.* First edition. Ann Arbor, MI: Tringa Press, 1986. 150 pp. $11.95, softcover.
Excellent initial effort, without bibliography or conspectus. VI.C., VIII.B.

Sloan, Harold S., and Arnold I. Zurcher. *Dictionary of Economics.* 5th ed. New York: Barnes and Noble Books, 1970. VIII.B.1.

Sloane, Sheila B. *Medical Abbreviations and Eponyms.* Philadelphia: W.B. Saunders, 1985. 410 pp. $19.95.

Sloane, Sheila B. *The Medical Word Book.* 2nd ed. Philadelphia: W.B. Saunders, 1982. 1008 pp. Illus. $22.95. VIII.B.

Sloane, Sheila B., and John Dusseau. *A Word Book in Pathology and Laboratory Medicine.* Philadelphia: W.B. Saunders, 1984. 610 pp. $19.95, softcover. III.C.

Special Studies Committee of the Michigan Occupational Therapy Association. *Medical Abbreviations: A Cross Reference Dictionary.* 2nd ed. Ann Arbor, MI: Michigan Occupational Therapy Association, 1967.
Lists abbreviations from all areas of medicine and allied health. Part I gives abbreviation and full meaning; part II indicates the full form followed by the accepted abbreviation.

Speert, Kathryn H., and Samuel M. Wishik. *Fertility Modification Thesaurus with Focus on Evaluation of Family Planning Programs.* New York: International Institute for the Study of Human Reproduction, Columbia University, 1973.

Thesaurus of terms relating to family planning program development and evaluation. Follows the MeSH tree structure. Nearly 2000 items divided in four sections. Includes three appendices; descriptors, categories, and hierarchy. Limited application; intended primarily as an indexing tool. I.B.1.

Staats, Elmer R. *Budgetary Definitions.* Pub. No. OPA-76-8. Washington: U.S. General Accounting Office, November 1975. VI.A.

Stafford, Peter. *Psychedelics Encyclopedia.* Berkeley, CA: And/Or Press, 1977.

Stedman's Medical Dictionary: A Vocabulary of Medicine and Its Allied Sciences With Pronunciations and Derivations. 23rd ed. Baltimore, MD: Williams & Wilkins, 1976. First edition, 1911.

Holds a lofty place among medical dictionaries with an exhaustive and current vocabulary, covering pharmacological, dental, and medical terms with pronunciations, derivations, and pertinent illustrations.

A goldmine of information is found in the indexes and appendices. Definitions are accurate, crisp, and technical. III.C.

Steen, Edwin B. *Bailliere's Abbreviations in Medicine.* 5th ed. London: Bailliere Tindall (distributed in the U.S. by W. B. Saunders), 1984. 264 pp. $12.95.

A more detailed list of acronyms than in this work, without definitions. Includes over 13,000 British, clinical, Latin prescription, military, organizational, and titular abbreviations.

Strauss, Maurice B. (ed.). *Familiar Medical Quotations.* Boston: Little, Brown and Company, 1968.

A medical Bartlett with over 7000 quotations organized by subject and indexed by author. VIII.A.1., VIII.B.

Studdard, Gloria J. *Common Environmental Terms: A Glossary.* Washington, DC: U.S. Environmental Protection Agency, 1973.

Over 400 terms with concise definitions of words and terms essential to understanding environmental issues, often gratefully used in preparing this work. I.C.

Subcommittee on NMR Nomenclature and Phantom Development, Committee on NMR Imaging Technology and Equipment, Commission on Nuclear Magnetic Resonance. *Glossary of NMR Terms.* Chicago: American College of Radiology, 1983. 32 pp. $4, softcover. III.B.2.

Tabery, Julia Jordan et al. *Communicating in Spanish for Medical Personnel: Communicion en Ingles para Personal Medico.* 2nd ed. Boston: Little, Brown and Company, 1984. 638 pp. VIII.B.

Thomas, Clayton L. (ed.). *Taber's Cyclopedic Medical Dictionary.* Philadelphia, PA: F.A. Davis, 1977. First edition, 1940.

High-quality dictionary for nurses and allied health professionals. Concise definitions with phonetic spellings, synonyms, derivations, and abbreviations where necessary. Some tables and two-color line drawings. Appendices cover first aid procedures, addresses of poison control centers, and common queries in several foreign languages. The simple, straightforward presentation should meet the demands of health professionals and laymen. III.A.4., III.C.

Thomson, William A.R. *Black's Medical Dictionary*. 31st ed. New York: Barnes and Noble Books, 1976. First edition, 1906.
>Literate, lay British medical dictionary. The numerous small differences in British and American perspectives are wonderful. Editions are frequently revised and updated. Definitions include information on diagnosis and therapy. Provides illustrations and tables. VII.B.2.b.

Tietjen, Gary L. *A Topical Dictionary of Statistics*. New York: Chapman and Hall (Methuen), 1986. 171 pp. $22.50. VIII.D.

Timmreck, Thomas. *Dictionary of Health Services Management*. Owings Mills, MD: National Health Publishing, 1982. 719 pp.
>Reproduces, with neither credit nor needed editing and updating, the entire first edition of this dictionary and similar derivative material. The only dictionary that mildewed during my last move. VI.

Tver, David F., and Howard F. Hunt. *Encyclopedic Dictionary of Sports Medicine*. New York: Chapman and Hall, 1986. 232 pp. III.C.

Tymchuk, Alexander J. *The Mental Retardation Dictionary*. Los Angeles, CA: Western Psychological Services, 1973.
>Contains 2000 entries with terse definitions selected from various disciplines concerned with exceptional children. Terms include persons, organizations, tests, abbreviations, eponyms, and acronyms. No pronunciations. A few references. II.B.2.

Uvarov, E.B., and Alan Isaacs. *The Penguin Dictionary of Science*. 6th ed. New York: Penguin, 1986. 468 pp. $7.95, softcover. I.

Vaisrub, Samuel. *Medicine's Metaphors: Messages and Menaces*. Oradell, NJ: Medical Economics Company, 1977.
>An exploration of the imagery of health and health care and of the sources of the language of the body and disease. VIII.B.

Veatch, Jethro Otto, and C.R. Humphreys. *Water and Water Use Terminology*. Kaukauna, WI: Thomas Printing and Publishing Company, Ltd., 1966.
>Good, dated. I.C.5.

Viseltear, Arthur J. "Review of *The Discursive Dictionary of Health Care*." *Medical Care*, 15: 446–9, 5/77.

Walker, Benjamin. *Encyclopedia of Metaphysical Medicine*. London: Routledge and Kegan Paul, 1978. 323 pp.
>Brief essays with references on some conditions (abulia, pain), aspects of medicine (diagnosis, iatrogenics), and irregular therapies (chromotherapy, touch healing). V.

Walton, John et al. (eds.). *The Oxford Companion to Medicine*. 2 vols. New York: Oxford University Press, 1986. 1524 pp. Illus. $95.
>A comprehensive reference book concerned with the theory, practice, and profession of medicine; a medical encyclopedia/history/dictionary with 150 essays. III.C.

Wasserman, Paul (ed.). *Encyclopedia of Health Information Sources*. Detroit: Gale Research Co., Book Tower, 1987. 483 pp. $135. VIII.A.

Weise, Frieda O. *Health Statistics: A Guide to Information Sources*. Vol. 4 in the Health Affairs Information Guide Series. Detroit: Gale Research Co., 1979.

An annotated bibliography of statistical sources (morbidity and mortality, specific diseases, health systems), covering recurrent and principal nonrecurring sources. II.C., VIII.D.

Werner, Arnold et al. *A Psychiatric Glossary.* 5th ed. Washington: American Psychiatric Association, 1980.
An excellent work written to suit both lay and professional readers and considered the work of a competent body by this author. III.C.

West, Geoffry P. (ed.). *Encyclopedia of Animal Care.* 12th ed. Baltimore, MD: Williams and Wilkins, 1977.
Modeled after *Black's Veterinary Dictionary,* a continually revised encyclopedia of veterinary science. Covers all major topics, cross-referenced. Includes drawings, photographs. III.C.

Wingate, Peter. *The Penguin Medical Encyclopedia.* 2nd ed. Baltimore: Penguin Books, Inc. 1976.
Another British lay dictionary. Idiosyncratic enough to be quite different from *Thomson, 1976.* VII.B.2.b.

Wolman, Benjamin B. (ed.). *Dictionary of Behavioral Science.* New York: Van Nostrand Reinhold, 1973. 478 pp. $22.50.
Covers terms used in psychology and related fields, as biochemistry, neurology, and endocrinology. Over 12,000 entries, by 29 international specialists. Concise definitions, cross-references, and disease classifications are provided. No pronunciations. I.A.2., III.C.

Wolman, Benjamin B. (ed.). *International Encyclopedia of Psychiatry, Psychology, Psychoanalysis, and Neurology.* 12 vols. New York: Van Nostrand Reinhold, 1977.
Contributions from 1500 international authorities. Articles are both biographical and conceptual in nature, and contain bibliographies. This is an extensive, specialized work with a clear and methodical format. III.C.

The World Book Illustrated Home Medical Encyclopedia. 4 vols. Chicago, IL: World Book, 1979. Vol. 1: *Medical Reference Guide (A-H) and Index of Symptoms;* vol. 2: *Medical Reference Guide (I-Z);* vol. 3: *First Aid, Safety, and Care of the Sick;* vol. 4: *Guide to Health and Fitness; Index.*
A family medical reference set with 2500 question-and-answer articles and 70 high-interest articles on cancer, arteriosclerosis, heart disease, etc. Color illustrations and anatomical drawings. Includes index and cross-references. VII.B.2.b.

World Health Organization (WHO). *Glossary of Mental Disorders and Guide to Their Classification.* 8th rev. Geneva: World Health Organization, 1974.
A WHO publication codifying the terminology and classification of mental disorders. Intended for use in conjunction with the *International Classification of Diseases.* Alphabetically arranged by category. Lists synonyms as well. II.B.2., III.C.

World Health Organization (WHO). "Guidelines to Terminology and Lexicography: Drafting of Definitions and Vocabularies." Terminology Circular No. 3. Technical Terminology Service. Geneva 27: WHO, June 1977. 23 pp.
Clear and concise instructions for preparation of vocabularies. VIII.B.

World Organization of National Colleges, Academies and Academic Associations of General Practitioners/Family Physicians (WONCA). *FAMLI: Family Medicine Literature Index.* Ontario (Canada M2K 2R9): Canadian Library of Family Medicine (4000 Leslie Street, Willowdale), M81.

A quarterly periodical with annual accumulation. Its thesaurus adds a defined family medicine vocabulary to MeSH. Also lists books, theses, and sources of material in family medicine. III.C.

Wren, R.C. *Potter's New Cyclopaedia of Medicinal Herbs and Preparations.* Reprint ed. New York: Harper & Row, 1972. Original edition, *New Cyclopaedia of Botanical Drugs and Preparations,* 1907.

A classic work on medicinal herbs with valuable information on herbal compounds and a glossary of botanical and medical terms. Indexed. I.A.2., V.

Yule, John-David (ed.). *Concise Encyclopedia of the Sciences.* New York: Facts on File, 1978. 590 pp. $29.95.

Definitions of 6000 key words and concepts, 1000 brief biographical essays, 600 illustrations. I.